Policy Responses to the COVID-19 Pandemic

This book examines why and how different countries developed different policy positions and responses to the COVID-19 pandemic, particularly in the early phase, by surveying a sample of countries that are geographically, politically, and culturally diverse, particularly those representing the East and the West.

Exploring nine countries, namely four Western countries (Finland, Germany, United States, and Sweden) and five Asia-Pacific countries (Japan, New Zealand, South Korea, Thailand, and Vietnam), contributors to this comprehensive new book compare and contrast similarities and differences in political systems, (de)centralization, policy responses, citizen engagement, and other factors. Written by experts on public policy within each of the counties explored, the chapters investigate how policy responses may be linked to the spread of the virus and fatalities in each location, drawing lessons from those experiences. Coercive tools (border control, school closure, movement constraints), incentive tools (emergency assistance, economic boosting assistance), and informative and facilitative tools (public information campaigns for social distancing, mask wearing) are all explored. In addition to policy responses, other contributing factors are carefully weighed, including national health care systems, applications of digital technology, institutional arrangements and governance systems, and political and civic culture.

This book is required reading for undergraduate and graduate students interested in comparative public policy and public governance, as well as policy-makers, government officials, and nonprofit workers in both developed and developing countries.

M. Jae Moon is Underwood Distinguished Professor of Public Administration as well as Director of the Institute for Future Government at Yonsei University, South Korea. He was the former Dean of the College of Social Sciences, Yonsei University, South Korea. He has been co-chairing the Infectious Disease Study Group of the National Research Council for Economics, Humanities, and Social Sciences under the Prime Minister's Office.

He is an elected Fellow of the National Academy of Public Administration (NAPA). He served as International Director of the American Society for Public Administration and Vice President of the Korean Association of Public Administration as well as the Korean Association of Policy Studies. He was selected as one of world's 100 most influential people in Digital Government 2018 and 2019 consecutively by Apolitical, which is a London-based leading nonprofit organization. He also received Order of Service Merit-Red Stripe from the Government of the Republic of Korea for his contribution to the public sector innovations as well as the Donald C. Stone Award from the American Society for Public Administration in 2020.

Dong-Young Kim is Associate Professor and Director of the Master's in Development Policy program at the KDI School of Public Policy and Management, South Korea. His research interests include theory and practice of public dispute resolution and negotiation in developing countries, participatory and collaborative governance, and environmental policy and sustainable development. Dr. Kim has 15 years of experience as a lecturer, researcher, and trainer on public dispute resolution, consensus building, negotiation, and participatory governance. He has extensive experience in training mid-career and senior government officials from many developing countries in Asia, Africa, Latin America, and the Middle East and in consulting various government institutions, such as the Prime Minister's Office, the Ministry of Environment, and the Ministry of Public Health and Welfare, public corporations, such as Korea Electric Power Corporation (KEPCO), private sectors, such as Nong-Hyup, Citi Bank, Industrial Bank of Korea, and Pfizer Korea, and non-governmental organizations in Korea.

Public Administration and Public Policy
A Comprehensive Publication Program
Editor-in-Chief
David H. Rosenbloom
Distinguished Professor of Public Administration
American University, Washington, DC

Recently Published Books

Contracting for Services in State and Local Government Agencies, Third Edition
Best Practices for Public Procurement
William Sims Curry

Public Management Reform in the Gulf Cooperation Council and Beyond
Mhamed Biygautane

The Politics of Collaborative Public Management
A Primer
Robert Agranoff and Aleksey Kolpakov

Deliberative Democracy, Public Policy, and Local Government
Joanna Podgórska-Rykała

Social Equity in a Post-Roe America
Gender, Race, and the Rule of Law
Lorenda A. Naylor and Heather Wyatt-Nichol

Policy Responses to the COVID-19 Pandemic
An International Comparative Approach
Edited by M. Jae Moon and Dong-Young Kim

For more information about this series please visit: https://www.routledge.com/Public-Administration-and-Public-Policy/book-series/AUEPUBADMPUP

Policy Responses to the COVID-19 Pandemic

An International Comparative Approach

Edited by
M. Jae Moon and Dong-Young Kim

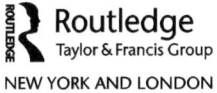

NEW YORK AND LONDON

Designed cover image: © Getty Images – Irina Shibanova

First published 2025
by Routledge
605 Third Avenue, New York, NY 10158

and by Routledge
4 Park Square, Milton Park, Abingdon, Oxon, OX14 4RN

Routledge is an imprint of the Taylor & Francis Group, an informa business

ISBN: 978-1-032-42439-2 (hbk)
ISBN: 978-1-003-36276-0 (ebk)

DOI: 10.4324/9781003362760

Typeset in Sabon
by codeMantra

Contents

Figures

Tables

Contributors

Pertti Ahonen is since 2021 Professor of Political Science on an Emeritus Contract at the Faculty of the Social Sciences of the University of Helsinki, Finland. He is also a Docent (Adjunct Professor) at the University of Tampere, Finland, the University of Vaasa, Finland, and the University of Jyväskylä, Finland. He has published on such topics in various public administration and policy journals.

Phanuphat Chattragul, CMU Proactive Researcher at Chiang Mai University [Grant Number 901/2566], Thailand, serves in the School of Public Policy. His interest lies in history, international relations, public policy, psychology, and Southeast Asian studies. Formerly an interpreter and research assistant, he holds a Master's in Political Science from Thammasat University.

Yoon Kyoung Cho is a visiting fellow of the Department of Public and International Affairs at the City University of Hong Kong. Her research focuses on empirical analysis of coproduction, natural language processing analysis in public finance on the local governments' level, and comparative public policy, especially in South Korea, Hong Kong, and the United States.

Louise K. Comfort is a Professor Emerita and former Director of the Center for Disaster Management, Graduate School of Public and International Affairs, University of Pittsburgh, Pittsburgh, PA, USA. She is also a Visiting Researcher at the Center for Information Technology Research in the Interest of Society, University of California, Berkeley. A Fellow of the National Academy of Public Administration, she received the 2020 Fred Riggs Award for Lifetime Achievement, Section on International Comparative Administration, American Society for Public Administration.

Carl Dahlström is a Professor of Political Science and Dean of the Faculty of Social Sciences at the University of Gothenburg, Sweden. His research is mainly concerned with bureaucratic structures and welfare state policy making from comparative perspectives. He is the author of books and papers on these topics, published by the *American Journal of Political Science* and *The Journal of Politics*, among others.

Jochen Franzke is a Senior Lecturer at the University of Potsdam, Germany, and a Member of the ICAPA Accreditation Committee of the International Association of Schools and Institutes of Administration (IASIA). His research focuses on empirical political and administrative research, especially on local and regional administrative reforms and citizen participation, as well as the transformation of public administrations in Eastern Germany and Central Eastern Europe.

Sophie Henderson is a Senior Researcher within the Country Research and Open Source Intelligence team at the Ministry of Business, Innovation and Employment, New Zealand. Her research interests revolve around global and regional governance of temporary labor migration and migrants' human and labor rights, with a comparative and empirical focus on the Asia-Pacific region.

Dong-Young Kim is a Professor and Director of the Master's in Development Policy program at the KDI School of Public Policy and Management, South Korea. His research interests include theory and practice of public dispute resolution and negotiation in developing countries, participatory and collaborative governance, and environmental policy and sustainable development.

Kilkon Ko is a Professor at the Graduate School of Public Administration at Seoul National University, South Korea. His research area is corruption, policy evaluation, and quantitative analysis. He has published his books and articles on efficiency analysis, categorical data analysis, Chinese corruption, and crisis management.

Sabine Kuhlmann is a Professor of Political Science, Public Administration and Organization at University of Potsdam, Germany, Vice President for Western Europe of the International Institute of Administrative Sciences (IIAS), and Holder of the Hedda Andersson Chair at Lund University, Sweden. Her areas of research include comparative public administration, public sector reforms, better regulation, digitalization of public administration, crisis governance and local government.

Johannes Lindvall is a Professor of Political Science at the University of Gothenburg, Sweden. His most recent book is *Inward Conquest: The Political Origins of Modern Public Services* (2021, with Ben Ansell). He is also the author of *Reform Capacity* (2017), *Mass Unemployment and the State* (2010), and articles in various journals.

M. Jae Moon is an Underwood Distinguished Professor of Public Administration at Yonsei University, South Korea. During the pandemic, he co-chaired the Infectious Disease Study Group of the National Research Council for Economics, Humanities, and Social Sciences under the Prime Minister's Office. The areas of his research include digital government, public sector reforms, and comparative public policy.

Trang (Mae) Nguyen is an Assistant Professor of Law at Temple University Beasley School of Law and an Affiliated Scholar at the U.S.-Asia Law Institute, New York University School of Law, USA. Her research takes an interdisciplinary approach to study transnational business governance, comparative law, and international business law, with a focus on Asia. Her work has appeared in the *American Journal of International Law Unbound*, *Stanford Law and Policy Review*, *Harvard Human Rights Journal*, and *New York University Law Review*, among others.

Ora-orn Poocharoen is the founding Director at the School of Public Policy at Chiang Mai University, Thailand. She's a former UN Committee of Experts in Public Administration (CEPA) (2018–2021). Her current interest lies in critical strategic foresight, empathy-based policy analysis, spirituality and public policy, holistic well-being, and just sustainability.

Kentaro Sakuwa is an Associate Professor in the Department of International Politics at Aoyama Gakuin University, Japan. He obtained his Ph.D. from Indiana University. He studies international relations, especially interstate conflict and foreign policy.

Kohei Suzuki is an Assistant Professor at the Institute of Public Administration, Leiden University, Netherlands. He mainly studies administrative reform and bureaucratic structures with a focus on cross-national settings and Japanese local municipalities. His research has been published in *Public Administration Review*, *Governance*, *Journal of European Public Policy*, *Public Management Review*, and several other peer-reviewed academic journals.

Matt Withers is a Research Fellow within the Department of Sociology at Macquarie University, Australia. His research examines the political economy of labor migration across the Indo-Pacific region, with an emphasis on social and public policymaking where migration, employment, and welfare regimes overlap.

Acknowledgments

This work was supported by the Office of Development Research & International Cooperation at the KDI School of Public Policy and Management as well as the Ministry of Education of the Republic of Korea and the National Research Foundation of Korea (NRF-2021S1A5A2A03065493).

1 International Comparative Analysis of Early COVID-19 Responses

Dong-Young Kim and M. Jae Moon

1.1 Introduction

The COVID-19 pandemic offers a very rare opportunity for scholars in comparative politics and administration to analyze (1) why many countries reacted differently (different timing and sequencing with different policy measures with different stringency) to this same external shock with equal epidemiological and biological susceptibility that occurred globally at virtually the same time, (2) how those policies led to different performance in rates of infection, testing, recovery and death, and (3) what the implications are for governments to be prepared for subsequent pandemic outbreaks. In the early wake of this pandemic, many universities and research organizations worldwide had already initiated projects to quickly gather data on the inventory of a comprehensive range of policy measures and tools used by various countries (Dong, Du, and Gardner, 2020; Hale, Angrist, Kira, Petherick, Phillips, and Webster, 2020). However, the interrelationships among important variables cannot be systematically teased out to answer the questions above with an array of policy tools in raw forms alone.

Fortunately, many scholarly efforts connected to the international comparison of a few countries have already been found in the global literature, which suggests multiple independent variables that might explain such variance among many countries. These variables include cultural orientation (An and Tang, 2020), regime type (Greer et al., 2020), centralization of power (Yan et al., 2020), policy learning from past experience (Lee et al., 2020; Moon, 2020), society's demographic structure (e.g., the share of the aged population) (Matsungo and Chopera, 2020), and citizens' compliance and voluntary support (Migdal, 2009).

However, it is not easy to answer the targeted questions above. First, there are so many variables and factors that interact with each other that it is difficult to control variables across many national cases. For example, high rates of deaths per population in a country may be influenced not only

DOI: 10.4324/9781003362760-1

by policy measures deployed by the government but also by lifestyle (e.g., smoking habits) and diet-related comorbidities, whose occurrence differs by country or based on environmental factors such as different levels of air pollution, which also affect people's respiration. Thus, it is important to find comparable cases appropriately.

Second, it is not easy often very challenging to judge the effect of policy measures and whether a country is successful at certain time frames during the ongoing evolution of this pandemic. Countries that were heralded as very successful in handling the pandemic in the early phase of the pandemic turned out to be less so or even disastrous at later stages. On the other hand, countries with less successful responses at the beginning of the pandemic proved reasonably successful in turning around outbreaks with vaccination of many population.

However, it is imperative to answer the questions raised above in any case but with more in-depth, detailed case studies that can supplement and improve large-n comparative empirical studies of national-level responses to COVID-19 (Toshkov, Yesilkagit, and Carroll, 2022). Particularly, it is important to understand how different countries responded to the pandemic in the early phase when governments were under tremendous challenges because of VUCA (volatility, uncertainty, complexity, and ambiguity) nature of the problem. In this vein, this book project was started to contribute to understanding similarities and differences in policy responses to the pandemic and their results in the early phase with detailed case studies of nine countries conducted by renowned scholars worldwide: South Korea, Japan, Thailand, Vietnam, and New Zealand (In Asia); Germany, Finland, and Sweden (Europe); and the United States (North America). The case studies of these nine countries focus only on identifying factors that led to different policy measures related to 'flattening the curve' and public health performance from the outbreak of the pandemic to early 2021 rather than on economic packages to rescue or boost the national economy.

In the next section, a systematic framework of crisis governance for the pandemic is suggested to provide a better understanding of the interrelationships among variables and factors that are identified in the case studies in this book. Then, significantly and potentially influential variables in the system will be introduced briefly. Afterward, with basic comparative statistics of the public health performances of these nine countries, the abstracts of nine chapters of case studies will be introduced. A set of various policy instruments were considered and adopted by different governments (see Table 1.1).

The simplest framework of infectious disease management includes two measures: the containment of the virus and the treatment of infected patients. The level of containment of the virus manifests in the number of confirmed cases through appropriate testing of potentially infected people. The treatment of infected patients affects the number of deaths per population.

Considering that the virus is transmitted through social contact among people in the population, containment without any vaccine can be achieved with both appropriate policy measures and citizens' appropriate behavior and compliance with government policies and guidelines. Various sorts of physical distancing among people can be maintained by ranges of measures including stringent lockdowns, border control, quarantine, school or shop closings, and social distancing in public spaces among people who wear a mask. Individual hygiene practices matter the most. In the meantime, containment should be done through the testing and tracing of people who might be infected by any social contacts.

Once infected patients are identified through tracing and testing, they should be treated medically to be cured or recovered in medical institutions without known medicines. Basic and advanced levels of public health institutions, such as hospitals and quarantine facilities with enough doctors, nurses, and staff with necessary equipment and facilities, such as ICU beds and oxygens, are critical for treating infected patients.

To answer the three key questions of sources of different policy measures (in terms of timing, sequences, and combinations of various policies with different levels of stringency) (Attwell and Navin, 2019; Knill, Schulze, and Tosun, 2012; Roser, Ritchie, Ortiz-Ospina, and Hasell, 2020; Schaffrin, Sewerin, and Seubert, 2015), and variables that affect public health performance, and policy implications for pandemic management in the future, we clarify a few categories of variables surrounding these containment and treatment schemes in general.

First, people in institutions, whether public or private, generate ideas and formulate and implement official plans. Thus, what is important is their capacity to assess a situation, make appropriate decisions, and implement them effectively (by communicating, networking, and coordinating with various actors including experts, private sectors, and public) in multiple levels of decision points and by acquiring necessary resources). In fighting the virus, which is transmitted so fast, the agility of actors may be the most important capacity. They need to quickly assess situations, make appropriate decisions, take action, learn from any mistakes, and adjust to new situations. Many countries took action too late and/or indecisively (with important exceptions such as Greece and Germany). They lost critical time, and these delays in action cost lives. Additionally, coordinating capacity may be very important since a few actors cannot address complicated issues alone but need help and support from different actors. Some of those capacities are already given or inherited in some countries and are the matter of system. Other kinds of capacities hinge on the personal traits of key politicians (or leaders) and top bureaucrats in governments.

Table 1.1 Policy instrument types during the COVID-19 pandemic

Types of policy instrument	*Instrument choices*
Testing	Geography: comprehensive vs. cluster-focused (i.e., hot spots)
	Coverage: any individuals with suspected symptoms vs. specific individuals with serious respiratory-related symptoms
	Eligibility: citizens vs. non-citizens; non-criminals vs. criminals
	Cost: free (universal) vs. cost sharing
	Accessibility: designated centers or drive/ walk-through sites vs. approval by doctors after consultation
Mobility restriction	Restriction degree: mandatory stay-at-home order vs. voluntary stay-at-home order vs. no restriction
	Geography: national lockdown vs. local lockdown
	Places: home, workplace, public transport
Border control	Entry ban target: all countries vs. select countries in high-risk groups vs. no border control
Quarantine and contact tracing	Surveillance: monitored vs. voluntary
	Locations: government facilities vs. hospitals vs. home
	Cost: self-pay vs. government assistance
	Methods: in-person interviews and visits vs. location-based application vs. electronic wristbands
Priority group for treatment	Groups: citizens vs. non-citizen; insurance holder vs. non-holder; elderly vs. non-elderly people
Social distancing and other hygiene practices	Enforcement: mandatory (by law) vs. determined by private enterprises vs. voluntary
Public information campaign	Sources: mobile text messages; newspapers; billboards; television ads; social media; government homepages
	Materials: cartoons; words; videos
Business (and school)	Operation: businesses opened as usual vs. essential industries only allowed to open vs. all closed; school opened vs. temporarily closed
Limits on mass gatherings	Threshold: universal number applied to the whole country vs. density-based restriction
	Type: all public gatherings banned vs. private gatherings also banned

Source: Adapted by the authors from An and Tang (2020)

Second, identifying background (contextual) factors are needed to understand why people in various institutions make different decisions and implement them differently in terms of containment and treatment. Contextual factors are given before the outbreak of the pandemic and maintained during the pandemic or changed abruptly in the process. These factors include (1) the cultural (or value) orientation of a country and its institutions, (2) the existing institutional setting or (public health) infrastructure, (3) financial and human resources, (4) preparedness by learning from the similar experience of infectious diseases in the past, (5) social structure (income inequality, racial discrimination, share of the older population, the level of public health), (6) the level of economic development of a country, (7) political situation (e.g., presidential election), (8) political regime type (autocratic vs. democratic government) (multiparty vs. single-party) and government structure (federal vs. unitary), and last but not least, (9) the size of the country (areas and population). Some background factors may influence both government responses and citizens' social and individual behaviors.

1.2 Variables

1.2.1 Background (Contextual) Factors

1.2.1.1 Institutional Infrastructure (that Existed before the COVID-19 Pandemic) and Policy Learning (Capano et al., 2020; Moon, 2020)

Some Asian countries, such as South Korea and Taiwan, that had previously experienced similar infectious diseases, such as SARS and MERS, overhauled and streamlined their public health systems with substantial staff, budget, critical health infrastructure, and necessary autonomy to prepare for similar rounds of epidemics in the future. For example, in South Korea, legislation was adjusted to facilitate the approval process for test-kit development and clinical trials. Lee et al. (2020) and Moon (2020) argue that quadruple-loop learning from past experience helped South Korea respond to COVID-19 more effectively and quickly.

However, Japan did not build the necessary health infrastructure although she experienced the H1N1 pandemic in 2009. The lack of preparedness for the pandemic in Japan was revealed when responsible agencies mishandled the inspection and quarantine of COVID-19-infected passengers on a cruise ship (Schumaker, 2020). In the United States, the Global Health Security and Biodefense Unit was established in 2015 by the Obama administration in the wake of the swine flu in the United States to prepare for a similar pandemic. However, that unit was abolished in

2018 by the Trump administration (Reuters, 2020). Ironically, wearing a mask during this pandemic was not controversial in South Korea because Korean people are already accustomed to this practice due to transboundary air pollution from China, the so-called "yellow dust."

1.2.1.2 Cultural Orientation

Culture matters in policy compliance and social behaviors. In East Asia, where collectivism prevails, individual freedom may be sacrificed for collective good during a crisis. Thus, stringent measures such as lockdowns that infringe on individual freedom may be acceptable and sustainable in such a culture. However, in Western culture, where individual freedom and self-responsibility are highly valued, stringent policy instruments may not be welcome or sustainable over a long period (Gelfand, 2012; Markus and Kitayama, 2003). Even different greeting styles in different cultures may affect the contagion of the virus. Bowing rather than kissing and hugging may be much safer in pandemic situations. Thus, some scholars argue that different national response strategies for COVID-19 are determined by the cultural orientation of each country since the most critical interventions facing uncertain viruses without medicine or vaccines are nonpharmaceutical interventions to modify individuals' behavior to contain and mitigate the COVID-19 pandemic (Wilder-Smith and Freedman, 2020; Yan et al., 2020).

1.2.1.3 Regime Type and Formal Political Institutions

In democratic regimes, taking decisive and forceful measures might have been more difficult compared with autocratic regimes since decision-making power is shared at different levels and leaders need to take multiple steps to consult citizens and stakeholders, and political parties may compete with each other with different positions. On the other hand, centralized, autocratic states may adopt and implement policies faster in a top-down fashion (León and Orriols, 2019). Thus, decentralized countries may prefer to provide recommendations and lax restrictions on citizens rather than stringent policy options. One formal institutional arrangement that is key to understanding different COVID-19 response strategies is the degree to which power and authority are centralized versus decentralized in a country.

In a similar vein, federal states, such as the United States, Germany, Brazil, and Russia, are often reproached for problems of coordination between federal governments and state or local governments. The question of who has which responsibilities and power becomes an important issue in risky situations. What is the ideal coordination between strong or weak federal or central government or independent, capable local government? The existence of multiple political parties and their ideological composition in a parliament may affect social policy decisions and impending decisions that may infringe on individual freedom. As Capano et al. (2020) argue, in the US case, as in Canada, federalism played a foundational role in structuring how the United States responded to the COVID-19 pandemic.

Other scholars emphasize that state capacity (not infrastructure or system) matters more than regime or institutional type or income level in responding to urgent risks. Improvements in government capacity to deliver services, implement policy measures, and communicate with the public matter.

1.2.2   Case Studies of COVID-19 Risk Governance of Nine Countries

The in-depth country case studies in this volume provide a more comprehensive assessment of risk governance for coping with the COVID-19 pandemic in nine countries: South Korea, Japan, New Zealand, Thailand, and Vietnam in Asia; Germany, Sweden, and Finland in Europe; and the United States in North America. Nine countries were selected so that there would be meaningful variation across multiple dimensions to increase the robustness of the findings from our international comparison. These dimensions include (1) existing institutions, such as organizations, laws, and regulations related to public health and infectious disease control as one of starting conditions, (2) size of the country in terms of areas and population, which may affect the efficiency and agility of decisions and the controllability of diseases, (3) civic culture manifest in relations between the government and citizens, (4) rules of law (5) use of technology (6) use of experts (7) political stability, (8) voluntarism vs. command and control (9) learning from the past experience (10) liberal, democratic, and autocratic rule and (11) federal, and unitary systems. For example, the United States and Germany are large countries with large populations and operate on the federal system, while some other countries, such as New Zealand and South Korea, are relatively smaller in size and population. We also selected some developing countries, such as Vietnam and Thailand, to be compared with other advanced countries in their efforts to cope with COVID-19.

1.2.3   Public Health Performance of Nine Countries during the COVID-19 Pandemic

In terms of performance, such as the number of confirmed cases and the number of deaths per million population, countries have shown relatively different levels of outcomes at different phases of pandemic outbreaks.

Some countries, such as South Korea, Vietnam, Thailand, New Zealand, Germany, and Finland, have coped with the pandemic situation relatively well, while the United States and Sweden have suffered relatively more confirmed cases and deaths than other countries.

References

An, Brian Y., and Shui-Yan Tang (2020). Lessons from COVID-19 Responses in East Asia: Institutional Infrastructure and Enduring Policy Instruments. *American Review of Public Administration*, 50(6–7), 790–800.

Attwell, Katie, and Mark Christopher Navin (2019). Childhood Vaccination Mandates: Scope, Sanctions, Severity, Selectivity, and Salience. *The Milbank Quarterly*, 97(4), 978–1014.

Capano, Giliberto, Michael Howlett, Darryl S.L. Jarvis, M. Ramesh, and Nihit Goyal (2020). Mobilizing Policy (In)Capacity to Fight COVID-19: Understanding Variations in State Responses. *Policy and Society*, 39(3), 285–308, https://doi.org/10.1080/14494035.2020.1787628.

Dong, Ensheng, Hongru Du, and Lauren Gardner. (2020). An Interactive Web-Based Dashboard to Track COVID-19 in Real Time. *The Lancet Infectious Diseases*, 20(5), 533–534.

Gelfand, Michele J. (2012). Culture's Constraints: International Differences in the Strength of Social Norms. *Current Directions in Psychological Science*, 21(6), 420–424.

Greer, Scott L., Elizabeth J. King, Elize Massard da Fonseca, and Andre Peralta-Santos (2020). The Comparative Politics of COVID-19: The Need to Understand Government Responses. *Global Public Health*, 15(9), 1413–1416.

Hale, Thomas, Noam Angrist, Beatriz Kira, Anna Petherick, Toby Phillps, and Samuel Webster. (2020). Variation in Government Responses to COVID-19.

Knill, Christoph, Kai Schulze, and Jale Tosun. (2012). Regulatory Policy Outputs and Impacts: Exploring a Complex Relationship. *Regulation & Governance*, 6(4), 427–444.

Lee, Sabinne, Changho Hwang, and M. Jae Moon (2020). Policy Learning and Crisis Policy-Making: Quadruple-Loop Learning and COVID-19 Responses in South Korea. *Policy and Society*, 39(3), 363–381, https://doi.org/10.1080/14494035.2020.1785195

León, Sandra, and Lluis Orriols. (2019). Attributing Responsibility in Devolved Contexts. Experimental Evidence from the UK. *Electoral Studies*, 59, 39–48.

Matsungo, Tonderayi Mathew, and Prosper Chopera. (2020). Effect of the COVID-19-Induced Lockdown on Nutrition, Health and Lifestyle Patterns among Adults in Zimbabwe. *BMJ Nutrition, Prevention & Health*, 3(2), 205.

Markus, Hazel Rose, and Shinobu Kitayama. (2003). Culture, Self, and the Reality of the Social. *Psychological inquiry*, 14(3–4), 277–283.

Migdal, Joel S. (2009). Researching the State. In *Comparative Politics: Rationality, Culture, and Structure*, 162–192.

Moon, M. Jae (2020). Fighting COVID-19 with Agility, Transparency, and Participation: Wicked Policy Problems and New Governance Challenges. *Public Administration Review*, 80(4), 651–656.

Schaffrin, André, Sebastian Sewerin, and Sibylle Seubert. (2015). Toward a Comparative Measure of Climate Policy Output. *Policy Studies Journal*, 43(2), 257–282.

Schumaker, E. (2020, February 19). Japanese Expert Who Sneaked onto Diamond Princess Cruise Ship Describes "Zero Infection Control" for Coronavirus. ABS News [Press release]. https://abcnews.go.com/Health/japanese-expert-sneaked diamondprincess-describes-infection-control/story?id=69071246.

Reuters. (2020). Partly False Claim: Trump Fired Entire Pandemic Response Team in 2018. *Reuters Fact Check*. https://www.reuters.com/article/world/partly-false -claim-trump-fired-entire-pandemic-response-team-in-2018-idUSKBN21C32C/.

Roser, Max, Hannah Ritchie, Esteban Ortiz-Ospina, and Joe Hasell (2020). Coronavirus Disease (COVID-19): Statistics and Research. *Our World in data*, 4, 1–45.

Toshkov, Dimiter, Brendan Carroll, and Kutsal Yesilkagit. (2022). Government Capacity, Societal Trust or Party Preferences: What Accounts for the Variety of National Policy Responses to the COVID-19 Pandemic in Europe?. *Journal of European Public Policy*, 29(7), 1009–1028.

Wilder-Smith, Annelies, and David O. Freedman (2020). Isolation, Quarantine, Social Distancing and Community Containment: Pivotal Role for Old-Style Public Health Measures in the Novel Coronavirus (2019-nCoV) Outbreak. *Journal of travel medicine*, 27(2), taaa020.

Yan, Bo, Xiaomin Zhang, Long Wu, Heng Zhu, and Bin Chen (2020). Why Do Countries Respond Differently to COVID-19? A Comparative Study of Sweden, China, France, and Japan. *American Review of Public Administration*, 50(6–7), 762–769.

2 Germany's Responses to COVID-19

Crisis Governance in a Multilevel System

Jochen Franzke and Sabine Kuhlmann

2.1 Introduction

This study analyzes how German public administration has coped with the COVID-19 pandemic. It analyzes crisis governance in the multilevel system, addressing in particular the role of intergovernmental coordination between the federal, Länder and local levels as well as how governments were advised by scientists, how data was generated and reported, how parliaments have responded to the crisis and what extent people supported the measures taken by governments. Concentrating on the developments in 2020, we will investigate how different actors in the intergovernmental setting have managed crisis mitigation, which challenges and tensions have become apparent, and which solutions have been chosen to overcome shortcomings. Doing so, we shed light on the institutional set-up and the legal framework of crisis management in the German federal system and assess the preparedness and capacities of the health system. Focusing on the developments in 2020, we make a distinction between four major phases of pandemic governance: (I) Phase I: reliance on local management; Phase II: unitarization and centralization; Phase III: reemphasis on local discretion and variance; Phase IV: "intergovernmental centralism." For the different phases of the pandemic, we outline the most important responses and measures adopted by the federal, Länder, and local governments as well as the (changing) coordination mechanisms at play. The study shows that while being well-prepared in terms of health capacities (ICUs, hospitals, etc.) and (local) public health service, a number of shortcomings and deficits have become apparent during the crisis, some of which originate in policy decision of previous years, such as understaffed hospitals and ill-prepared care facilities for the elderly. Furthermore, the analysis reveals multiple governance problems that have occurred over the course of the crisis, such as weakened parliamentary control mechanisms and checks and balances, the poor digital preparedness of local health authorities, shortcomings in data transmission and reporting, and insufficient interdisciplinarity and

DOI: 10.4324/9781003362760-2

openness in policy advice. Regarding intergovernmental coordination, we show that there was a general trend toward more unitarization and centralization in pandemic-related decision-making up to what we label "intergovernmental centralism," while at the same time, major implementation and coordination functions remained with the – increasingly overburdened – local levels as key actors in pandemic management.

In the following, we first present some basic statistical data on COVID-19 and how it affected the German health system (Section 2.2). Afterwards key features of the German system of crisis management and its preparedness in regards to pandemics will be outlined (Section 2.3). This is followed by an in-depth analysis of crisis governance and management at the federal, Länder, and local levels (Section 2.4), the governments' responses to the crisis (Section 2.5), and the policy advice (Section 2.6). Finally, we provide some survey data on institutional trust, the populations' support of the measures, and emerging opposition to governments' crisis management (Section 2.7). The concluding Section (2.8) summarizes major characteristics, strengths, and weaknesses of Germany's COVID-19 governance and gives an outlook on future developments.

2.2   Basic Statistical Information on COVID-19 in Germany

Since the detection of the first COVID-19 case on January 28, 2020, until December 31, 2020, a total of 1,719,737 people were positively tested on SARS-COV2[1] in Germany with a population of app. Eighty-three million people, about 1.4 million had recovered or finished quarantine, and 33,071 died in association with COVID-19 (see RKI 2020a). After an initial period of significant growth from the end of February to the end of March 2020 (the first COVID-19 wave), when the rate of positively tested persons was highest (about 9% in week 14), a substantial decline was registered to a quota of about 1% by the end of May. Since then, the quota has remained more or less stable until the end of September, when it progressively climbed again up to about 12% at the end of December (second COVID-19 wave) as the highest level in 2020 (Statista 2020b) (Figure 2.1).

The testing capacity and policy have changed significantly over time in Germany. At the beginning of the pandemic, the testing frequency was limited to between 125,000 (March) and 400,000 (April) weekly tests (see Figure 2.2). These were predominantly concentrated on people with symptoms and those in contact with positively tested persons. The German testing policy was adapted quantitatively by expanding the testing capacity to about 1.6 million by November 2020. It was altered by increasingly including people without symptoms or contacts to be positively tested (particularly travelers returning home) and shifting to a mass testing strategy. The extended testing activity was accompanied by increasing absolute

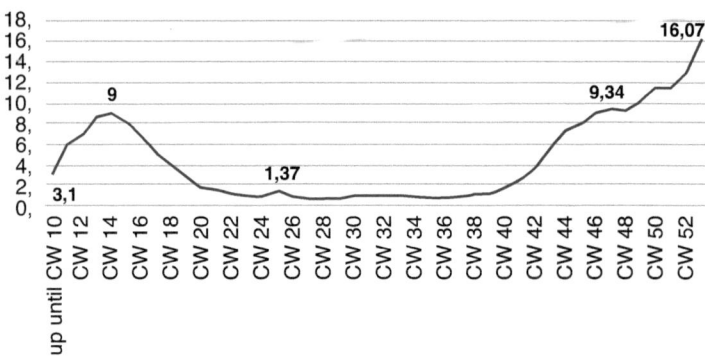

Figure 2.1 Quota of SARS-CoV-2 positive persons in Germany (March–December 2020).

Source: Adapted from Statista 2020b. CW short for Calendar week.

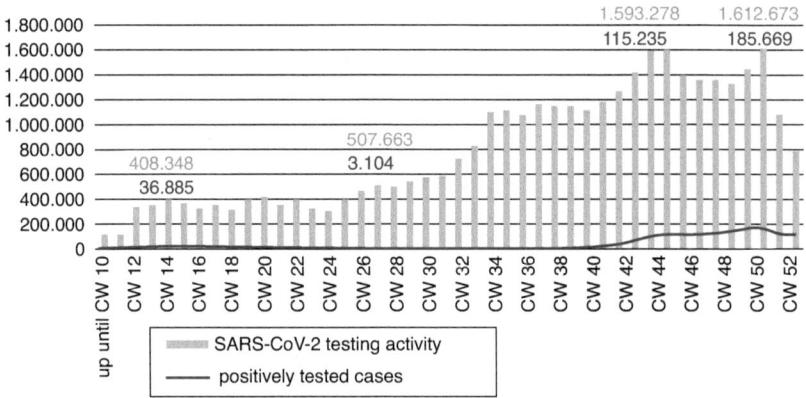

Figure 2.2 SARS-CoV-2 tests and positive cases in Germany (March–December 2020).

Source: Adapted from Statista 2020a. CW short for Calendar week.

case numbers, yet also a quite stable quota of positively tested from July to September while since then the quote of positively tested climbed, too (see Figure 2.1). From an international comparative perspective, the German testing intensity was with about 400,000 tests per million inhabitants by the end of 2020 at a medium/lower level.

Regarding hospitalized cases (see Figure 2.4), a first peak was reached in April with a total of 6,064 patients, which corresponds to a 20% COVID-19-associated hospitalization rate (inpatient treatment). Since then, the number of hospitalized continuously shrank to about 244 at the beginning of July (11% hospitalization rate). From September to the end of the year, the number of hospitalized cases climbed again up to a second peak in December (8,899 cases in week 51) while the hospitalization rate remained quite stable at about 6%–9%. The first peak utilization of the intensive care units in Germany was reached on 18 April, with 2,922 cases (75% of them ventilated) based on a total capacity of about 30,077 places available in ICUs at that time (see DIVI 2021; Deutsches Netzwerk Evidenzbasierte Medizin 2020). Since then, the number of cases in ICUs has constantly shrunk, reaching a level of about 200 cases by September (DIVI 2020). The total amount of hospitalized and ICU cases thus remains below 400. Since June revealed that the increasing number of people positively tested for SARS-CoV-2 did not correspond to soaring numbers of seriously ill people at that time. However, with hospitalizations increasing from September onwards, the number of COVID-19 patients in need of ICU treatment jumped up to 5,639 cases by end of December which was the highest peak in 2020. At the same time the total ICU bed capacities had been reduced from 33,367 in July to 26,576 by December for still unclear reasons. However, German hospitals dispose of a so-called "emergency reserve" of ICUs to be activated within 7 days (10,900 emergency ICUs in December). Thus, even at the peak of hospitalizations in December, still 15,646 ICUs were available, including the "emergency reserve." About 15% of them were used by COVID-19 patients. The general occupancy of ICU beds in Germany remained quite stable at about 22,000 from September to December 2020. In general, the much-feared overburdening of the German health system did not become apparent (see Deutsches Netzwerk Evidenzbasierte Medizin 2020: 2) (Figures 2.3 and 2.4).

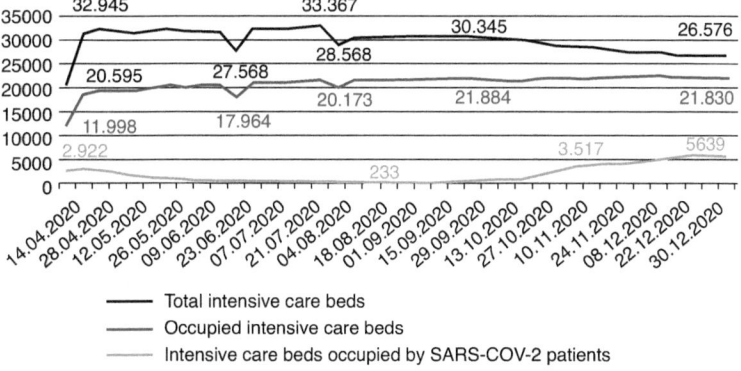

Figure 2.3 Intensive Care Units (ICU), occupation by COVID-19 patients in Germany

Source: Adapted from DIVI 2020. CW short for Calendar week.

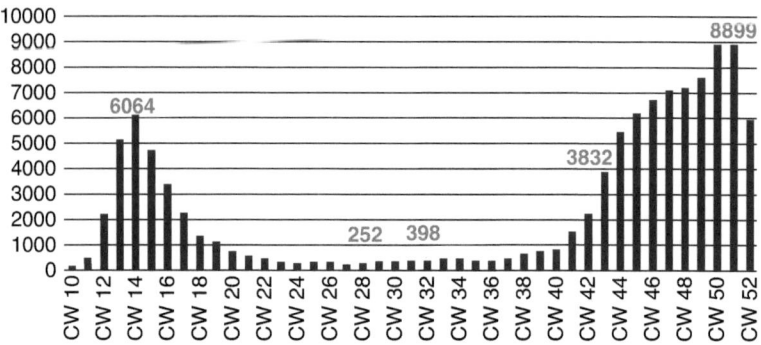

Figure 2.4 COVID-19 associated hospitalizations in Germany in 2020.
Source: Adapted from RKI 2020b. CW short for Calendar week.

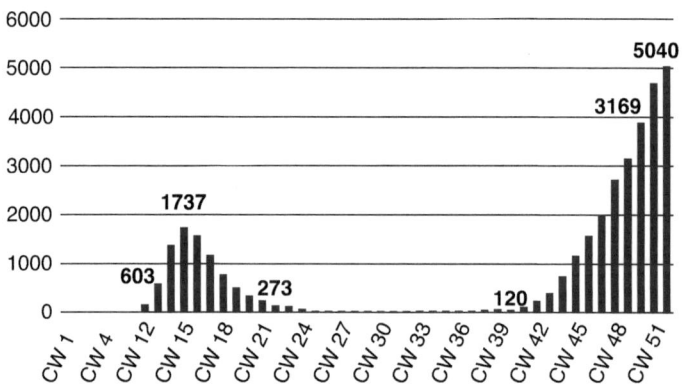

Figure 2.5 Weekly deaths associated with COVID-19 in Germany in 2020.
Source: Adapted from RKI 2020c. CW short for Calendar week.

The first cases of death in association with COVID-19 were registered in Germany on 9 March 2020, to a total of 33,071 until 31 December. Corona-associated weekly deaths reached a first climax from March (with 603 deaths in CW 13) to May (with 273 deaths in CW 21), with a peak in April (1,737 deaths in CW 15). There was also an excess mortality from March to May (see Figure 2.5). Over the summer, the number of deaths associated with COVID-19 decreased and stabilized at a level between 30 and 60 weekly cases from July to September (the average number of daily deaths in Germany is about 2,600). In the subsequent time period, the number of COVID-19-associated weekly deaths progressively climbed from 120 at the beginning of October (CW 41) to a maximum of 3,169 in December

(CW 49) (see RKI 2020c). The median death age remained stable at about 82 years, which is above the average life expectancy for men in Germany (79 years; women: 84 years) (Statista 2020b). The share of COVID-19-related deaths that happened in care homes or others in outpatient care was specified at 50% (see Streeck 2021) to 60% (see Rothgang et al. 2020).

Regarding COVID-19-associated deaths per 1 million inhabitants, Germany ranks significantly lower by the end of December than other countries (not only in Belgium, the United Kingdom, Italy, Spain, and France but also in Sweden, Austria, Switzerland, and the Netherlands), yet higher than Denmark and Norway (see Figure 2.6). There was registered excess mortality in Germany compared to the 2016–2019 average, specifically from March to May, with a peak in week 15 (15%), in August with a peak in week 33 (21%), and December with a maximum of 25% in week 50 (see Figure 2.7). Excess mortality was partly (especially in March/April and November/December) paralleled by an increase in COVID-19-associated deaths (see Destatis 2020a). In total, 39,201 deaths were indicated as being associated with COVID-19, by and of 2020 (which is about 4% of all deaths). Overall, in 2020, about 48,100 deaths were registered than the 2016–2019 average, which is just under a 5% increase (see Destatis 2020b). However, this should not be interpreted as "excess mortality" because an increase in deaths by about 50,000 cases had been expected for 2020 in Germany anyway (compared to 2019), inter alia due to the changing age structure of the population which consists of an increasing proportion of inhabitants aged 80 years and beyond. Therefore, experts do not see a noticeable excess mortality in Germany for 2020 (see Der Spiegel 2021, FOCUS 2021a).

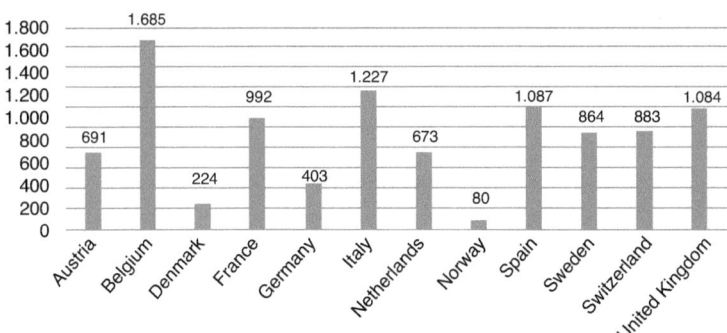

Figure 2.6 Deaths associated with COVID-19 per Mio. Inhabitants in selected European Countries (as of December 31, 2020).

Source: Adapted from Our World in Data. 2021. Please note: The comparability of these numbers is limited due to different methods of registration and counting of COVID-19 associated deaths in European countries.

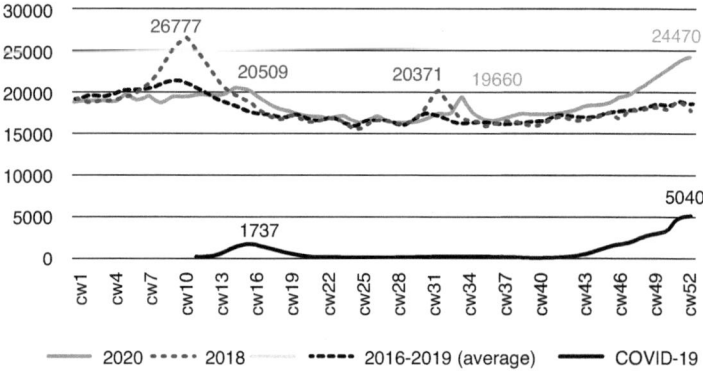

Figure 2.7 Mortality in Germany (deaths per week in 2016–2019 average, 2018, 2020).

Source: Adapted from Destatis 2020c. CW short for Calendar week.

2.3   National Context and Starting Conditions

2.3.1   *Intergovernmental Set-up*

In Germany, the pandemic encounters a politico-administrative system of "unitary federalism" (unitarischer Föderalismus), which is based on two potentially opposing principles. On the one hand, the 16 federal states (Länder) enjoy a powerful autonomy in having their own legislatives, executives, and judicative bodies as well as a high degree of discretion, specifically regarding the execution of federal, EU and its own laws. On the other hand, the unity of law, economy and living conditions are constitutionally protected. Multiple mechanisms provide for an enforcement of collaboration and joint decision-making across levels and jurisdictions in order to guarantee federal unity (see Fuhr et al. 2018; Kuhlmann 2020; Kuhlmann et al. 2021d).

Manifold intergovernmental collaboration mechanisms have been institutionalized, some of which involving the Länder only (horizontal collaboration), whereas others involve the federal and the Länder level (vertical collaboration). Within this setting the principle of an "executive federalism" is another important key feature, which also played out during the pandemic. According to this principle, the federal level is mainly responsible for policy formulation, whereas the Länder and the local governments as parts of Länder administration are mostly engaged in policy implementation (see Kuhlmann and Wollmann 2019). Under these circumstances, the federal level has no hierarchical control, no legal supervision, and also no financial appropriation over the Länder level. As a consequence, the federal executive has only very little direct involvement in implementation and service delivery and thus does not operate with regional or local offices (exceptions include defense, customs, inland waterways, and the federal police).

As part of the Länder administration, the 10,790 municipalities[2] and the 294 counties (to a somewhat lesser degree) have the constitutional right "to regulate all matters relevant for the local community under their own responsibility within the limits set by the laws." Their wide range of self-government and delegated functions makes up 70%–80% of all legal provisions (federal, Land, and EU) applied and implemented by the local authorities (Fuhr et al. 2018). Within this multi-purpose profile, the local executive acts as a politically accountable local politician, rather than as "agent of the State," even in the conduct of delegated state tasks. From a comparative perspective, the German local government system can be regarded as one of the functionally and politically strongest in Europe, possessing a broad multi-purpose task profile, robust administrative structures, and manifold competencies, inter alia in public health issues and implementing the protection measures of the federal and Länder governments.

2.3.2   Health System

The German health service consists of three pillars: the public health service (Öffentlicher Gesundheitsdienst, ÖGD), the outpatient medical care (Ambulante medizinische Versorgung) and the inpatient medical care (Stationäre medizinsche Versorgung). This corporate system is highly decentralized, involving a multitude of subnational and local institutional actors, self-governing bodies and sub-state authorities (see Kuhlmann et al. 2021c, 2021d). Whereas the federal level is basically limited within the system to monitoring, surveillance, research and legislative functions, the lion's share of health-related tasks is assigned to the Länder and local governments. This goes especially for health protection and aid, supervision of professions and health care facilities, based on specific Länder health service laws. These tasks are institutionally assigned to the Länder ministries of health, most of which have subordinated health authorities (mostly combined with other related tasks like social affairs). The management and financing of hospitals is assumed by the Länder and local governments. The Länder must ensure investments and elaborate hospital plans for their territory, which determine the number, the location, and the medical specializations of hospitals in different parts of the Land as well as the number of hospital beds. Local governments are responsible for the management of local hospitals, where roughly 30% of all clinic doctors are employed (Vereinigung der kommunalen Arbeitgeberverbände 2020).

In quantitative terms Germany belongs to the top-scorer in the European Union, especially regarding health expenditures (see Bouckaert et al. 2020;

Kuhlmann et al. 2021c). With 4,300 € per capita or 11.2% of the GDP, they are the highest in Europe and approximately 50% above the EU average (see European Commission 2019). Additionally, Germany has "some of the highest rates of beds, doctors and nurses per inhabitants in the EU" (OECD/European Observatory on Health Systems and Policies 2019: 3). Around 84.4% of the total German health expenditure is financed by government programs and compulsory insurance, including statutory and private health insurance, additionally private households contributing 12.5%. Health care industry is one of the largest sectors of the German economy with 11.2% of GDP. Around 85% of the population is covered by statutory health insurance, the rest by private ones (European Commission 2019: 9). With eight hospital beds per 1,000 inhabitants, the number is the highest in Europe (see European Commission 2019). In March 2020, the roughly 2,000 public, private, and non-profit hospitals provided about 500,000 beds, 28,000 of which had intensive care equipment and 25,000 with respiratory devices. The occupancy quote of ICUs during the first year of the pandemic was never beyond 85%.

With regard to the qualitative indicators, by contrast, a number of deficits in the German health system have revealed, which have been criticized since many years without being resolved. These shortcomings have become acute and visible to the wider public during the pandemic. The major problem lies with the severe staffing deficits in hospitals and nursing services as well as with their inadequate technical equipment. The OECD therefore valued the German health system as only "moderately effective" (OECD/European Observatory on Health Systems and Policies 2019: 22). Since the 1990s, the German hospital system has in the focus of New Public Management (NPM) driven privatization and marketization. Since 2009, the number of publicly owned hospitals has been lower than the number of hospitals in private or profit-oriented ownership.[3] One consequence of this NPM-driven trend has been that efficiency and profitability concerns have become increasingly important in hospital management – partly at the expense of employees and patients, although, in total, the investment volume has increased as a result of more private investments (see Klenk and Reiter 2012: 410). Since 2003, treatments in German hospitals have been billed based on state-financed lump sums, which creates cost pressure without systematic consideration of quality and non-transparent redistribution effects in and between clinics[4] (Simon 2020: 12). Significant economic and financial malfunctions have resulted from this mode of financing. Another consequence has been staff reductions leading to shortages and bottlenecks in the care sector. Since a long, German hospitals, especially the nursing services, have been understaffed, 12,000 full-time positions were vacant in the nursing sector (including 4,700 in intensive care) and about 3,300 for medical doctors (Blum et al. 2019). From a comparative perspective,

Germany is one of the countries with the lowest number of care personnel per capita in Europe. This so-called "state of emergency in the care sector" (Pflegenotstand) has been increasingly debated, however, without effective solutions so far.

Some critics see the causes for these dramatic deficits more deeply, in the inflexible corporatist structure of the German health care system, especially in the role of the Federal Joint Committee (Gemeinsamer Bundesausschuss, G-BA) as an organ of self-administration in the health care system, in which the general interests of society as a whole hardly play a role. (Reinhart et al. 2020). Like a legislator, the G-BA adopts guidelines and other standards that everyone in the healthcare system must adhere to.

2.4   Crisis Governance

2.4.1   *Pandemic Governance in the Multilevel System*

In times of peace, the central state (federal level) has no legal means to impose pandemic emergency measures (such as shutdowns and lockdowns) at the subnational levels (see Franzke and Kuhlmann 2021; Kuhlmann 2020; Franzke 2021a). Since the Federal Government did not make use of its constitutional emergency regulations on defense (Art. 91, 35 Basic law) but based its crisis strategy mainly on the Federal Infection Protection Act (Infektionsschutzgesetz IfSG), which is executed by the Länder and local governments, the intervention powers of the federal government in the pandemic remained rather limited. Based on the general clause (§28) of the IfSG (Drittes Gesetz zum Schutz der Bevölkerung bei einer epidemischen Lage von nationaler Tragweite 2020), only the Länder can enact executive orders to temporarily suspend fundamental civil rights, such as the right to free assembly, free movement, free development of the individual, free exercise of religion and free exercise of profession. The Federal Government could only give recommendations to the Länder and push for coordinated measures. Consequently, the German containment policies were mainly based on executive orders by the Länder and local governments imposing lockdowns, contact bans, shutdowns, and closures of public facilities.

However, the predominance of sub-national actors does not mean disconnected and completely discretionary actions – quite on the contrary (see section above). According to the principles of "unitary" and "cooperative federalism" (see Behnke and Kropp 2021), intense coordination and collaboration across levels and jurisdictions were extensively practiced during the pandemic, at times even tending to the peculiar and untypical feature of informal executive centralism. Drawing on well-trained intergovernmental coordination mechanisms, horizontal and vertical coordination of the federal and 16 Länder governments ("Bund-Länder Koordination") was used to achieve nationwide standards of pandemic containment, particularly in phases with rising case numbers (March/April; October onwards). Over the course of the crisis, phases of intense coordination and "unitarization" of decision-making, especially when the pandemic situation was perceived as aggravating, alternated with phases of looser intergovernmental collaboration and more discretionary regulatory powers of the Länder and local governments, particularly when the situation was perceived as more relaxed and a lifting of measures as justifiable. To put it exaggeratedly, the lockdown-yoyo was paralleled by a centralization-yoyo with subsequent phases and repeated re-balancing of localized/discretionary and centralized/uniform containment regulation. Interestingly, regulatory unitarization and negotiated alignment of measures were predominant in phases of perceived crisis aggravation whereas in times of perceived relief, subnational discretion and more regional variance of containment rules appeared to be appropriate. As a result, the regulatory landscape (lockdown rules etc.) looked quite homogeneous in different German regions, some criticism about an alleged federal mess in the Länder-specific details of containment notwithstanding.

So-called "Bund-Länder-Summits," consisting of the Federal Chancellor and the 16 Länder Prime Ministers, have developed as the main mechanism of intergovernmental coordination in the pandemic. In 2020, 16 of these "Summits" have taken place between 12 March, and 13 December whereas in previous (non-crisis) periods, these conferences only took place twice a year. By far the majority of Germany's key decisions in pandemic containment were adopted in these intergovernmental "Summits" by way of legally non-binding framework agreements. The latter were transposed later on into legally binding regulations by each Land individually. The intergovernmental Summits represent however only an informal coordination body without constitutional foundation, direct political accountability or the legal power of enacting binding decisions. As the relevance and importance of this body have increased immensely during the crisis, we can observe a new quality and intensity of intergovernmental coordination and executive federalism, which we have pointedly labeled "intergovernmental centralism."[5]

While, initially, the Länder differed widely in their approaches regarding lockdowns, shutdowns, school closures, etc., later on, as a result of this coordination mechanism, but also following court decisions, the regulatory landscape of pandemic containment became more homogeneous, with however some remaining variance in degrees of strictness and details of execution. Hence, federal harmonization by way of intergovernmental coordination, with a conspicuous centralizing and unifying impetus, became an ever-more crucial feature of pandemic management, specifically regarding high-stakes decisions on containment. At the same time, local governments remained at the major implementation level of these decisions jointly taken by the Länder and Federal Governments.

2.4.2   *Phases of Pandemic Containment*

Regarding the intergovernmental coordination of pandemic containment, four phases can be distinguished from January until December 2020 (see Franzke and Kuhlmann 2021; see Figure 2.8):

- **First Phase:** From detection of the first COVID-19 case on the 28 January, 2020, in Bavaria until the 17 March, when the infection risk level was rated "high" by the Federal Authority for Disease Surveillance and Prevention (Robert-Koch-Institut, RKI), the logic of the pandemic management was predominantly local or at least decentralized. Besides the cancellation of mass events by the Länder governments, no country-wide measures of containment were considered necessary. During this first phase the sub-national administrations (Länder, local governments) managed the pandemic on their own discretion according to the pertinent provisions of the IfSG. When on 8 March the Federal Minister of Health recommended to cancel all public events with more than 1,000 participants, all Länder governments followed. During this phase, local governments were key actors of pandemic mitigation and took responsibility for enacting containment measures tailored to the local necessities. Besides contact tracing and domestic quarantining, local health authorities enacted punctual containment regulations, such as school closures or shutdowns of facilities. The county of Heinsberg in North-Rhine Westphalia (NRW), for instance, where the first German COVID-19 hotspot was identified, was the first local government to enact the closure of all schools and kindergartens, on the 26 February.
- **Second Phase:** After the RKI adjusted the infection risk level from "low/medium" to "high" on 17 March (it remained "high" over the rest of the year), discretionary containment by the sub-national governments was not considered appropriate anymore. Instead, more intergovernmental coordination of measures and a uniform national strategy of containment was seen as necessary accompanied by centralizing attempts to allocate more powers to the federal executive. In this phase – the first peak of the pandemic in terms of case numbers – containment measures were intensely coordinated and streamlined in order to achieve uniform regulations across levels and to avoid a "federal patchwork" which was criticized by some. "Speaking with one voice" became the predominant narrative of an increasing and rapid tightening of containment measures and a (temporal) suspension of a number of fundamental rights. With the "joint guidelines to slow down the spread of the Coronavirus" adopted on the 16 March, the Federal and the Länder Governments attempted a harmonized proceeding in pandemic containment across the entire country. Nationwide shutdowns were enacted by all Länder

and, step by step, all schools and kindergartens were closed, nationwide contact-bans (limited lockdowns) imposed and subsequently extended (see Section 2.4). In general, this phase was a "race to the top" regarding the Länder responses to the pandemic (Eckhard and Lenz 2020: 7): after the lockdown was decided in Bavaria and Saarland on the 21 March, all other Länder followed suit only a day later. The same applies to the introduction of monetary fines for those people disregarding the regulations, which were first introduced in NRW on the 27 March, followed by all other Länder in April (ibid.). As a consequence of vertical and horizontal (self-) coordination, local governments' discretion in deciding on mitigation measures in their territories tailored to their specific epidemic situation shrunk.

- **Third phase:** With the numbers of cases, hospitalizations and deaths decreasing and then remaining stable on a very low level over spring and summer, the pendulum swung back again, toward more sub-national discretion and variance. Thus, between the extremes of unity and variance within the "unitary federalism," the features of variance and competition regained importance in this third phase. The debates and decisions regarding regulations on how to exit lockdown and how to deal with new cases in the long term became more diverse and less coordinated (thus linking up to the first phase). NRW and Bavaria represented two extremes here, with the former standing for a more permissive approach and the latter supporting a stricter one during this time period. Although the Länder prime ministers and the Federal Government decided on the 15 April to extend most of the containment measures (apart from the re-opening of smaller shops and schools for higher classes in compliance with the Corona hygiene regulations), much discretion and leeway was granted to the Länder. Consequently, they could decide about possible deviations from the general rule, stipulate more relaxed or stricter rules for their respective territories and determine the concrete timing of school re-openings. As a result, increasing variation and complexity occurred in the concrete details of the "exit regulations" in the different Länder and cities, with some of them enacting stricter and some looser rules according to regional particularities and political preferences. Whereas in the second phase of the pandemic, the Federal Government had assumed a leading role in coordinating and moderating the intergovernmental agreements to ensure federal unity (see above), this position was largely given up from the 6 May onwards. The further process left up to the Länder and local governments, except for some basic rules which continued or newly started to apply nationwide (see Section 2.4).
- **Fourth phase:** When from October 2020 onwards incidences raised again (see Section 2.2) the intergovernmental coordination between the

federal and the Länder governments intensified. Containment regulations were tightened step by step until the end of the year. Drawing on the experiences of the second phase (see above), the density and frequency of joint executive decision-making were even accelerated in the fourth phase. Thus, the heads of the Länder and federal governments met biweekly to reassess the situation and to deliberate on the further continuation and tightening of containment. This high meeting frequency might also be explained by the fact that, apart from the "incidence rule," no long-term strategy of pandemic mitigation was defined and thus all measures had to be adjusted ad hoc based on the just occurring incidence numbers. To put it pointedly, the intergovernmental body of federal and Länder executives tended to get the status of a "substitute government" where all key pandemic decisions were taken to be ratified and formalized later on by the Länder. With the agreement of 14 October, the "hotspot-strategy"[6] introduced in May was concretized. Thus, the leeway for the Länder and local governments to autonomously decide about containment concepts in local hotspots of their territories was trimmed, based on some standardized nationwide rules.[7] Arguing that only below a threshold of 50 new incidences per 100,000 inhabitants within one week contact tracing by the local health authorities would still be manageable which in turn was seen as a precondition to avoid a crash down of the health system, this "incidence rule" continued to be the key indicator for all governmental decisions over the course of the pandemic.

When the fairly soft measures failed to stop case numbers climbing in the whole country and about 75% of all cases were not traceable anymore, stricter measures were seen to be necessary by end of October. With the agreements of 28 October, 16 November, 25 November, and 13 December progressively tighter restrictions were jointly agreed upon by the Länder and federal governments, initially limited in time and then subsequently prolonged, with the aim of making case numbers shrink below the incidence margin of 50. These efforts climaxed in a "light" and then "hard" lockdown decided on 28 October and 13 December respectively (for details see Section 2.4), including inter alia the re-closing of schools, kindergartens, shops, and restaurants. In contrast to the spring lockdown, the winter lockdown included even formal curfews in some Länder (e.g. Brandenburg), indicating stricter containment than in the first wave. Critics also labeled the repeated alternation of lockdown and relief as a kind of "Lockdown Yoyo" severely questioning the long-term effectiveness of this approach (see FOCUS, 2021b). Although according to the "hotspot strategy," the Länder still could enact stricter or looser rules adapted to their regional circumstances and political preferences, the intergovernmental

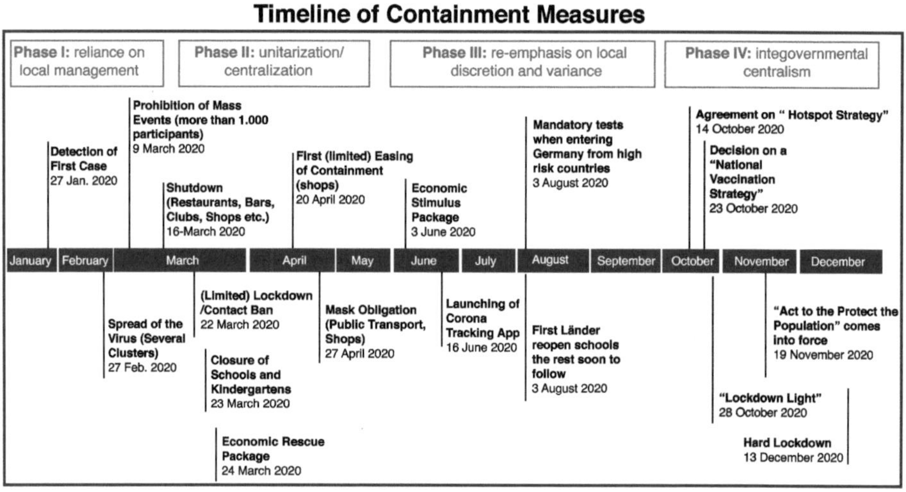

Timeline of Containment Measures

Phase I: reliance on local management	Phase II: unitarization/ centralization	Phase III: re-emphasis on local discretion and variance	Phase IV: integovernmental centralism

Figure 2.8 Timeline of containment measures.

Source: Own compilation of the authors.

containment agreements have resulted in growing national uniformity, standardization and harmonization of pandemic measures whereas the local discretion and variance shrank considerably. "Normal" subnational crisis governance was largely substituted by intergovernmental arrangements at central state level composed by the heads of the federal and the Länder governments. The peculiar pattern of an informal executive centralism thus became characteristic during the peaks of the pandemic with negotiations and agreements as predominant modes of governance formalized later on by the Länder as legally binding executive orders. Although within the model of unitary and executive federalism in Germany, various federal-Länder coordination bodies are well-known and multilevel agreements much practiced, the centralizing impetus of pandemic intergovernmental arrangements appears to be quite exceptional.

2.4.3 Establishing an Emergency Regime

As the Federal Government's intervention options in managing emergencies and governing the pandemic are limited, the Federal Minister of Health strived to strengthen his institutional position by shifting powers in the institutional system and gaining additional competencies regarding sub-national pandemic management (see also Kuhlmann et al. 2021c). Based on a new law on "the protection of the population in the event of an epidemic emergency of national concern," which was passed with a broad cross-party consensus in parliament, the Bundestag became empowered to declare (and stop) this kind of emergency. According to the amended §5 of the IfSG (Erstes Bevölkerungsschutzgesetz), during an "emergency of national concern," declared on the 27 March and further extended beyond 2020, the Federal Minister of Health gains considerable additional powers and discretion to decide measures unilaterally and to issue orders in the (otherwise decentralized) system of public health governance as long as the emergency legally persists. He is then authorized to enact exceptions from the federal law (IfSG) by way of statutory ordinances without parliamentary approval and without consulting the Länder and their parliamentary chamber (Bundesrat).[8] This is a highly controversial issue which some lawyers considered as unconstitutional (Thielbörger and Behlert 2020) or at least constitutionally questionable (see Deutscher Bundestag 2020a: 6).

Drawing on the new pandemic "emergency rule," the Ministry of Health made widely use of its upgraded regulatory competencies. A range of new ordinances were enacted which in a "non-emergency situation" would not fall under the regulatory competence of the Minister of Health, for instance new ordinances regarding stock increases of medicaments for intensive care, licensing regulations for doctors, dentists and pharmacists, securing training in the health professions, compensating financial burdens of dentists, drug providers and maternal health care facilities, procurement of medical products and personal protective equipment, ensuring the supply of the population with medical products as well as on international travel. The "carte blanche" authorization of the Ministry of Health concerns substantial parts of federal regulations that are actually or could potentially be affected.[9] Besides the upgrading of the operative powers of the Federal Ministry of Health regarding the pandemic management system and the national regulation of pandemic emergency issues, further centralizing steps were taken by upgrading the institutional position of the RKI to a "national authority for disease monitoring and prevention" charged with new intervention powers and capacities to coordinate mitigation strategies between the Länder and the federal level.

The second amendment of the IfSG (Zweites Bevölkerungsschutzgesetz) of 19 May referred to some practical issues of pandemic management, for example regarding support for the public health service, increasing testing, track and trace capacities and granting financial means to staff in care facilities. The third amendment of the IfSG was passed by the Bundestag on 18th of November with the third law on civil defense (Drittes Bevölkerungsschutzgesetz). This law was an important step to legally consolidate and secure the pandemic containment policies of the Länder. Given that the IfSG general clause § 28 was the sole legal basis for suspending civil liberties and that some executive orders had been repealed by the courts due to unconstitutionality (e.g., the "lodging ban") a necessity was seen to create a more solid legal basis for pandemic containment. The new law was adopted with the votes of the parliamentary parties in government (CDU/CSU, SPD) and the Greens whereas the other opposition parties rejected the proposal. With this law, the legal foundation of the Länder executive orders, was enhanced based on a new §28a in the IfSG. By "listing" (or "copy and pasting") (see Matuschek et al., 2020) the Länder executives' containment measures (lockdowns, shutdowns, curfews, physical distancing rules, mask obligation etc.) explicitly in the IfSG, the federal parliament "certified" their lawfulness (see Kießling 2020: 4). The same applied to the "incidence rule" (50 cases per 100,000 inhabitants) of the Bund-Länder agreements defined in the law as the general threshold value for the suspension of civil rights (see above). With this, on the one hand, the parliament reacted to a major critique raised by lawyers according to which the "old" IfSG was not sufficient to justify comprehensive suspensions of civil rights enacted by the Länder executives. These interventions were regarded as requiring a direct parliamentary legitimation (see inter alia Papier 2020). Accordingly, the new law provided a solid statutory basis for the suspension of constitutional rights by the Länder executives.

As a consequence, the legal basis of pandemic containment was fortified and the position of the Länder executives to suspend constitutional rights during a pandemic legally consolidated while possibilities for citizens to successfully sue against the restrictions were reduced. The legislative proposal was heavily criticized by many experts in the parliamentary hearings and beyond. It was claimed that the legislator had failed to weight different constitutionally affected interests, to formulate the regulations clearly, precisely and unambiguously (Bestimmheitsgrundsatz), to respect the principle of parliamentary reservation (Parlamentsvorbehalt), to specify the conditions under which mild, sever and highly restrictive containment measures must be adopted and to respect the administrative autonomy of the Länder when stipulating nationwide uniform measures under certain conditions (see Klafki 2020: 8; Kießling 2020: 2). Against this background the third civil defense law was regarded as "deficient in many respects" (Klafki 2020: 8) and criticized as one-sidedly legitimizing the pandemic policies of the Länder executives without balancing interests (see Kießling 2020: 2). Some experts in the parliamentary hearing therefore dissuaded from adopting the law and warned it would bring about more harm than benefit (Klafki 2020: 8). Many civil society groups, too, protested against the law, for example, "Mehr Demokratie" (see Deutscher Bundestag 2020b).

In terms of checks and balances, the overall result of the various legal amendments was a weakening of the federal legislative (Bundestag) and (partly) the Länder in an "epidemic emergency of national concern" while the central-state executive, specifically the Minister of Health, was conspicuously upgraded. The balance between the legislative and the executive branches has clearly shifted toward the latter. The pandemic can therefore undoubtedly be referred to as the "moment of the executive" leading to what could be labeled as an (informal) executive centralism as a peculiar feature of crisis governance. As the pandemic progressed, parliaments became increasingly adept at reducing this deficit.

2.4.4   Interdepartmental Coordination

Although in times of peace hazard control and danger prevention are essentially subnational tasks assumed by the German Länder (see Art. 30 Basic Law), in risk situations of national concern the federal Government can grant support to the Länder (information, advice, provision of resources). Additionally, it has to make sure that a coordination between the Länder and the federal level is ensured regarding risk assessments and protective measures. In the case of national emergencies, the establishment of inter-ministerial emergency task forces on the federal level of government is provided as a pertinent tool of coordination across departments. This type of cross-departmental organization represents an exception to the normal departmental principle (Ressortprinzip) which is constitutionally enshrined and otherwise predominant in German federal governmental coordination. The cross-departmental composition of the emergency task forces is meant to bundle various departmental interests and to guarantee horizontal coordination and a joint approach of central-level emergency management in cases of large-scale risk situations, such as a pandemic.

During the COVID-19 pandemic, this task was assumed, from February 27 onwards, collaboratively by the Federal Ministries of Health and of Interior as lead ministries of the task force which met twice a week. Furthermore, representatives of the Ministries of Economy, Finance and Social Affairs and other departments were included to take into account adequately the high risk of collateral damages for the economy and society. Apart from that, two - a small and a large one - federal-level "Corona Cabinets" were established, which met twice a week, especially during the shutdowns.[10] By mid-March 2020, all Länder governments, too, set up emergency task forces to cope with the pandemic crisis in their territories. These worked in close collaboration with Länder-level inter-ministerial coordination groups to ensure an intergovernmental and interdepartmental coordination.

2.4.5   The Role of Local Governments

The backbone of the German public health service is made up by the 375 local health authorities (Kommunale Gesundheitsämter) located in the counties and county free cities (see Franzke and Kuhlmann 2021). Quickly beefed up with additional money and manpower during the pandemic, they have become "one of the central pillars of Germany's crisis response"

(Financial Times 2020). However, their most important task during the COVID-19 was to implement the IfSG on their own discretion and under the supervision of the Länder. Dealing with epidemic crises is nothing new to the local health authorities as they can draw on longstanding experiences in managing health threats and containing local outbreaks, for example, of measles and other infectious diseases. They have proven to be institutionally resilient and viable in coping with major health crises. "Every public health officer of a county has more powers than the Federal Minister of Health" stated a leading German newspaper (Der Tagesspiegel 2020; see Franzke 2020), illustrating the outstanding importance of the local public health service in initiating pandemic-related emergency measures.

Local governments assumed a number of key functions regarding local pandemic containment and health protection (see Franzke 2020, 2021b; Kuhlmann and Franzke 2022). Within their broad multi-purpose task portfolio, local governments were not only responsible for health-related issues but, more generally, for pandemic crisis management within their territories, the horizontal coordination of various crisis-related administrative units at local level as well as for vertical coordination between the respective Länder authorities and the federal level (specifically the RKI). They made important decisions on crisis mitigation and pandemic containment and were also in charge of organizing related administrative processes and communication with the local public. For the cross-sectoral coordination of emergency management, on the local level, too, specific emergency task forces were established in all counties and county-free cities in mid-February 2020. They were meant to support the local executives in all crisis-related issues, internally coordinating mitigation measures and guaranteeing coherence of crisis management across administrative units and with other local jurisdictions. The composition of these Corona emergency task forces varied across jurisdictions, yet in general, they reflected the multi-functionality and the cross-cutting horizontal coordination capacities of local governments in Germany.[11]

The local Corona emergency task forces had to take over a couple of key functions in local pandemic management: (1) Bundling and coordinating all local activities on pandemic containment, drawing up process plans and developing scenarios for further crisis mitigation; (2) Collecting all available information on the local pandemic situation, evaluating and distributing it to the responsible local administrative units; (3) Organization of temporary staff transfers and resource reallocations within local administrations, mainly from various sectoral units to local health departments; (4) Providing information and communication about pandemic management to the local public; (5) Procurement of protective equipment for staff of local health authorities, such as high-quality respiratory masks, protective clothes, disposable suits and disinfectants.[12]

A major concern during the crisis was the precarious staff situation and the shortage of resources in the local health authorities criticized for a long time (see Bayer 2020).[13] Against this background it comes as no surprise that many local health authorities were hardly able to fulfill their regular tasks even before the crisis and in urgent need of additional resources, manpower and subsidies when the pandemic began. Although these resources were partly been granted by the federal and Länder governments, the pure number of activities related to tracking and tracing of infection chains, quarantining persons and, in case of untraceable "infection chains," closing facilities conspicuously overburdened the local health authorities. Not at least because of the amended testing strategy (see Section 2.1) more cases (also without symptoms or clinical findings) were identified and thus the "infection chains" to be traced and tracked amounted to a magnitude hardly manageable anymore. As a result, many local health authorities reached their capacity limits in October 2020 at the latest. After the case numbers had soared again, in about 75% of all cases the infections chains were not traceable anymore by the local health authorities, which was a major justification for the second lockdown in Germany enacted on 29 October. The federal army (Bundeswehr) was called by some overburdened local health authorities in April to support them in tracing "infection chains" and supervising quarantining, however with limited success only. The same applies to the Corona Warning App meant to support the local health authorities, yet failing in significantly relieving local health authorities from their trace and track burdens.

2.5 Government Responses and Crisis-Related Policies

2.5.1 *Pandemic Plans and Risk Analyses*

German health authorities can draw on longstanding experiences in managing health threats, such as SARS in 2003, bird and swine flu in the 2000s, belonging to their traditional portfolio of functions. They have proven to be institutionally resilient and viable in coping with them. Over the course of previous epidemics, the German local health authorities became more and more experienced in tracking infection chains, tracing contacts and containing virus spread, which proved to be particularly useful in the COVID-19 pandemic. This institutional legacy might be an important difference to unitary centralized countries (such as the UK) where subnational and local expertise and know-how in pandemic mitigation are less valued and trusted by central governments.

In Germany, the first national pandemic plan was published by the RKI in 2005. This plan was updated several times, including at the beginning of the pandemic on 4 March 2020 (see RKI 2016, 2020g). It forms the general procedural framework for prospective pandemic preparation and containment measures, based on the on the global pandemic plan of the WHO and the still mentioned German pandemic experiences in the last few decades. Furthermore, all German Länder established pandemic plans for their territory based on the national plan, whereas many local authorities have not done so. In the crisis, these plans served as salient sources for national and sub-national policy makers as well as for local professionals and managers to take concrete actions, establish necessary governance structures (e.g., crisis task forces), and to decide upon appropriate measures of crisis management during the various phases of the pandemic (like containment, protection, mitigation and recovery). However, crisis management practice has shown, that the various pandemic plans are not always compatible, but sometimes rather conflicting which has made coordinating containment measures across jurisdictions difficult.

Risk analyses have become important instruments to prepare German public organizations to disasters, specifically in the context of emergencies caused by floods. They have been implemented at all levels of government, however to varying degrees and with different impacts regarding the current COVID-19 pandemic. According to the Federal Law on Civil Protection and Emergency Aid (Zivilschutz und Katastrophenhilfegesetz des Bundes, ZSKG), the federal government is obliged to conduct risk analyses in the field of civil protection. On this basis, in 2012 a comprehensive risk analysis was conducted by the Federal Agency for Civil Protection and Disaster Assistance (Bundesamt für Bevölkerungsschutz und Katastrophenhilfe, BBK) and other federal offices, which was approved by the federal Parliament in 2013 (Deutscher Bundestag 2012). In this analysis, various scenarios of possible disasters were modeled (including pandemics) based on previous experiences with comparable emergencies.

Although this analysis included a scenario of a pandemic caused by virus SARS, the predicted damage for Germany (e.g., millions of deaths, similar affectedness of all age groups by the virus) does not correspond to the current pandemic. It turned out to be up to now much milder in its health-related effects than the modeled one, but some of the envisaged protective measures and the modeled collateral damages (e.g., economic and societal impacts) partly do reflect the situation during the actual pandemic. Interestingly, however, this risk analysis of a SARS virus pandemic has not explicitly been taken into account by decision-makers at all political-administrative levels, specifically to meet preparatory measures and establish appropriate governance arrangements in preparation of the predicted event. Therefore, Germany was not as well-prepared for the COVID-19 pandemic as it could have been.

The poor functioning of risk analysis as a tool of emergency management does not only apply to the ex-ante and ongoing assessment of first-round crisis effects, that is the immediate health-related damages to be measured by numbers of infected, hospitalized and deaths. It even more applies to the so-called "risk-risk trade-offs" (see Collins et al. 2020) of crisis management to be calculated in a comprehensive multi-dimensional risk assessment. This analysis is meant to explore the expected collateral damages of the crisis mitigation measures themselves. These so-called "second-round effects" are related to any type of coping strategy and which can be economic, social, political, mental, environmental but also health-related on the longer run. Such an assessment which, by including un-intended side-effects of pandemic containment measures, would be intended to lead to a more balanced multi-dimensional risk analysis and correspond to the constitutionally required proportionality principle of crisis mitigation policies (especially when accompanied by a mid-/long-term suspension of fundamental rights on a nationwide scale). However, multi-dimensional risk assessments, have been applied during the crisis only rudimentary if at all (see Leopoldina 2020a: 11) and not been taken into account systematically by governments when enacting and extending restrictions.

2.5.2   Key Measures of the Containment Approach

As already mentioned further above, the German COVID-19 containment strategy was mainly based on an execution of the general clause (§28) of the IfSG by the Länder and local governments. With their executive orders on lockdowns, contact-bans, shutdowns and closures of public facilities (for details see below), the Länder governments temporarily suspended a number of fundamental civil rights.

The following measures have been key to the COVID-19 strategy in Germany (see also appendix)

- *Lockdowns and contact-bans*: The first measure of pandemic mitigation in Germany was the cancellation of mass events with more than 1,000 participants recommended to the Länder governments by the Federal Minister of Health on 8 March 2020. All Länder followed this advice with varying delays. In the meantime, this ban was extended by 2021. From mid-March until June 2020 a considerably tighter containment strategy was pursued based on a Federal-Länder-Agreement adopted on 22 March. The most severe measures of this nationwide containment approach were (limited) lockdowns (March to April), shutdowns, contact-bans and closures of public facilities, including schools and kindergartens (see below). On 22 March, all 16 Länder Prime Ministers and the Chancellor agreed upon a fairly coherent and uniform containment strategy with a number of common key measures to enforce physical distancing nationwide. All agreed upon a limited lockdown and contact-ban (instead of a strict lockdown, such as in France, Italy, Spain etc.) which provided that people were generally allowed to leave their homes but they had to keep a distance of 1.5 meters minimum and must not appear in groups of more than two persons (except for families or domestic partnerships). Groups of people partying or assembling in the public were forbidden, any contacts to persons outside one's own household were to be minimized. Playing grounds for children were closed. Indoor private events and family gatherings clashing with these rules were prohibited, too. The compliance to these rules was supervised by the local authorities for public safety and order and by the police. Monetary fines were introduced by the Länder governments for punishing non-compliance. In the first lockdown, on 20 March 2020, almost all German Länder closed restaurants and shops. Large parts of the economy were shut down on a nationwide scale for roughly one month (first liftings on 15 April). The shutdown specifically affected the catering trade, shops, "body-related" services, cinemas, theaters, discotheques, bars, clubs, sports facilities. Furthermore museums, galleries, exhibitions, public memorials, zoos and botanic gardens were closed (first lifting of restrictions on 30 April). The assembly of people in churches, mosques, and synagogues for worship was prohibited. A second lockdown was decided on 28 October by the Länder prime ministers and the chancellor. It was expected to be a "breakwater lockdown" to stop virus spread, which actually did not work out by end of the year. The intention was to strictly limit social contacts outside one's own family. Therefore, from 2 November onwards, social contacts with other people outside the members of one's own household were meant to be reduced to a minimum. Staying in public was only permitted with members of one's own household + members of one additional household, yet not exceeding the maximum of ten people in total. Later this was reduced to one household + one member of another household. Citizens were requested to refrain from unnecessary private trips and visits, including their own relatives. A court in Thuringia stating the unconstitutionality of this contact ban (see Amtsgericht Weimar[14]), which was however contradicted by other courts later on (see Thüringer Allgemeine 2021).

- *Closing intra-federal borders and internal travel restrictions*: Besides closing external borders as decided by the federal government on 15 March, some Länder also closed their internal borders for non-residents coming from other Länder. In Mecklenburg-Vorpommern, for instance, non-residents, including those with a secondary holiday home, were not allowed to cross the border of the Land anymore. Only on 4 September, this Land opened up its internal borders again for external day tourists and citizens from other German Länder. Per RKI countries/regions with more than 50 new cases on 100,000 inhabitants over a period of 7 days ("incidence rule") were defined as corona "risk zones." In October 2020, most of the Länder enacted travel restrictions for inhabitants coming from "risk zones." Citizens having their permanent residence in "risk zones" were not allowed there to be hosted in hotels or holiday apartments (so-called "lodging ban"). This measure was highly controversial and the courts repealed it. However, with the second lockdown, hotels were closed again for tourist purposes.

- *Closure of schools and kindergartens*: From mid-March, some local governments enacted directives for single schools in the event of detected cases. This was followed by the Länder to debate school shutdowns for their entire jurisdiction and finally fairly homogeneous approaches of the Länder regarding countrywide school shutdowns and a general turn to home and remote. As schools are an exclusive competency of the Länder and kindergartens falling with the portfolio of local governments, joint federal-Länder guidelines did not include their shutdown. Despite some attempts at coordinating school policy during the pandemic across the Länder by the so-called "conference of the Länder ministers for education" (Kultusministerkonferenz, KMK), a uniform agreement on school closures could not be reached. Although formally no harmonized solution was passed, after the 16 March, step by step, all Länder enacted ordinances regarding the closure of schools and kindergartens accompanied by specific regulations on emergency childcare. In September 2020, the federal and Länder governments agreed to avoid general school closings in the event of a second wave of corona infections. However, from December onwards kindergartens and schools closed were closed again combined with emergency care in day-care centers and online learning in schools.
- *"Incidence rule" as a national indicator and yard stick:* With the aim to ensure nationally uniform standards in pandemic containment, the so-called "incidence rule" was agreed by the federal and Länder governments on 6 May 2020 which is monitored by the RKI. According to this rule counties and county-free cities with more than 50 new cases per 100,000 inhabitants registered within seven days, must elaborate a severe containment concept including contact-bans and possible local lockdowns. The limits of this regional hotspot approach became apparent in the second wave of infections, when at the end of 2020 all Länder were temporarily above the incidence of 50.
- *Mask obligations:* The wearing of face masks in public transport, shops and other public spaces were made obligatory – a measure which most Länder subsequently extended to other public spaces, such as restaurants, cultural and sports facilities, public buildings, stations, platforms, hotels, office buildings etc. The wearing of face masks in public was

initially (on 15 April) only a joint recommendation (and not binding decision) by the Länder and the Federal Government based on the advice of the RKI. However, in the aftermath, Saxony, Mecklenburg-Vorpommern and Bavaria were the first three Länder to stipulate a general mask obligation in public transport and shops. All other Länder followed suit and from 27 April onwards, so this became a nationwide obligation. The City of Jena had been the first sub-national jurisdiction to introduce a mask obligation already on 3 April. This, again, shows the predominant trend of a "race to the top" and the diffusion of containment measures across the country without centrally steering it.

- *Testing, tracking, tracing, quarantining*: As still mentioned in Figure 2.2, testing was significantly extended from roughly 125,000 weekly tests in March to more than one million in September. For instance, Bavaria launched a comprehensive publicly financed mass testing strategy as part of its strict containment approach. Tightened quarantining rules were applied and controlled by the local health authorities, including all persons with a positive PCR test and his/her direct contacts to be identified by the authorities based on their track and trace system. The 14 days domestic quarantining did not only apply to all persons of an "infection chain" but also to returners from internal or external "risk areas" irrespective of symptoms. The comprehensive track and trace system increasingly faced the local health authorities with capacity problems, because they had to scrutinize each individual case (irrespective of symptoms) with the aim of tracing and quarantining all possible direct contact persons or, in case of major clusters or untraceable "infection chains," closing the respective facilities. Because of the amended testing strategy more cases (also without clinical findings) were identified and thus the "infection chains" to be traced and tracked amounted to a magnitude only hardly manageable. As a result, many local health authorities reached their capacity limits. Since April 2020, the federal army (Bundeswehr) helped overburdened local health authorities in tracing "infection chains" and supervising quarantining. In mid-October, around 1,550 soldiers provided administrative assistance for local authorities in combating the pandemic, 1,100 soldiers supported 98 health authorities in tracking and tracing. Up to 5,000 soldiers were available at short notice (MDR 2020).

In Germany, patients were mostly tested and cared for outside the hospitals which relieved the latter from being overrun and saved capacities for critical cases. It is assumed that outpatient care structures play a key role when it comes to explaining varying degrees of crisis affectedness and severity (see Beerheide 2020). Lastly, yet importantly, there has never been a decision (as, for instance, in Italy, UK, US) to send infectious COVID-19 patients from hospitals to care homes.

The "Corona Warning App" launched by the federal government in June 2020 was meant to support the pandemic containment and specifically to relieve local health authorities from at least some burdens in tracing infections chains. The download was to be completely voluntary. The official Corona app of the RKI is based on a decentralized solution with data storage locally on the smartphones based on the Privacy-Preserving Contact Tracing Protocol (PPCP) from Apple and Google via Bluetooth and was developed by Telekom and SAP. Until the end of 2020, app. 24 million Germans (one-third of the population) had downloaded the App, although not everyone actually uses it. The doubts about its effectiveness in pandemic mitigation are growing. Above all, criticism is leveled at the app's overly strict data protection, which makes it impossible to effectively track the chains of infection. The German Ethics Council chair Alena Buyx assumes that data protection should be restricted in order to combat the pandemic (ZDF, 19.10.2020).

The severe containment approach, the comprehensive tracing system and the strong focus on the "incidence rule" were criticized by some public health experts (see also Sections 2.6 and 2.7). These claimed that the overall emphasis on the "incidence rule" (counting of cases), the extensive contact tracing and mass quarantining of large parts of the population were not to be considered appropriate strategies anymore. They pointed to the fact that the disease mostly proceeds mild or even without symptoms for the largest majority of cases and that no excess mortality has been observed in Germany so far. Furthermore, the continued predominance of the containment approach instead of shifting to a more balanced protection and mitigation strategy, likewise provided by the RKI pandemic plan (e.g., giving the protection of vulnerable groups and targeted testing a higher priority), was criticized. The containment approach was also criticized for threatening the societal and economic structures of the country and the operational procedures in the local health authorities who were entirely absorbed by corona management and could not fulfill other obligations anymore, such as important prevention tasks.

Vaccination strategy: When ordering vaccines, Germany, like the other EU member states, deliberately opted for a multilateral European approach. A race between the 27 member states for the scarce vaccine would have meant new explosives for the EU. If the financially strong Germany had bought the vaccine itself, conflicts, especially with less prosperous EU member states, would have been inevitable. In addition, there is the market power of the EU Commission, which was able to achieve better prices than single states because of the large quantities. Regarding vaccine approval, the decisions of the European Commission, which are based on the recommendations of the European Medicines Agency (EMA), apply for the EU and thus also for Germany. The EMA granted the first preliminary approval for the Pfizer-Biontech's vaccine on December 21, 2020. On 7 November, the federal and Länder health ministers decided on a joint German vaccination strategy. The resolution stipulates that the federal government procures and finances the vaccines and the Länder set up a total of 60 vaccination centers. The vaccination is voluntary. Risk groups were to be treated first. The distribution of the vaccine was based on recommendations of the Standing Vaccination Commission (Ständige Impfkommission, Stiko) at the RKI, the German Ethics Council and the National Academy of Sciences Leopoldina (see Ständige Impfkommission et al. 2020). The vaccinations in Germany started at 26 December 2020 with care homes residents. The vaccination campaign proved to be a key to the permanent containment of COVID-19 in the long term.

2.5.3   *Measures in the Health and Care Sector*

At all levels of government, efforts were taken to increase hospital capacities and anticipate a crises-related overburdening of public health institutions. However, these efforts were mainly concentrated on financial compensations and material investments in facilities, beds, ICUs etc. without taking human resources and working conditions for the care and nursing personnel and particularly the poor preparedness of many care homes into account. On the one hand, the federal government passed a legislative proposal aimed at financially supporting hospitals and medical practitioners and reducing red-tape for special-care homes. The new federal law on "COVID-19 hospital relief" adopted on 25 March 2020 granted inter alia financial support to hospitals facing economic problems due to the postponement of regular operations (€2.8 billion) and for the purchase of protective equipment (financial supplement of €50 per patient). Furthermore, measures were enacted to increase the liquidity of hospitals, to compensate medical practitioners for income losses resulting from decreasing numbers of patients, and to temporarily abstain from strict quality assessments and site visits in special-care homes. Generous lump sums for each bed kept clear and additional financial support for newly created intensive care beds were meant to anticipate the expected inrush of COVID-19 patients. But, the effects of these financial aids turned out to be very unequal. While clinics focusing on corona patients hardly benefited from these grants, it was more lucrative for other clinics, for example psychiatric and psychosomatic clinics, to keep beds free.

Additionally, the Länder took various measures to enhance their hospital capacities in preparation of an expected increase in case numbers. Their strategies were based on an agreement of the Federal and the Länder chancelleries passed on 17 March 2020 stipulating an emergency plan for the German hospitals. The plan included a doubling of the 28,000 places in intensive care units (25,000 of which with ventilation) and the conversion of rehabilitation facilities, hotels and bigger halls into care centers for mild corona cases. The Länder were responsible to elaborate local plans with their clinics regarding the creation of provisional care capacities for expected corona patients, if necessary, with the support of the German Red Cross (Deutsches Rotes Kreuz, DRK) or the Technical Aid Organization (Technisches Hilfswerk, THW). Furthermore, local governments developed concepts together with their health authorities and corona task forces directed at converting local real estates into hospital-like structures or re-activating vacant or old clinic estates or even construct completely new corona care center. Last but not least, the hospitals started to re-organize their internal processes in order to be prepared organizationally for the inrush of corona patients. These immediate reactions to increase hospital capacities notwithstanding, the long-term trend to close smaller hospitals has not stopped in the pandemic. Twenty hospitals with 2,144 beds and 4,000 jobs were closed in 2020, twice as many as on average in recent years ().

Two particularly critical problem areas must be emphasized at this point: ICU capacities and the role of care homes. The availability of sufficient ICUs for COVID-19 patients was a major concern from the beginning of the crisis (see Figure 2.3 in Section 2.2). Therefore, the Federal Government funded the creation of thousands of new ICUs with more than half a billion euros. An emergency ordinance was adopted in April 2020 providing for a daily notification of ICU's occupancy to allow the federal ministry of health to react quickly to impending bottlenecks. In general, the much-feared overburdening of the German health system, as measured by the nationwide availability of ICU beds (leaving aside some regional bottlenecks), did not become apparent. However, as said before, this comparatively relaxed situation did not apply to care and nursing personnel which turned out to be a major shortage in the crisis.

Taking into account, that more than 10,000 new beds have been newly created since the beginning of the pandemic, there was a surplus in bed capacities for (expected) COVID-19 patients rather than a shortage. Against this background, the federal policy which obliged the hospitals to keep considerable parts of their capacities clear for expected corona patients became increasingly criticized by experts. Paired with the generally shrinking non-COVID surgery in hospitals during the pandemic and the compulsory postponement of plannable operations (agreed by the federal and Länder governments) this policy led to a situation in which hospital capacities became even (temporarily) under-utilized, at least in some clinic departments, and hospital employment sank below capacity in some medical fields. In general, the already existing economic problems of many clinics have been exacerbated by the pandemic (see Deutsche Krankenhausgesellschaft 2020).

According to their Hospital Barometer 2020, the clinics are experiencing the effects of health-related policy measures especially with regard to (postponed) operations and resulting financial income (losses). From the mid-March 2020, planned interventions and operations were temporarily postponed or suspended. More than 908,000 plannable operations were canceled by May 2020. Regarding inpatient care, the number of surgical interventions fell by 41% on average, in outpatient care by 58% (Deutsche Krankenhausgesellschaft 2020: 8). "On average, each clinic lost around 2.5 million euros due to the decline in inpatient interventions and 250,000 euros due to the lower number of outpatient measures" (ibid.: 14). After an interim "normalization" during the summer months, since beginning of October, German hospitals have restarted to postpone operations to keep ICUs clear for COVID-19 patients, thus similar effects can be expected. As a result, almost half of all German hospitals (47%) expect an annual deficit in 2020. For 2021, only a quarter of all hospitals expect a positive development, while 40 percent expect their economic situation to deteriorate. Under these circumstances, hospitals are claiming government compensation for their financial losses in 2021 and beyond.

Another problematic area is care homes, where the protection of vulnerable groups, elderly people failed. About 40% of COVID-19 related deaths in Germany (3,736 residents and 41 employees) have happened in various types of care facilities (see RKI 2020d: 5) and between 50% and 60% in care homes for the elderly or other in outpatient care (see Rothgang et al. 2020; Beneker 2020) Because of the median death age of COVID-19 patients of 82 years in Germany (Statista 2020b), the focused protection of care homes is key to pandemic management. However, the situation in German care homes was from the beginning much worse than that of hospitals. Whereas a general containment approach for the population was in the center of pandemic management, the focused protection of vulnerable groups, specifically elderly people with pre-existing illnesses, was less emphatically pursued by policy makers. This is all the more puzzling as the dramatic problems regarding the staff situation in care homes, the chronic underpayment, overburdening und poor qualification of the employees have been well-known since many years. Furthermore, serious hygiene problems in some homes have also been discussed publicly since decades. Care homes were conspicuously ill prepared, which dramatically popped up in the pandemic. In addition, there is the permanent overload situation of the nursing staff in the pandemic that has been going on for one year.

2.5.4 *Impacts on the Economy and Economic Stimulus Packages*

In the first half of 2020, the German economy found itself in the deepest recession in its post-war history. Following a decline of 2.0% in the first quarter of 2020, the German GDP shrank by 9.7% in the second quarter, which represents a historical quarterly decline never seen before. Three in four German companies were negatively affected by the COVID-19 pandemic (see KANTAR 2020a, 2020b). The economic sectors that have been hit mostly are hospitals, social services, vehicles and machinery, and food production. Companies were most frequently affected by a loss in demand and cash-flow problems. During the first shutdown approximately half of all German private companies had to shut down their operations temporarily, either partly or fully. In the third quarter of 2020, the GDP grew again by 8.5%. Despite the second shutdown, the GDP grew by 0.3% in the fourth quarter 2020. For the whole year 2020 the GDP declined by - 4.9%. Germany is thus well above the decline in GDP in the euro zone (–7.5%) and significantly better than France and Italy (–9.1%) (OECD 2020).

Because of the intensive use of an extended short-term allowance, the unemployment rate rose from 5.1% to the peak with 6.4% in August, then falling down to 5.9% in December 2020 (Bundesagentur für Arbeit 2020). Approximately 25% of this increase was corona-related, mostly because unemployed people under the pandemic conditions have more difficulties to find a new job (Frankfurter Allgemeine Zeitung, 1.10.2020). Since July 2020, there has been "no corona-related increase in unemployment on the labour market" (Bundesministerium für Wirtschaft und Energie 2020).

Several instruments, some of which already known from previous crisis periods (e.g., financial crisis 2008/2009), have been applied to remedy the economic impacts of pandemic containment. The most important are:

- *Short-time allowance (Kurzarbeitergeld)* which is in Germany a "classical" instrument of economic crisis mitigation played a decisive role in the pandemic in order to temporarily saving jobs and securing the existence of companies. Temporary regulations were introduced, on 1 March 2020 until the end of the year, to simplify and increase the receipt of short-time allowance, which have been extended until the end of 2021. Employees whose wages are reduced by at least half receive up to 70% of the lost net wage from the fourth month of receipt (77% for employees with at least one child) and from the seventh month on 80% (87% for employees with at least one child). The maximum duration of short-time allowance, paid by the Federal Employment Agency (Bundesagentur für Arbeit), is 24 months. So far, the federal government has approved a total of 25 billion euros for short-time working benefits during the pandemic. The number of short-time allowances peaked in April 2020 with 5.95 million recipients and then sank up until December 2020 around 2.2 million. This tool has proved to be quite effective because it relieves employers of the salary costs for their employees, which helps to avoid immediate dismissals and facilitates to keep employees in the companies (Pusch and Seifert 2021).

- *Economic rescue packages with multiple corona emergency funding schemes*: The economic rescue package (Rettungspaket) enacted by the federal government in March 2020 represents the most comprehensive state aid provided to the economy in German history so far. The package included a rescue fund of about 600 billion Euros for medium-sized and larger companies, which consisted of loan guarantees amounting to 400 billion Euros, 100 billion Euros for state holdings in companies and 100 billion Euro to finance easier access for bridging loans from the state-owned German reconstruction bank (Kreditanstalt für Wiederaufbau, KfW). Furthermore, aids for small businesses and solo-entrepreneurs worth around €50 billion were enacted. The measures embraced a total value of around 750 billion Euros (Bundesministerium für Wirtschaft und Energie 2021). In addition, VAT was reduced from 1 July to 31 December 2020. The regular tax rate drops from 19% to 16%, the reduced tax rate from 7% to 5%. With the second lockdown since end of October 2020, companies, businesses, self-employed persons, associations and institutions affected were supported by a specific "Package of measures to combat the impact of coronavirus on companies" (Bundesministerium für Wirtschaft und Energie 2021). Some examples of its instruments. A special economic assistance for November and December is granted in the form of a one-off grant covering the period of closure in this time. A specific Coronavirus Bridging Assistance III for small and medium-sized companies runs from November 2020 to the end of June 2021. The suspension of the obligation to file for insolvency will be extended until 30 April 2021 for debtors who have file d applications for financial assistance under government assistance programs between 1 November 2020 and 28 February 2021 in order to mitigate the fallout/consequences of the COVID-19 pandemic. This support program was largely welcomed by the business community, but there is increasing criticism of the bureaucratic application process and the slow payment of the funds. This additional state corona aid for companies since October 2020 will cost at least ten billion euros. The corona crisis has cost the German state according to the Federal Minister of Finance more than 1.4 trillion Euros so far. The size of the aid packages corresponds to 42% of 2019 German GDP. This tremendous sum is made up of many expenditure points. In addition to the guarantees, which make up the largest part, this includes short-time working benefits, immediate and bridging aid for companies that had to close in lockdowns, but also the increased costs in the health system and international aid, such as the 750 billion Euro Corona aid fund the EU (FOCUS 2021c).

* *Social protection:* On March 23, 2020, the federal Ministries of Labor and Social Affairs and Health put forward the first package of social protection measures directed at absorbing situations of social hardship and existence threatening circumstances caused by the pandemic. The major aim of the social protection package was declared as follows "no one shall face a threat of existence due to the economic impacts of the crisis" (Bundesministerium für Arbeit und Soziales 2020). For one, the access to basic security benefits for job seekers (so-called Hartz IV) was simplified, in order to offer quick support to the employees which lost their jobs during the crises, many of whom coming from small businesses, freelancers or so-called "solo-entrepreneurs." These groups belong to the most seriously hit economic actors because in many cases the shutdown entailed a complete cancellation of all orders and a breakdown of all business activities. In addition, owners and employees of small businesses and solo-entrepreneurs usually have no access to unemployment benefits or other social security measures and do not have noteworthy financial reserves at their disposal to bridge income losses over longer periods of time. Furthermore, a moratorium for rents was enacted in aid of those tenants who were not in the position anymore to pay their rents as a result of income losses caused by crisis-related shutdowns and lockdowns. The moratorium was to be valid from 1 April until 30 September 2020 and provided the deferred amount of rent to be paid back by the tenants later on. Finally, for parents of small children who face income losses because of the shutdowns of school and kindergartens an entitlement for compensation was introduced. On May 28, the law on Law on social measures to combat the corona pandemic (Social Protection Package II) came into force. This package includes a number of individual measures, including, for example, improved conditions for drawing short-time work benefits, and extending the period of entitlement to unemployment benefits.

* *Paradigm shift in financial policy and new debts:* The pandemic has profound financial consequences for Germany (see Bundesministerium der Finanzen 2020a, 2020b, Gebhardt and Siemers 2020). To finance the economic crisis mitigation programs, the federal government decided to run up new debts of app. 140 billion Euro which represents the biggest new indebtedness ever seen in this country. With the economic rescue package, the federal budget in 2020 will exceed the permitted credit limit of app. 83 billion euros. This clashes with the constitutionally enshrined debt brake and represents a fundamental paradigm shift in German financial policy. For the first time, the constitutional option

was used of temporarily suspending the debt brake. This is possible in the event of natural disasters or exceptional emergency situations which are beyond the control of the state and have a significant negative impact on the state's financial position. To make the suspension of the debt brake legally possible, the Bundestag decided, in an urgent procedure on March 25, 2020, that the exceptional emergency situation according Article 115 Basic Law applied and that on this basis the constitutional debt brake was to be lifted for the 2020 budget year.

With the first and second supplementary budgets for 2020, the federal government was countering the effects of the pandemic, both in terms of health and economic challenges. The additional expenditure volume decided in the supplementary budgets amounts to around €146.5 billion, including around €28.9 billion for additional investments. To finance this, the BMF was authorized to take out loans amounting to around € 217.8 billion (Bundesministerium der Finanzen 2020a). With the federal budget 2021 with expenditures amounting to 498.62 billion euros, the federal government wants to create the financial prerequisites to powerfully overcome the effects of the corona crisis so that the acute pandemic is over. However, in this exceptional emergency situation, the upper limit for new borrowing permitted under the debt rule will be exceeded by around 164.2 billion euros. The federal government is thus continuing its two-pillar strategy in the pandemic: The first pillar is intended to stabilize the economy with emergency aid, liquidity aid, bridging measures and short-time work benefits. The second pillar is to combine overcoming the pandemic with modernizing the economy in the 2020s.

2.6   Policy-Advice, Knowledge Generation, and Scientific Controversy

2.6.1   *Role and Organization of Policy Advice in the Pandemic*

Given the severity and magnitude of mitigation measures in the pandemic and the fact that a firm support and broad acceptance by the population were key to implement them (see Section 2.6), a major concern of politicians was to create legitimacy, ensure public trust in their strategies and to avoid contestation regarding their actions. Against this background government decisions were justified and legitimized first and foremost by referring to the recommendations of experts. Politicians at all governmental levels emphasized their decisions to be firmly based on the professional advice of scientists, even though – as usual in science – knowledge is uncertain, controversial, contested and initial assessments changed over time (see Van Dooren and Noordegraaf 2020). Science and experts' opinions were thus crucial sources of policy justification and legitimization. Typical headlines of newspapers even suggested that politics was in the backseat whereas the experts were assumed to govern the crisis.[15]

However, having a closer look, there can be some doubts as to whether this interpretation holds true. Especially from a comparative perspective (see Kuhlmann et al. 2021a, 2021b, 2021c) it becomes apparent that, in Germany, the political rationality was very crucial in the pandemic and executive politics was not – as in Sweden for instance – in the backseat but in the driver seat of decision-making. Although experts' recommendations were a key source for generating legitimacy and trust, political preferences and interests played a major role in pandemic management, too, and executive actor's power-seeking strategies provide important explanations for their crises' decisions. In addition, internal policy advisors (particularly the RKI as a directly subordinated authority of the Federal Ministry of Health) assumed an institutionally less independent position than national health authorities in some other countries, for example, in Sweden (see Kuhlmann et al. 2021c; Franzke and Kuhlmann 2021). Direct interventions by executive leaders (Minister of Health) into the internal advisors' work were potentially possible. However, so far, empirical evidence is lacking about whether and to what extent such interventions actually happened.

Regarding health-related policy advice, a distinction must be made between internal or institutionalized (governmental) advisers on the one hand (see Gerlinger 2019: 15) and external (non-governmental) advisers on the other. The former was provided by the federal authority for disease monitoring and prevention (RKI) which is a higher federal authority (Bundesoberbehörde) and directly subordinated to the Federal Ministry of Health. Due to its hierarchical integration in the federal ministerial administration, the RKI enjoys less autonomy and discretion than, for instance, the Swedish National Public Health Agency (see Kuhlmann et al. 2021c) and is legally bound to the ministry's directives. The advisory function of the RKI basically referred to three major fields: (1) Pre-crisis risk prognosis, including the elaboration of a national pandemic plan; (2) Monitoring and publication of infection cases (positively tested by a PCR test), number of hospitalized cases, recoveries, and deaths; (3) Epidemic risk assessment based on which measures of containment, protection, mitigation, and recovery were recommended to politics and communicated to the public.

During the corona crisis, the RKI has become the most important player in institutionalized policy expertise not only on the part of the federal government but also regarding containment strategies developed by the Länder and local governments. Although it could not impose decisions, its recommendations were followed thoroughly by the Länder and local governments, who transformed them into legally binding rules for their territories. Thus, internal policy advice in the pandemic was clearly dominated, in Germany, by the RKI as a federal authority and thus framed and practiced in a rather centralized manner.

In addition, some of the Länder also mobilized own policy advice for pandemic management in their jurisdictions, such as the interdisciplinary corona experts' council set up by the government of North Rhine-Westphalia on 1 April 2020, consisting of 12 experts from medicine, law, economics, philosophy, psychology, sociology and social work. The council is meant to develop a more holistic approach toward pandemic management, also taking economic and social consequences of COVID-19 crisis management into account, in addition to the usual short-term health-related and epidemiological aspects. Based on systematic and transparent criteria, the council aims to develop strategies for returning to social and public life.[16] Another example of sub-national pandemic policy advice is the Land of Thuringia, where on 26 May 2020, a scientific advisory board on corona management was formed composed of 12 members from different disciplines. Similar to NRW, this board is expected to approach the complexity of pandemic management from an interdisciplinary perspective and draw up a work program to address the broader consequences of pandemic management.[17] These efforts by some Länder governments notwithstanding, the executive orders enacted by the Länder (e.g., regarding the "incidence rule," the extension of lockdowns etc.) did not fundamentally diverge from the central-level provisions proclaimed by the RKI and agreed in the intergovernmental meetings.

The RKI's internal policy advice was combined with external expertise, which the Federal Government on the one hand obtained from the well-known Charité virologist,[18] Christian Drosten, who has served as a direct advisor to the federal government from the beginning of the pandemic.[19] He reached considerable prominence during the COVID-19 pandemic as the "Corona educator of the nation" (Süddeutsche Zeitung, 13.3.2020). On the other hand, the Federal Government based its containment policy on public statements by the National Academy of Science Leopoldina,[20] which consists of renowned academics predominantly coming from natural sciences and medicine, but also including expertise in economics, history, and other fields. When the Leopoldina, in its seventh ad hoc statement of December 2020 (Leopoldina 2021b), recommended a hard lockdown to the Federal Government based on a four pages document, legitimizing draconian measures and societal incisions from December onwards, the quality of the Academy's advisory role came however to be contested by some critics.[21]

Unlike other policy discourses in the German federal system (see Kuhlmann and Wollmann 2019: 139 et seq.), the scientific discourse about COVID-19 mitigation measures did not unfold in a vertically decentralized and fragmented manner which, in Germany, usually gears to slow and incremental change. Instead, the discourse was clearly dominated by few central-level internal and external advisors all of whom more or less favoring a quite incisive containment approach. According to their advice, from November 2020 onwards, ever stricter measures for the whole population were inevitable to slow down the spread of the virus, "flatten the curve," (re)enable contact tracing by local health authorities and thereby avoid a crash down of the health system. Milder measures (e.g., recommendations and voluntariness instead of restrictions and sanctions) and alternative solutions (e.g., a focused protection of vulnerable groups instead of general lockdowns) to avoiding negative long-term societal impacts were not supported by the experts who had been selected to advise the Federal Government.

2.6.2   *Reporting and Transmission of Information*

Germany disposes of a comprehensive system of health surveillance and reporting. Since many years, the RKI collects and publishes data on contagious infection diseases, including seasonal influenza, and surveils in particular the development of serious acute respiratory infections (SARI), including the seasonal influenza and most recently COVID-19. In particular, the RKI based "Working group on influenza" (Arbeitsgemeinschaft Influenza, AGI), founded in 1992, collects data on SARI using a so-called "sentinel system" in which 689 doctors' practices voluntarily report their clinical information about SARI to the AGI. It also collaborates with the health surveillance systems at the level of the Länder who collect data regionally and share it (voluntarily) with the AGI. The German National Reference Centre for Influenza Viruses (Nationales Referenzzentrum für Influenzaviren, NRZ) supports the examination of the SARI viruses by the AGI. Finally, there is the "Grippe-web" ("influenza web"), a data basis for SARI with about 8,000 participants which surveils the spread of SARI in the population, which was assessed as one of the best in Europe.

The obligation to report COVID-19 as an infectious disease was stipulated in the IfSG already end of January 2020. It includes not only all confirmed COVID-19 cases with a positive PCR test (irrespective of symptoms) but also suspected cases of COVID-19. Physicians, laboratories, care and nursing personnel as well as heads of various public institutions (schools, universities, kindergartens, hostels, lodging houses, mass dormitories) are obliged to report confirmed and suspected cases within 24 hours to their local health authorities. In the next step, they report their data (without personal information of patients) several times per day to the Länder health authorities which in turn is responsible to transmit the data to the RKI electronically. However, in some Länder (e.g., Brandenburg), the local health authorities are allowed to directly report their data to the

RKI and in addition to the respective Länder health authority, thus a kind of double reporting. This led to some confusion because incidence data differed between the RKI and the Länder authority with the consequence that data about the correct number of corona hotspots and thus the containment measures (e.g., in hotspots) to be applied differed considerably. Furthermore, the RKI reporting procedures were criticized by some local health authorities as being rather complex, time consuming and bureaucratic which also contributed to some reluctance in completing the files and thus diverging data sets on incidences at Länder and federal levels.

Finally, a major issue of criticism concerned the missing digitalization in health administration which turned out to be a crucial bottleneck in the reporting of cases across jurisdictions and levels. Thus, particularly direct reporting from the local health authorities to the RKI was oftentimes proceeded by fax or telephone. Data transmission was impaired by many media discontinuities and not machine-readable, which led to delays and faults in data transfer (see Normenkontrollrat 2020: 12). Despite several projects and initiatives aimed at modernizing and digitalizing public health related data sharing, a comprehensive nationwide digital reporting system has not been established yet, which led to a number of reporting failures from December onwards, when the reported data was officially declared to be unreliable (see RKI 2020e) yet continued to be the basis for (tightened) containment decisions. It can be assumed that these failures and inconsistencies have also negatively impacted on the population's trust regarding pandemic management.

On November 16, 2020, the federal and state governments had stipulated that the local health authorities should network with the SORMAS digital system in order to be able to more easily understand the contacts of corona infected people and to prevent hotspots from developing. The goal of connecting 90% of the health authorities to this system by the end of 2020 has not been achieved. Many local health authorities refuse to change their self-developed digital reporting system in the middle of the pandemic and because of technical interface problems (Frankfurter Allgemeine Zeitung 2021).

The RKI publishes a huge amount of information and data on the pandemic over time, the regional spread of the disease, the development of cases and the capacity situation in hospitals. This information is based on locally collected data (see above) and published online in The RKI status reports (see RKI 2020f) provide a detailed picture on the pandemic situation in the country on a daily basis since March 2020. In addition, a new data resource was created in April 2020 with the DIVI-Registry for Intensive Care (see Section 2.2). This registry captures the capacity situation regarding ICUs in about 1,300 German hospitals for acute surgery in real time and thus helps to identify regional shortfalls. It enables governments and hospital staff to react quickly to changing circumstances in order to avoid supply bottlenecks for patients and to early detect local overloads of hospitals. Besides the data generated at national scale (RKI, DIVI), the Länder produce their own information bases and status reports on the pandemic situation in their territories, which sometimes however differed from the RKI data due to reporting problems and deficiencies in data sharing.

The information provided by the RKI and other institutions notwithstanding, there was also criticism regarding the lack of representative studies on the nature of the COVID-19 pandemic (based on age groups, morbidity indicators, regions etc.). It was claimed that representative cohort studies would be necessary to understand the dangerousness of the virus for various groups in the society and thus to decide containment measures in a more differentiated manner and on an evidence base. However, these kinds of studies have not been conducted yet in Germany at time of writing which was criticized as a serious default of the government (see inter alia the interview with Hendrik Streeck (Streeck 2021).

2.6.3 *Scientific Controversies and Contestation*

Over the course of the crisis, the scientific positions of how to deal with the pandemic have become more differentiated, but also controversial, partly polarized. In general, an increasing number of experts expressed their discontent with the governments' approach publicly,[22] while in the first phase of the pandemic these voices had been rather weak. Toward the second half of the year, there was more openness and controversy in the public debate regarding the appropriate assessment and handling of the crisis in the long run. It became visible that among specialists the opinions about the dangerousness of the virus and the effectiveness of measures were controversial and had also changed over time.

Leaving apart the extreme position of some experts who claimed a "non-COVID" or "zero-COVID" strategy (Expertengruppe No-Covid-Strategie 2021)[23] by way of tightening containment and reinforcing the stringency of lockdowns, the scientific opinions oscillated around various degrees of strictness or permeability of mitigation measures, with some experts more in line with the governmental approach in supporting a (modified) extension of containment and others claiming a profound change in strategy by inter alia demanding a more focused protection of vulnerable groups and criticizing the political neglect of (mid- and long term) societal and health effects of governmental response measures (see inter alia Schrappe et al. 2020b).[24] In a joint experts' statement published by the Association of Statutory Health Insurance Physicians and renowned virologists with the support of about 30 professional associations, major criticism was raised regarding the general pandemic approach. The experts questioned the appropriateness and effectiveness of comprehensive contact tracing as well as the predominance of authoritative prohibitions, unspecific mass quarantining, and lacking evaluative knowledge about pandemic mitigation measures (see Kassenärztliche Bundesvereinigung 2020). Furthermore, the group of specialists appealed to the government to shift its pandemic approach from a rather unspecified mass containment to a more targeted protection of high-risk populations,[25] also preferring recommendations and encouragement of the population instead of bans, prohibitions and fear and putting more emphasis on evidence and evaluations. They also suggested to not only base political decisions on sheer case numbers and incidences ("incidence rule"), but to include additional key indicators when enacting measures, particularly the number of tests, hospital capacities, number of hospitalizations and intensive care treatments. Many other experts[26] shared this critique also pointing to the collateral damages, for example, the fact that the containment measures would threat the societal and economic structures of the country and cause additional health damages in the long run and increase some population group's death risks, due to lost livelihoods, socio-economic downturn, the neglect of health authorities' important prevention tasks, and postponed medical treatments and (elective) operations, the number of which accumulated to 851,000 in May 2020, including around 52,000 cancer operations (WELT 2020a; Berliner Zeitung 2020).

On the other hand, increasing concerns were raised over the lacking interdisciplinary approach, the missing multi-dimensional ("risk-risk trade-off") impact assessments and the fact that the containment policy appeared to be predominantly based on medical specialists', particularly virologists', recommendations, largely ignoring other aspects and second round effects of crisis mitigation. Experts from outside the narrow circle of governmental policy advice claimed that the protection of interests other than short term prevention of corona deaths must also be taken into account by policy makers in order to ensure the proportionality of measures. They claimed an imperative of multi-dimensional/-disciplinary risk assessment and a plurality of disciplines in pandemic policy advice instead of a mono-thematic containment strategy.[27] Furthermore, they raised concerns about the overly narrowed discourse pointing to the necessity of a more balanced, rational, and enlightened deliberation and a more democratic competition of opinions when it comes to determine proportional measures (see Schrappe et al. 2020a: 7). Some also warned of a further politicization of the pandemic and the instrumentalization of science for political aims[28]; see also further above on the critique raised toward the Leopoldina).

As a consequence, in the public debate and in politics, the awareness of an overly narrowed discourse being detrimental for a multi-dimensional risk assessment and proportionate decision-making in the crisis increased.

Besides virologists, epidemiologists and modelers representatives from other disciplines (economists, psychologists, pedagogues, social scientists etc.) publicly took the floor to address the non-virus-related long-term impacts of crisis management, particularly pointing to the societally and economically devastating effects of repeated lockdowns, but also of the insufficient focused protection of vulnerable groups. This partial shift in the public debate notwithstanding, the government apparently relied on the expertise of virologists, epidemiologists, but also physics, the latter particularly consulted for modeling and forecasting epidemic scenarios (see Streeck 2021). Key decisions were largely lacking a broader interdisciplinary discussion and controversy. Against this background, the Federal Government was also criticized of being "resistant against advice"[29] and of showing a kind of "bunker mentality."[30] Alternative proposals, such as the establishment of an "independent scientific pandemic council" at the Federal Chancellery, which the Bundestag faction of Bündnis 90/Die Grünen (Deutscher Bundestag 2020c) had proposed in July 2020, have not yet been implemented. This also applies to the proposals to locate such a pandemic council at the RKI[31] or to strengthen the unsatisfactory interdisciplinary expertise of the RKI (see Deutsche Krankenhausgesellschaft 2020).

2.7   Institutional Trust, Acceptance of and Opposition to Containment Measures

2.7.1   *Institutional Trust and Citizens' Satisfaction with Public Administration in the Pandemic*

Trust in government and in public authorities oscillated over the year with an initial peak followed by a decline from April to December. After a substantial increase at the beginning of the pandemic (see Figure 2.9; Frankfurter Allgemeine Zeitung 2020a), trust levels progressively shrank toward the end of the year. Thus, the share of respondents with (rather) low trust in the Federal Government climbed from 25% (in April) to 39% (in December), while still a relative majority (44%) had high trust in the Federal Government by December (Cosmo 2021[32]). It is also striking that the trust in local public health authorities declined quite significantly since November, which also applies to the Federal Ministry of Health and to the Länder ministries of Health. While trust levels for the RKI were in general comparatively high over the course of the pandemic, it also registered a clear decline in trust until the end of the year, most significantly from April to June, and from November onwards. One reason for this could be that many citizens consider government's response to the increase in the number of infections since October 2020 to be too late and insufficient.

Very high or high Trust regarding the following institutions
(in brackets change since January 2020):

Federal President 76% (+3)	Chancellor 72% (+22)
Federal Government 60% (+26)	Mayors 58% (+10)
Länder Government 58% (+11)	Municipal Councils 57% (+9)
City Administrations 56% (+9)	Bundestag 54% (+13)
European Union 37% (–3)	Political Parties 25% (+9)

Figure 2.9 Trust in political institutions (May 2020).

Source: Adapted from forsa 2020 according to Frankfurter Allgemeine Zeitung, 16.5.2020. In brackets difference to forsa-survey as of January 2020.

A relative majority of citizens assessed German public administrations' responses to the COVID-19 pandemic as "very good" or "rather good" with the Länder authorities receiving highest support (45% "good" or "rather good"), followed by the federal authorities (43%), the local health authorities (40%), and the municipal/county administrations in general (36% (see Eckhard and Lenz 2020).[33] By contrast, the European Commission was perceived rather critically with only 25% positive ratings in March/April 2020. According to a more recent representative survey (Wagschal et al. 2020), by the end of the year (November 2020), German citizens were still very satisfied with the Federal Government in managing the pandemic, even more than with other levels of government, which could indicate an increasingly critical stance toward the performance of subnational administrations. The share of respondents who stated to be "very" or "rather satisfied" with the Federal Government's pandemic management amounted to about 56% while other levels received lower satisfaction values (45% for the Länder governments; 47% for the mayors). Yet, these finding also imply that, by the end of the year, significant parts of the population were only partly or not satisfied with the with the governments' performance in handling the pandemic; thus, roughly one-third indicated to be "very" or "rather unsatisfied" (30% with the Federal Government, 28% with the Länder governments, 28% with the mayors).

In the March/April survey (see Eckhard and Lenz 2020) it was also asked whether citizens believe that the German federal system helps to cope with the COVID-19 pandemic. Interestingly more than 40% negated this statement whereas only about 24% supported it (24% "partially agree/disagree"; 11% answered "don't know"). Citizen's assessments regarding the functioning of public administration during the pandemic were rather critical as well. According to a survey conducted in July 2020 (see Next: Public 2020) about 41% of the citizens evaluated the general functioning of public administration during the (first wave of) the pandemic as poor ("administration was functioning rather poorly" or "not functioning at all") while 44% perceived it as "well-functioning."

2.7.2   *Acceptance of Containment Measures*

The acceptance of containment measures is an important indicator and precondition for implementation success and compliance with these rules. Regarding various types of measures, a longitudinal study of the University of Mannheim revealed in a representative survey that the degree of acceptance to these measures declined over time since the beginning of the pandemic until July (Blom et al. 2020: 7). Whereas the acceptance rate regarding the prohibition of mass events, the closure of public facilities and the closure of borders was at almost 100% in March the support shrank to between 30% (borders) and 20% (public facilities) by July. Only the prohibition of mass events was still accepted by a clear majority of the German population (64%). Other containment measures, too, which from the beginning did not receive extremely high acceptance rates, were increasingly rejected by the population. Thus, the acceptance of a general lockdown decreased from more than 50% to around 10%.

At the same time, the proportion of people who did not accept any of these measures increased from almost zero in March to roughly one-quarter in July. In November 2020, only a few containment measures continued to receive support by a majority of the population (e.g., general mask obligation: 66% in favor; closing off COVID-19 hot spots: 60%; prohibition of religious festivities/services: 60%) (see Wagschal et al. 2020).[34] Most of the other measures were only supported by a minority of citizens. For all measures a clear decreasing trend in acceptance rates was noticeable from May to November.[35]

Asked about the general appropriateness of containment measures, however, one-third of the respondents considered them as exaggerated, whereas still a clear majority (54%) regarded them as appropriate (see Wagschal et al. 2020: 10). Nevertheless, at the beginning of January 2021, only one-third trusted in the effectiveness of the containment measures, while more than half of the population believed that the measures would finally not succeed in reducing case numbers (see forsa survey of RTL 2021). Furthermore, with the case numbers rising from October onwards the share of the population in favor of more restrictive containment measures regarding the pandemic rose substantially (see Kirsch et al. 2020).[36] In November/December, almost half of respondents (44%) believed the measures were far from enough, which marks a clear increase compared to June/July when only 15% supported more stringent measures. At the same time, the proportion of those who regard the scope of the measures as appropriate dropped from 65% to 35%. Those who thought the scope being excessive have remained fairly unchanged over time at about 20%. In general, the perceived severity of the pandemic situation appears to affect people's acceptance of containment stringency (see also Cosmo 2021).

Regarding the extension of Federal Government's powers, there was on the one hand a clear decline in public support from March, when almost 80% were in favor of such an upgrade, to April when this support had almost halved and shrunk to roughly 40% (see Juhl et al. 2020: 6). On the other hand, from May to November people's support of the government to enact laws without involving the parliament increased from 13% to 20% (Wagschal et al. 2020: 16). In general, the public satisfaction with pandemic management has decreased substantially over time (see Kirsch et al. 2020). Thus, in November/December only around 55% respondents were still satisfied with government efforts to fight the pandemic, 13% less than in summer, while dissatisfaction has risen substantially.

2.7.3   Opposition to Containment

Whereas at the beginning of the crisis, there was no noticeable opposition to the measures taken and protests were very rare, over the course of the pandemic, an increasing number of platforms and social movements flourished directed at criticizing governments' response measures. The support of the party groups in parliament regarding the general containment approach of the government continued to be very high, with the only few exceptions. Against this background, more fundamental opposition to the governments' containment policies mainly formed outside government and parliament. The most prominent movement of extra-parliamentary "corona-opposition" in Germany are the so-called Querdenker ("lateral thinkers") which is an ideologically and socially rather heterogeneous movement of protest against the containment measures and for the re-establishment of suspended constitutional rights.[37] From the Easter weekend onwards, the Querdenker (and their predecessor organizations[38]) organized demonstrations against the containment measures in various German cities (Stuttgart, Leipzig, Dresden, Munich) with a peak of about 38,000 participants, end of August in Berlin and 45,000 in November in Leipzig (see Wikipedia 2021). After some bans at the end of 2020, their demonstrations in the meantime came to a halt. However, it seems likely that new protests will restart in 2021, so the future of this kind of new social movement, including its possible radicalization,[39] is still open.

Critical voices toward the governments' pandemic containment approach also came from some scientists,[40] health experts,[41] local government practitioners[42] (see also Section 2.7), and politicians.[43] Their critique ranged from questioning the effectiveness of the governmental stop-and-go approach, the appropriateness of the "incidence rule" as key indicator for decisions (see Section 2.5), the comprehensive contact tracing and the neglect of the vulnerable groups in pandemic mitigation to the lack of a clear policy strategy and reliable representative data to base mitigation measures on. Furthermore, the government's communication strategy was criticized as being too much focused on "incidences" (instead of health capacities and serious illness cases) and provoking people's fear. Some experts also claimed that scientific policy advice was biased or qualitatively poor.[44]

Resistance also came from the economy, predominantly from the associations of the gastronomy and hotel business and representatives of small and medium-sized enterprises, some of whom (e.g., the former president of the professional association of medium-sized businesses, BVMV) announced to bring the occupational bans imposed on enterprises to the courts. Many entrepreneurs sued against the closure of their businesses to achieve their annulment, which was partially successful when in October the so-called "lodging prohibition" (for hotel guests coming from regions with high incidences) had to be repealed due to a lacking evidence-base of the respective executive orders. However, thousands of other lawsuits put forward from November onwards against the shutdown of businesses or against the suspension of the constitutional rights for free assembly and free movement were rejected.

Last but not least, the growing importance of social media channels must be mentioned as a platform of protests. Some scientists also criticized the official media to have partly failed in presenting pandemic-related information soberly, un-emotionally, fact-based and in a well-balanced manner (see Schrappe et al. 2020a). It was criticized that an open and controversial debate about the crisis was not encouraged and relevant data not put in proportion but instead the corridor of opinions narrowed down and the broadcasting of alarming news and emotional pictures preferred to neutral reporting (ibid.). This might partially explain the growing relevance of "alternative media" channels during the pandemic. It has become apparent that over the course of the pandemic an open public debate, about possible alternatives to the governmental response measures and about future perspectives of crisis governance, including greater parliamentary participation and a more open (scientific) debate, is requested by growing parts of the population.

2.8   Conclusions

Our study has shown that the German approach of COVID-19 governance in the first year of the pandemic features, on the one hand, a number of strengths and assets which are closely related to the fairly comfortable starting conditions, for instance in terms of hospital capacities, economic prosperity, and an overall stable institutional set-up. Germany belongs to the top-scorers in the European Union regarding health expenditures, ICU equipment, medical specialization and quality of (public) health services. Even at the peak of hospitalizations in December 2020, there were still more than 15,000 ICUs available and its occupancy quote during the first year of the pandemic was never beyond 85% and remained quite stable at about 22,000 from September onwards. In general, the much-feared over-burdening of the German health system did not take place. Experts do not see a noticeable excess mortality in Germany for 2020.

On the other hand, some important weaknesses and shortcomings have become apparent. In particular, the precarious staff situation in the health and care sectors, the institutional overload of local health authorities and their ill digital readiness, the (disciplinary) narrowness of the scientific debate and policy advice, and the peculiar shifts in vertical and horizontal checks and balances during the pandemic. Criticism was also raised with respect to the containment approach as such, the back-and-forth logic ("lockdown-yoyo") as well as the basis and consistency of decisions. Some of these problems originated in policy decisions of previous years, such as understaffed hospitals and care facilities, NPM-driven privatization and marketization in the hospital and care sector as well as the missed digital transformation in public administration. Others resulted from crisis-related decisions and political actors' "opportunity management" (Kuhlmann et al. 2021a; Kuhlmann et al. 2021b), that is, the way actors used the crisis as an opportunity for more far-reaching changes in the institutional setting.

Institutionally, Germany's pandemic governance stands out for its highly decentralized and organizationally fragmented character which is enshrined in administrative federalism with the Länder and local governments as key actors of crisis management and epidemic mitigation. The lacking executive power of the center to enact containment measures and impose crisis responses to the sub-national levels is a peculiar feature of the German approach. We have shown that these decentralized patterns of pandemic governance, with the local health authorities as key actors of pandemic management, have in many respects turned out to be supportive for crisis mitigation. They ensured institutional reactivity, agility, proximity, and territorial adequacy of the responses tailored to the specific local circumstances and varying degrees of crisis affectedness. Furthermore, local governments' comprehensive task portfolio and their mandate to execute all territorially relevant policies proved to be favorable for horizontal coordination across various policy sectors and task areas of crisis management. Yet, the missing digital readiness of (local) administration and resulting service constraints during the lockdown have revealed as salient shortcomings in crisis management. Lacking digital tools and channels to proceed transactions with citizens (see Kuhlmann and Bogumil 2021), many citizen-related services (e.g., in local one-stop shops, building supervisory boards and other licensing authorities) could not be provided during the pandemic (see Kuhlmann and Franzke 2022, Franzke 2021b). Furthermore, local health authorities became increasingly overloaded as a result of the general containment approach, particularly the comprehensive tracking and tracing obligations, seen by the Federal and Länder governments as an indispensable basis for containing the pandemic and preventing a crash of the health system. When many local health authorities reached their capacity limits in October 2020 and in about 75% of all cases could not trace the infection chains anymore, this was interpreted by many as a major failure of (local) administration. However, some experts also questioned the appropriateness and effectiveness of the crisis responses (the "policy theory") as such, specifically the overemphasis of the "incidence rule" as major basis for containment decisions, the mass contact tracing, testing, and quarantining, all of which had to be executed by local health authorities. Therefore, this approach was also criticized as putting a wrong emphasis and thereby threatening the operational procedures in the local health authorities who were entirely absorbed by containment management while other duties, such as important prevention tasks or the protection of vulnerable groups by way of supporting care homes, could not be assumed by them.

Regarding intergovernmental relations, there was a clear trend toward more unitarization and centralization during the pandemic up to what we label here as "intergovernmental centralism," while at the same time major implementation and management functions remained with the – increasingly overburdened - local levels. As our analysis has shown, over the course of the crisis, phases of intense coordination and "unitarization" of decision-making alternated with phases of looser intergovernmental collaboration and more discretionary regulatory powers of the Länder and local governments, especially when the situation was considered as being more relaxed and a lifting of measures justifiable. To put it exaggeratedly, the lockdown-yoyo was paralleled by a centralization-yoyo with subsequent phases and repeated re-balancing of localized/discretionary and centralized/uniform containment regulation. The increased relevance and importance of intergovernmental coordination is thus a key property of pandemic governance in Germany. Although, formally, no nationwide containment was provided by the pertinent legislation, in fact it was achieved when the federal and Länder executives established a kind of informal "substitute government" ("Bund-Länder Summits"), also labeled by some critics as the German intergovernmental "conclave" or "super-corona-government" (Der Tagesspiegel 2021), which took all major decisions. The result was a quickly harmonized containment landscape in different German regions, while variation across Länder and local jurisdictions primarily concerned details and nuances of regulations, which some observers misinterpreted as a "federal mess." It remains to be seen whether this new feature of intergovernmental centralization, which has also provoked many critical assessments, not only regarding its (lacking) constitutional basis, but also more general issues of legitimacy, accountability, transparency and checks and balances, will leave some longer lasting marks in Germany's institutional system.

In terms of checks and balances, the overall result of the various legal amendments during the crisis was a weakening of the federal legislative (Bundestag) and (partly) the Länder during an "epidemic emergency of national concern" while the central-state executive, specifically the Minister of Health, was conspicuously upgraded. The balance between the legislative and the executive branches has clearly shifted toward the latter. The pandemic can therefore undoubtedly be referred to as the "moment of the executive." This does not only apply to the federal executive, in particular the Minister of Health, but also to the Länder governments. Their power to enact containment measures by way of suspending civil liberties during a pandemic was clearly enhanced by the third pandemic law, which now provides a more solid statutory basis for Länder executive orders, while possibilities for citizens to successfully sue against them were reduced.

While the major emphasis of the German approach was on general containment, the focused protection of vulnerable groups and elderly people with pre-existing illnesses, particularly in care homes, has been considered by many as a failure. Whereas unspecified containment for the whole population was in the center of pandemic management, the focused protection of vulnerable groups was less emphatically pursued by policy makers. This is all the more puzzling as the dramatic problems regarding the staff situation in care homes, the chronic underpayment, overburdening and poor qualification of the employees have been well-known since many years. These shortcomings dramatically popped up during the pandemic, especially when it became clear, early in 2020, that care homes would need focused protection.

From a comparative perspective (see Kuhlmann et al. 2021a, 2021b, 2021c; Bouckaert et al. 2020) it becomes apparent that, in Germany, the political rationality in crisis-related decision-making was very crucial in the pandemic. Executive politics was not in the backseat or only executing scientific recommendations but in the driver seat of decision-making. While experts' recommendations were key for generating legitimacy and trust in pandemic management, the major basis and source of crisis decisions were political preferences, interests, and executive actor's political choices. Unlike other policy discourses in the German federal system, the COVID-19 related discourse was clearly dominated by few central-level internal and external advisors who were more or less in favor of strict containment while milder measures and alternative solutions were much less prominently staged. Nevertheless, over the course of the crisis, the scientific positions of how to deal with the pandemic have become more differentiated, controversial, partly even polarized. An increasing number of experts expressed their discontent with the governments' approach publicly, while in the first phase of the pandemic these voices had been rather weak. Toward the second half of the year, there was also more openness in the public debate regarding the appropriate assessment and handling of the crisis in the long run. It became visible that among specialists the opinions about the dangerousness of the virus and the effectiveness of measures were controversial and had also changed over time. The scientific opinions oscillated around various degrees of strictness or permeability of mitigation measures, with some experts more in line with the governmental approach and others claiming a change in strategy inter alia demanding a more focused protection of vulnerable groups, a systematic assessment of "collateral damages" and of (mid- and long term) societal and health effects of the response measures ("second round effects"). Some also warned of a further politicization of the pandemic and the instrumentalization of science by politics.

The pandemic has meanwhile developed from an initial mainly health-related challenge to a universal presumably long-term societal and economic crisis. As this study has focused on the states and public administration's role in mitigating the crisis, it only addresses one – although we assume important – factor of the overall picture. For an interim assessment of Germany's "success" or "failure" in governing the crisis some empirical and conceptual questions remain open which cannot be resolved in this contribution. For one, we cannot isolate governments and administrations' influence on crisis mitigation from other (external, environmental, medical, demographic, epidemiological, societal etc.) variables. To what extent is the overall "pandemic outcome" a result of governments and administrations' actions or/and of other (potentially even more important?) factors which cannot not be controlled by governments? What actually constitutes the so-called "pandemic outcome"? Second and closely related, what is "success" or "failure" in this pandemic, including the post-pandemic phase not yet reached at time of writing? It is a myth to believe that "indicators of success and failure are clear and outcomes can be well defined and objectively measured" (Jasanoff et al. 2021: 11). Outcome measures are always value-laden, contested, and erase important features of their context. Performance measures are contradictory and experts disagree about which ones are appropriate and relevant: "Choosing indicators to evaluate policies is therefore a political decision" (Jasanoff et al. 2021: 11). Finally, to evaluate "success" or "failure," multiple dimensions must be taken into account. For instance, the effects of health-related emergency measures ("first round effects") must be set in a proportion to the (likewise public health-related) societal, economic etc. longer-term consequences of governments' response measures ("second round effects"). What will be an appropriate time horizon to do so? And which (comparative) data and indicators can we draw on to conduct these kinds of (interdisciplinary) studies? Explanations of (partial) "failures" must also differentiate between "false theories" (e.g., political decisions on how to mitigate the crisis) and "bad implementation" (e.g., ill preparedness of administrations). Finally, from a normative perspective: is "success"/ "failure" of a country in one area of assessment more important than in another? Obviously, it is up to future research to provide sufficient concepts, measures and empirical data on these multiple evaluative questions and to create a solid basis for comparative assessments of pandemic outcomes and governmental success. This chapter is meant to contribute to the establishment of such a comparative knowledge basis. The key issue of which concepts, indicators and measures to adopt for a comprehensive "corona evaluation" cannot be decided however solely from a technical or methodological point of view, but will remain, in the end, also a normative and political question.

Notes

1 We use the term "cases" for people with a positive PCR laboratory test result on SARS-CoV-2.
2 As independent cities (kreisfreie Städte), 107 of them, also have the competencies of a county.
3 In 2017, 37% of German hospitals were in private ownership, 29% publicly owned and 34% managed by non-profit providers (Statista 2020c).
4 In this context, additionally the dense network of health facilities throughout the country which guarantees for proximity and short distances was also criticized for reasons of efficiency by some health economists.
5 All decisions of these intergovernmental Summits can be found in the appendix.
6 This strategy was agreed between the *Länder* and the federal governments on 6 May obliged the former to make sure that in counties or county-free cities with more than 50 new incidences per 100,000 inhabitants within 7 days strict containment concepts will be implemented (see Bundesregierung 2020b).
7 They include inter alia an extended obligation for wearing faced masks, the limitation of participants in events to 100, including 1.5 m physical distance, and the limit of public gatherings to a maximum of 10 persons as well as a closing hour for restaurants from 11 pm.
8 The new intervention powers of the Minister of Health under this pandemic emergency rule include inter alia the right to order physical examinations for travellers, travel bans for specific countries, and to secure the purchase of medicaments and cures, medical products, and materials for disinfection and laboratory prognostics. This authorization is limited in time, but must be withdrawn on 31 March 2021 or 31 March 2022 (IfSG, version of November 2020) or when epidemic emergency does not persist anymore.

9 Data regarding the number of regulations concerned by the Minister's "carte blanche" vary. According to the official information of the Federal Ministry of Health about 34 ordinances were concerned (Bundesministerium für Gesundheit 2021). The legal expertise of the FDP fraction identified however more than 1,000 regulations potentially affected by this authorization (Kingreen 2020: 7; experts' hearing of the German Bundestag, committee for health, 9.9.2020).

10 The so-called small Corona Cabinet, headed by the Federal Chancellor, included the federal ministers of defense, finance, the interior, foreign affairs, health, and the head of the Federal Chancellery. The so-called large Corona Cabinet additionally included all specialist federal ministers who are responsible for the topics on the agenda. If, for example, the matter of organizing enough harvest workers was on the table, the federal Minister of Agriculture was included (see Bundesregierung 2020a).

11 In the county of Neuss (North-Rhine-Westphalia), for instance, the task force comprised the heads of the following departments: local health authority, local board for public safety and public order office (*Ordnungsamt*), school and youth offices, social welfare board, personnel office, municipal supervisory authority (Kommunalaufsicht), county press office, county fire brigade control center (Kreisleitstelle der Feuerwehr) and county liaison command of the Bundeswehr (Kreisverbindungskommando) as well as the medical director of the rescue service and the county fire brigade chief (see Rhein-Kreis Neuss 2020). The crisis team is headed by the general representative of the head of the county. Depending on local circumstances, additional external experts were involved, e.g., from the police or from municipal hospitals.

12 This task originally not belonging to the local task portfolio shows the failure of the Federal and the *Länder* Governments in anticipating pandemic-related procurement functions and preparing for prospective health threats.

13 The number of doctors had fallen by about 1/3 between 2000 and 2018 due to staff cuts, a shortage of skilled doctors and long-time vacant positions (see Bundesverband der Ärztinnen und Ärzte des öffentlichen Gesundheitsdienstes 2020; Bayer 2020).

14 See Az.: 6 OWi - 523 Js 202518/20.

15 Examples are: "The virologists govern" (Der Spiegel 2020) or "The power of virologists" (Handelsblatt 2020).

16 The expert advisory board submitted three statements by end of 2020 (see Staatskanzlei des Landes Nordrhein-Westfalen 2021, Viewed on March 10, 2021)

17 Until End of 2020, the board had submitted several statements, e.g., on pandemic management in schools and day-care centers and on risk communication (see Wissenschaftlicher Beirat Corona Landesregierung Thüringen 2020).

18 The Berlin Charité is an association of university clinics with 290 professors and more than 8,000 students organized in the legal form of a public corporation owned by the Land Berlin.

19 Drosten is a German virologist heading the Institute of Virology at the Berlin university hospital Charité. He became known internationally when he was the first to decode the genome of the SARS virus from the group of corona viruses, which in early 2003 triggered several epidemics of atypical pneumonia, especially in Asia. He also became nationally famous during the Swine Flu pandemic of 2009. As an external advisor, Drosten is formally not affiliated to the federal government.

20 The Leopoldina was founded as a natural sciences academy in 1652 and appointed as the National Academy of Science by the federal and Länder governments in 2008. It officially represents German science in international bodies and provides advice to politics and society on various subjects, from climate change, energy provision, and digitalization to demographic challenges, natural resources, and health. During the pandemic, the Leopoldina published seven ad hoc statements (until January 2021).

21 The former member of the Academy of Science Mainz (Thomas Aigner), for instance, publicly resigned from his Academy position because of severe discontent with the Leopoldina's role and scientific statements he claimed to be seriously biased and qualitatively poor. He accused the Leopoldina's statement as being "unworthy of an honest and critically reflecting science in dedication of human well-being" (see Schwäbisches Tagblatt 2021).

22 For instance, the biochemist and director of the institute for medical microbiology of the university clinic Halle, Alexander Kekulé, the director of the institute for virology in Bonn, Hendrik Streeck, and the virologist of the Bernhard-Nocht Institute for tropical medicine at Hamburg University, Jonas Schmidt-Canasit.

23 The respective statement was published by a group of scientists, including inter alia the director of the university clinic in Cologne, Prof. Dr. Michael Hallek.

24 This applies inter alia to the virologist, Hendrik Streeck (university clinic Bonn), who criticized the drastic containment measures as overly rushed by politicians and claimed a broader evidence and evaluative knowledge regarding the various measures (see Streeck 2021).

25 Although the protection of vulnerable groups (care homes) without totally isolating people had been jointly decided by the federal and Länder governments on 15 April, this strategy played a less dominant role in the public debate as compared to the general containment approach.

26 An interdisciplinary expert's group, based in the universities of Berlin, Bremen and Cologne, composed by renowned German scientists, inter alia the former vice-president of the Experts' Council for Health (Prof. Dr. Schrappe, University of Cologne), lawyers specialized in public health (e.g. Prof. Dr. Hart, University of Bremen), public health experts (e.g. Prof. Dr. Glaeske, University of Bremen), a specialist in forensic medicine (Prof. Dr. Püschel, University Clinic Bremen) and a political scientist (Prof. Dr. Manow, University of Bremen) is worth mentioning here. Until January 2021, this group published seven ad hoc statements in which the experts challenged the governmental approach and outlining possible alternatives of pandemic management. In addition, various practitioners, e.g., the heads of the local health authorities in Frankfurt, in Aichach-Friedberg, and the head of the Charité institute for forensic medicine (see Berliner Zeitung 2020; BR24 2020; Landesärztekammer Hessen 2020) publicly questioned the appropriateness of the measures in managing the crisis.

27 One example is the third statement of the Leopoldina National Academy of Science (see Leopoldina 2020a: 11 et seq.) which was also consulted by the German Federal government. Another example is the Berlin/Bremen/Cologne experts' group, mentioned above, which was however not formally consulted by the government.

28 "The politicization and medialization of scientists is as problematic as substituting politics by virology – politics engrosses science for its decisions and scientists slip into the role of political decision-makers" (Schrappe et al. 2020a: 66).

29 Stated by the former vice-president of the Experts' Council for Health, Matthias Schrappe (see Welt 19.11.2020).
30 Claimed by the president of the association of company health insurance funds and former head of department in the Ministry of Health, Franz Knieps (see Epoch Times 2021).
31 Stellungnahme der Bundesärztekammer zum Antrag der Fraktion BÜNDNIS 90/DIE GRÜNEN „Pandemierat jetzt gründen. Mit breiterer wissenschaftlicher Perspektive besser durch die Corona-Krise" (Deutscher Bundestag 2020c) anlässlich der öffentlichen Anhörung im Ausschuss für Gesundheit des Bundestages am 9.9.2020.
32 The survey was part of the bigger COSMO project within which since March 2020 about 1,000 citizens are contacted in weekly or be-weekly cycles (see Cosmo 2021)
33 Data basis: representative survey from March/April 2020; N = 2.336.
34 The survey was conducted in two waves: May (N =7,651–7,693) and November 2020 (N=6563–6641); see Wagschaal et al. (2020: 16).
35 This includes e.g. closing borders with decline from 65% to 47%; contact bans declining from 60% to 46%; closing shops declining from 55% to 30% and closing schools and kindergartens declining from 62% to 27%). With the only exception of tracing apps ("use of citizens' mobile phone data to trace infections) which remained more or less stable (from 40.4% to 40.9%).
36 This trend was identified by a study of the University of Heidelberg, in which the public support of pandemic containment was measured in June/July (N = 1,351) and November/December (N = 1,099). Participants were surveyed from an online access panel. See Kirch et al. 2020.
37 According to a (non-representative) study of the University of Basel, 21% of the "Querdenker" had voted for the Green party, 15% for the Left party and 14% for the (right wing) AfD in the last general elections (see WELT 2020b). Another study which analyzed the socio-economic and political composition of protests against the corona regulations in the City of Constance (N=138) found out that 55% of the surveyed did not lean towards any political party, 14% towards the Greens, 7% CDU, 6% the Left, 3% FDP, 2% SPD, 2% AfD (Koos 2021: 8).
38 One of these predecessor organizations was „Widerstand 2020" which was dissolved by summer (see Deutschlandfunk Nova 2020).
39 The Constance-survey mentioned above revealed however that 75% of the surveyed participants rejected a further radicalization of corona-related protests (Koos 2021: 11).
40 Among them the chief virologist of the university clinic of Bonn Hendrik Streeck; see Frankfurter Rundschau 2020.
41 Among them the former vice-president of the experts' council on health, Matthias Schrappe; see Welt 2020c.
42 As example the local health authority head of Aichach-Friedberg, Friedrich Pürner (see Süddeutsche Zeitung, 4.11.2020), and his colleague in the City of Frankfurt René Gottschalk (see Frankfurter Allgemeine Zeitung 2020b).
43 As example the Mayor of the City of Tübingen, Boris Palmer (see Frankfurter Rundschau 2021).
44 Against this background, the former member of the Academy of Science Mainz (Thomas Aigner), for instance, publicly resigned from his Academy position decrying its uncritical stance towards the National Academy of Science Leopoldina accused to be "unworthy of an honest and critically reflecting science in dedication of human well-being" (see Section 2.6). A similar critique was raised

by the Leopoldina member, Michael Esfeld (University of Lausanne), who, in a protest letter, accused the Leopoldina of accepting an "instrumentalization" by the Federal Government and thus causing damage the overall reputation of science (see MDR 2021). In its 7th statement, the Leopoldina had recommended a second (hard) lockdown and with this legitimized the government's decision (see Leopoldina 2020b).

References

Bayer, S. 2020. *Intervention statt Prävention als politisches Paradigma? GID Statement 2/2020.* Hamburg: German Institute for Defense and Strategic Studies.

Beerheide, R. 2020. Ambulante Versorgung: Systemvorteil in der Pandemie. *Deutsches Ärzteblatt*, 117(41): A-1903/B-1621.

Behnke, N. and S. Kropp. 2021. Administrative Federalism. In S. Kuhlmann, I. Proeller, D. Schimanke and J. Ziekow (Eds.), *Public Administration in Germany*, 35–51. Houndmills Basingstoke: Palgrave Macmillan.

Beneker, C. 2020. COVID-19. Jedes zweite Corona-Opfer lebte im Heim. https://www.aerztezeitung.de/Politik/Jedes-zweite-Corona-Opfer-lebte-im-Heim-410389.html. Accessed: 4 March 2021.

Berliner Zeitung. 2020. Keine Übersterblichkeit durch COVID-19: Chef von Gesundheitsamt vergleicht Corona mit Grippe und Hitzewellen, 1.10.2020. https://www.berliner-zeitung.de/news/keine-uebersterblichkeit-trotz-corona-amtsarzt-fordert-diskussion-ueber-die-mittel-der-pandemie-bekaempfung-li.108672. Accessed: 4 March 2021.

Blom, A., C. Cornesse, S. Friedel, U. Krieger, M. Fikel, T. Rettig, A. Wenz, S. Juhl, R. Lehrer, K. Möhring, E. Naumann and M. Reifenscheid. 2020. High-Frequency and High-Quality Survey Data Collection: The Mannheim Corona Study. *Survey Research Methods.* 14(2): 171–178.

Blum, K., S. Löffert, M. Offermanns and P. Steffen. 2019. *Krankenhaus Barometer.* Düsseldorf: DKI.

Bouckaert, G., D. Galli, S. Kuhlmann, R. Reiter and S. van Hecke. 2020. European Coronationalism? A Hot Spot Governing a Pandemic Crisis. *Public Administration Review.* 80(5): 765–773.

BR24. 2020. Corona: Gesundheitsamtsleiter kritisiert Staatsregierung, 5.10.2020.

Bundesagentur für Arbeit. 2020. Monatsbericht zum Arbeits- und Ausbildungsmarkt. September 2020. https://www.arbeitsagentur.de/datei/arbeitsmarktbericht-september-2020-_ba146655.pdf. Accessed: 4 March 2021.

Bundesministerium der Finanzen. 2020a. Nachtragshaushalt 2020 des Bundes (Sollbericht). https://www.bundesfinanzministerium.de/Monatsberichte/2020/08/Inhalte/Kapitel-3-Analysen/3-1-nachtragshaushalte-2020-des-bundes-sollbericht-pdf.pdf?—blob=publicationFile&v=2. Accessed: 2 March 2021.

Bundesministerium der Finanzen. 2020b. Eckwerte: Bundeshaushalt 2021 und Finanzplan bis 2024, Berlin.

Bundesministerium für Arbeit und Soziales. 2020. Sozialschutz-Pakete. https://www.bmas.de/DE/Corona/sozialschutz-paket.html. Accessed: 4 March 2021.

Bundesministerium für Gesundheit. 2021. Gesetze und Verordnungen. https://www.bundesgesundheitsministerium.de/service/gesetze-und-verordnungen.html. Accessed: 9 March 2021.

Bundesministerium für Wirtschaft und Energie. 2020. Die wirtschaftliche Lage in Deutschland im September 2020. https://www.bmwi.de/Redaktion/DE/ Pressemitteilungen/Wirtschaftliche-Lage/2020/20200914-die-wirtschaftliche-lage-in-deutschland-im-september-2020.html. Accessed: 4 March 2021.

Bundesministerium für Wirtschaft und Energie. 2021. Package of Measures to Combat the Impact of Coronavirus on Companies. https://www.bmwi.de/Redaktion/ EN/Downloads/P/package-of-measures-to-combat-the-impact-of-coronavirus-on-companies.pdf?—blob=publicationFile&v=29. Accessed: 2 March 2021.

Bundesregierung. 2020a. Kanzlerin nach Corona-Kabinett. Jetzt nicht nachlassen. https://www.bundeskanzlerin.de/bkin-de/aktuelles/merkel-corona-kabinett-1742676. Accessed: 4 March 2021.

Bundesregierung. 2020b. Telefonschaltkonferenz der Bundeskanzlerin mit den Regierungschefinnen und Regierungschefs der Länder am 6. Mai 2020. https:// www.bundesregierung.de/resource/blob/975226/1750986/fc61b6eb1fc1d39 8d66cfea79b565129/2020-05-06-mpk-beschluss-data.pdf?download=1,%20 12.1.2021. Accessed: 2 March 2021.

Bundesverband der Ärztinnen und Ärzte des Öffentlichen Gesundheitsdienstes. 2020. *Coronaviren in Deutschland – Gesundheitsämter in Bedrängnis wegen Ärztemangel*. Berlin: BVÖGD.

Collins, A., M.V. Florin and O. Renn. 2020. COVID-19 Risk Governance: Drivers, Responses and Lessons to be Learned. *Journal of Risk Research*, 23(7–8): 1073–1082.

Cosmo. 2021. Vertrauen in Institutionen. https://projekte.uni-erfurt.de/cosmo2020/ web/topic/vertrauen-ablehnung-demos/10-vertrauen/. Accessed: 2 March 2021.

Der Spiegel. 2020. Plötzlich regieren und die Virologen, 23.3.2020. www. spiegel.de/politik/deutschland/corona-krise-wie-virologen-ploetzlich-zu-einer-nebenregierung-werden-a-00000000-0002-0001-0000-000170114611, Accessed: 15 March 2021.

Der Spiegel. 2021. Keine deutliche Übersterblichkeit in Deutschland, 1.2.2021. https://www.spiegel.de/wissenschaft/mensch/corona-jahr-2020-keine-deutliche-uebersterblichkeit-in-deutschland-a-e4524a2e-cc59-44ff-b63a-86ed8bbcf81d.

Der Tagesspiegel 2021. Vergeblicher Kampf gegen Corona: Merkels Superregierung, die es nicht bringt, 11.1.2021.

Destatis. 2020a. Sonderauswertung zu Sterbefallzahlen der Jahre 2020/2021. https://www.destatis.de/DE/Themen/Gesellschaft-Umwelt/Bevoelkerung/Sterbefaelle-Lebenserwartung/sterbefallzahlen.html. Accessed: 2 March 2021.

Destatis. 2020b. Sterbefallzahlen in der 52. Kalenderwoche 2020: 31% über dem Durchschnitt der Vorjahre. https://www.destatis.de/DE/Presse/Pressemitteilungen/ 2021/01/PD21_032_12621.html. Accessed: 2 March 2021.

Destatis. 2020c. Sterbefälle – Fallzahlen nach Tagen, Wochen, Monaten, Altersgruppen, Geschlecht und Bundesländern für Deutschland 2016-2021. www. destatis.de/DE/Themen/Gesellschaft-Umwelt/Bevoelkerung/Sterbefaelle-Lebenserwartung/Publikationen/Downloads-Sterbefaelle/statistischer-bericht-sterbefaelle-tage-wochen-monate-aktuell-5126109.html.

Deutsche Krankenhausgesellschaft. 2020. Stellungnahme der Deutschen Krankenhausgesellschaft. https://www.bundestag.de/resource/blob/711300/aba64e39cb428b194 bb2aabbecac7d8f/19_14_0197-6-_Deutsche-Krankenhausgesellschaft-e-V-_COVID19-data.pdf. Accessed: 9 March 2021.

Deutscher Bundestag. 2012. Unterrichtung durch die Bundesregierung, Bericht zur Risikoanalyse im Bevölkerungsschutz 2012. Drucksache 17/12051, 3.1.2013.

Deutscher Bundestag. 2020a. Virtuelles Parlament. Verfassungsrechtliche Bewertung und mögliche Grudgesetzänderung. https://www.bundestag.de/resource/blob/690270/07e7b1aff547a62bbc7477281574de2c/WD-3-084-20-pdf-data.pdf. Accessed: 2 March 2021.

Deutscher Bundestag. 2020b. Gesetzentwurf der Fraktionen der CDU/CSU und SPD. Entwurf eines Dritten Gesetzes zum Schutz der Bevölkerung bei einer epidemischen Lage von nationaler Tragweite. http://dip21.bundestag.de/dip21/btd/19/239/1923944.pdf. Accessed: 9 March 2021.

Deutscher Bundestag. 2020c. Pandemierat jetzt gründen – Mit breiterer wissenschaftlicher Perspektive besser durch die Corona-Krise. https://dip21.bundestag.de/dip21/btd/19/205/1920565.pdf. Accessed: 9 March.

Deutsches Netzwerk Evidenzbasierte Medizin. 2020. COVID-19: Wo ist die Evidenz? https://www.ebm-netzwerk.de/de/veroeffentlichungen/pdf/stn-20200903-covid19-update.pdf. Accessed: 2 March 2021.

Deutschlandfunk Nova. 2020. Gruppierung offenbar aufgelöst. Corona-Pandemie: „Widerstand 2020" ist wohl abgesagt, 7.7.2020. https://www.deutschlandfunknova.de/beitrag/widerstand-2020-die-gruppierung-gegen-anti-corona-ma%C3%9Fnahmen-scheint-sich-aufzuloesen. Accessed: 2 March 2021.

DIVI. 2020. Tagesreport 15.09.2020.

DIVI. 2021. DIVI-Intensivregister Tagesreport 20.04.2021. https://www.divi.de/divi-intensivregister-tagesreport-archiv/viewdocument/3824/divi-intensivregistertagesreport-2020-04-20. Accessed: 2 March 2021.

Eckhard, S. and A. Lenz. 2020. *Die öffentliche Wahrnehmung des Krisenmanagements in der Covid-19 Pandemie*. Konstanz: Universität Konstanz.

Epoch Times. 2021. BKK-Chef Knieps kritisiert Corona-Politik von Bund und Ländern – „Bunkermentalität im Kanzleramt", 18.1.2021. www.epochtimes.de/politik/deutschland/bkk-chef-knieps-kritisiert-corona-politik-von-bund-und-laendern-rasche-oeffnung-der-schulen-und-kitas-a3426494.html. Accessed: 2 February 2021.

European Commission. 2019. *State of Health in the EU. Companion Report 2019*. Luxembourg: Publications Office of the European Union.

Expertengruppe No-Covid-Strategie. 2021. Eine neue proaktive Zielsetzung für Deutschland zur Bekämpfung von SARS-CoV-2 (Stand 18. Januar 2021, Version 1.0) See www.zeit.de/wissen/gesundheit/2021-01/no-covid-strategie.pdf.

Financial Times. 2020. How Germany Got Coronavirus Right, 4.6.2020, www.ft.com/content/cc1f650a-91c0-4e1f-b990-ee8ceb5339ea?shareType=nongift, Accessed: 15 March 2021.

FOCUS. 2021a. Massive Kritik an Pandemie-Behörde. Statistiker holt zur RKI-Schelte aus: Corona-Daten "eine einzige Katastrophe", 1.2.2021. https://m.focus.de/gesundheit/news/massive-kritik-an-pandemie-behoerde-statistiker-holt-zur-rki-schelte-aus-corona-daten-eine-einzige-katastrophe_id_12927819.html. Accessed: 15 March 2021.

FOCUS. 2021b. Medizinprofessor: Das ständige Lockdown-Jojo ist "völlig wirkungslos", 13.1.2021. https://www.focus.de/gesundheit/coronavirus/aeltere-weiter-ungeschuetzt-scharfe-kritik-an-corona-politik-aneinanderreihungvon-lockdowns-voellig-wirkungslos_id_12856904.html, Accessed: 15 March 2021.

FOCUS. 2021c. IW: Corona-Verlust in Höhe von 250 Milliarden Euro, 22.1.2021, Accessed: 15 March 2021.

Frankfurter Allgemeine Zeitung. 2020a. Vertrauen in deutsche Politik stark gewachsen, 16.5.2020. www.faz.net/aktuell/politik/inland/umfrage-vertrauen-in-deutsche-politik-stark-gewachsen-16772693.html, Accessed: 15 March 2021.

Frankfurter Allgemeine Zeitung. 2020b. Frankfurter Gesundheitsamtsleiter: Corona-Strategie überdenken. https://www.faz.net/aktuell/rhein-main/frankfurt/frankfurter-gesundheitsamtsleiter-corona-strategie-ueberdenken-16981161.html. Accessed: 2 March 2021.

Frankfurter Allgemeine Zeitung. 2021. Jeder kämpft für sich allein, 2.1.2021. www.faz.net/aktuell/wirtschaft/gesundheitsaemter-in-der-krise-jeder-kaempft-fuer-sich-allein-17126600.html.

Frankfurter Rundschau. 2020. Virologe Hendrik Streeck übt scharfe Kritik an Corona-Politik:„EchteStrategie"fehlt,4.11.2020.https://www.fr.de/politik/virologe-hendrik-streeck-corona-deutschland-interview-fr-impfstoff-covid19-coronavirus-pandemie-neuinfektionen-90082318.html. Accessed: 16 March 2020.

Frankfurter Rundschau. 2021. Boris Palmer fordert Kursänderung im Corona-Lockdown: „Es reicht jetzt, wir müssen leben", 14.1.2021. www.fr.de/politik/boris-palmer-lockdown-ende-corona-virus-lockerungen-covid19-inzidenz-50-karl-lauterbach-90165038.html. Accessed: 15 March 2021.

Franzke, J. 2020. German Municipalities in the COVID-19 Pandemic Crisis. Challenges and Adjustments. A Preliminary Analysis. *International Geographical Union*, 30 April 2020.

Franzke, J. 2021a. Deutschlands Krisenmanagement in der CORONA-Pandemie. Herausforderungen eines föderalen politisch-administrativen Systems. In: *Rocznik Integracji Europejskiej (Jahrbuch der Europäischen Integration)*. S. 321–339. Poznań, Jahrgang 2021, Nr. 14.

Franzke, J. 2021b. German Local Authorities in the COVID-19 Pandemic. Challenges, Impacts and Adaptions, Paper angenommen für den 34. International Geographical Congress in Istanbul (Türkei) vom 16–20 August 2021, Session "Local Government Response Toward COVID-19 Pandemic."

Franzke, J. and S. Kuhlmann. 2021. COVID-19 Governance in Germany. Published as "Tyskland og covid-19-krisen. Bilag 5. Landerapport in *Folketinget: Håndteringen af covid-19 I foråret 2020. Rapport af givet af den af Folketingets Udvalg for Forretnignsordenen nedsatte udredningsgruppe vedr. håndteringen af Covid-19.* 630–676. Copenhagen: Folketinget.

Fuhr, H., J. Fleischer and S. Kuhlmann. 2018. *Federalism and Decentralization in Germany. Basic Features and Principles for German Development Cooperation.* Bonn/Eschborn: GIZ.

Gebhardt, H. and L.H. Siemers. 2020. Wirkung der Corona-Krise auf die Staatsfinanzen. *Wirtschaftsdienst*, 2020(7): 468–470.

Gerlinger, T. 2019. Wissenschaftliche Politikberatung im Gesundheitswesen. *Gesundheit und Gesellschaft – Wissenschaft*, 19(1): 15–22.

Handelsblatt. 2020. Die neue Macht der Virologen, 26.3.2020. amp2.handelsblatt.com/meinung/kommentar-die-neue-macht-der-virologen/25684390.html, Accessed: 15 March 2021.

Jasanoff, S., S. Hilgartner, J.B. Hurlbut, O. Özgöde and M. Rayzberg. 2021. *Comparative Covid Response: Crisis, Knowledge, Politics*. Interim Report. 12.1.2021. https://assets.website-files.com/5fdfca1c14b4b91eeaa7196a/5ffda00d50fca2e6f 8782aed_Harvard-Cornell%20Report%202020.pdf. Accessed: 16 March 2021.

Juhl, S., R. Lehrer, A. Blom, A. Wenz, T. Rettig, M. Reifenscheid, E. Naumann, K. Möhring, U. Krieger, S. Friedel, M. Fikel and C. Cornesse. 2020. *Die Mannheimer Corona-Stuide: Demokratiesche Kontrolle in der Corona-Krise*. Mannheim: MZES.

Kantar. 2020a. *Betroffenheit deutscher Unternehmen durch die Corona-Pandemie. Mai 2020*. Berlin: Bundesministerium für Wirtschaft und Energie.

Kantar. 2020b. *Betroffenheit deutscher Unternehmen durch die Corona-Pandemie. Zweite Erhebungswelle, Juli 2020*. Berlin: Bundesministerium für Wirtschaft und Energie.

Kassenärztliche Bundesvereinigung. 2020. *Gemeinsame Position von Wissenschaft und Ärzteschaft. Evidenz- und Erfahrungsgewinn im weiteren Management der covid-19-Pandemie berücksichtigen*. Berlin: KBV.

Kießling, A. 2020. *Stellungnahme als eingeladene Einzelsachverständige für die öffentliche Anhörung im Gesundheitsausschuss des Deutschen Bundestages am 12.11.2020*. Bochum: Ruhr-Universität Bochum.

Kingreen, T. 2020. Whatever It Takes? Der demokratische Rechtsstaat in Zeiten von Corona. https://verfassungsblog.de/whatever-it-takes/. Accessed: 4 March 2021.

Kirsch, P., H. Kube and R. Zohlnhöfer. 2020. Gesellschaftliche Selbstermächtigung. Die Akzeptanz der Maßnahmen zur Eindämmung der Corona-Pandemie in der deutschen Bevölkerung im dezember 2020 – Zusammenfassung der Ergebnisse. https://www.marsilius-kolleg.uni-heidelberg.de/fellows/Publikationfellows2020. html. Accessed: 2 March 2021.

Klafki, A. 2020. Stellungnahme als Einzelsachverständige zum Entwurf des Dritten Gesetzes zum Schutz der Bevölkerung bei einer epidemischen Lage von nationaler Tragweite. www.bundestag.de/resource/blob/870654/fa66cd7a9b-630f9eea5726f686cd920c/Stellungnahme-Klafki-data.pdf. Accessed: 31 October 2024.

Klenk, T. and R. Reiter. 2012. Öffentliche Daseinsvorsorge, privat organisiert? Ein deutsch-französischer Vergleich der Bereitstellung der Krankenhausinfrastruktur. *Zeitschrift für Sozialreform*, 58(4): 401–426.

Koos, S. 2021. Die „Querdenker". Wer nimmt an Corona-Protesten teil und warum? Ergebnisse einer Befragung der „Corona-Proteste" am 4.10.2020 in Konstanz. https://kops.uni-konstanz.de/bitstream/handle/123456789/52497/ Koos_2-bnrddxo8opad0.pdf?sequence=1. Accessed: 4 March 2021.

Kuhlmann, S. 2020. Between Unity and Variety: Germany's Responses to the COVID-19 Pandemic. In M. Joyce, F. Maron and R. Purshottama Sivanarain (Eds.), *Good Public Governance in a Global Pandemic*. IIAS Public Governance Series. 291–304. Brussels: IAS-IISA.

Kuhlmann, S. and J. Bogumil. 2021. The Digitalisation of Local Public Services. Evidence from the German Case. In T. Bergström, J. Franzke, S. Kuhlmann and E. Wayenberg (Eds.), *The Future of Local Self-Government. European Trends in Autonomy, Innovations and Central-Local Relations.* 101–113. Basingstoke: Palgrave Macmillan. https://doi.org/10.1007/978-3-030-56059-1.

Kuhlmann, S. and J. Franzke. 2022. Multi-Level Responses to COVID-19: Crisis Coordination in Germany from an Intergovernmental Perspective. *Local Government Studies* 48(2), 312–334.

Kuhlmann, S., G. Bouckaert, D. Galli, R. Reiter and S. van Hecke. 2021a. *Opportunity Management of the COVID-19 Pandemic: Testing the Crisis from a Global Perspective.* IRAS Special Issue.

Kuhlmann, S., G. Bouckaert, D. Galli, R. Reiter and S. van Hecke. 2021b. *The Governance of the COVID-19 Pandemic Compared.* IRAS Special Issue.

Kuhlmann, S., M. Hellström, U. Ramberg, and R. Reiter. 2021. Tracing Divergence in Crisis Governance: Responses to the COVID-19 Pandemic in France, Germany and Sweden Compared. *International Review of Administrative Sciences,* 87(3), 556–575.

Kuhlmann, S., I. Proeller, D. Schimanke and J. Ziekow. 2021d. *Public Administration in Germany: Institutions, Reforms, Governance.* Basingstoke: Palgrave Macmillan.

Kuhlmann, S. and H. Wollmann. 2019. *Introduction to Comparative Public Administration: Administrative Systems and Reforms in Europe.* Cheltenham/Northampton: Edward Elgar.

Landesärztekammer Hessen. 2020. *Schwerpunkt Schlafmedizin.* Hessisches Ärzteblatt. 2020(10).

Leopoldina. 2020a. Coronavirus-Pandemie. Die Krise nachhaltig überwinden, 3. Ad-hoc-Stellungnahme zur Coronavirus-Pandemie, 13.4.2020.

Leopoldina. 2020b. Coronavirus-Pandemie: Die Feriertage und den Jahrewwechsel für einen harten Lockdown nutzen. https://www.leopoldina.org/uploads/tx_leopublication/2020_12_08_Stellungnahme_Corona_Feiertage_final.pdf. Accessed: 2 March 2021.

Matuschek, C., F. Moll, H. Fangerau, J.C. Fischer, K. Zänker, M. van Griensven, ... and J. Haussmann. 2020. Face Masks: Benefits and Risks During the COVID-19 Crisis. *European journal of medical research,* 25, 1–8.

MDR. 2020. Bundeswehr unterstützt immer mehr Gesundheitsämter, 18.10.2020.

MDR. 2021. Wird die Leopoldina politisch instrumentalisiert? 19.2.2021. www.mdr.de/wissen/leopoldina-politisch-instrumentalisiert-100.html Accessed: 14 March 2021.

Nationaler Normenkontrollrat. 2020. *Krise als Weckruf: Verwaltung modernisieren, Digitalisierungsschub nutzen, Gesetze praxistauglich machen.* Berlin: NKR.

Next:Public. 2020. *Verwaltung in Krisenzeiten. Eine Bestandsaufnahme der Auswirkungen der Corona-Pandemie auf den Öffentlichen Dienst.* Berlin.

OECD. 2020. Turning Hope into Reality. *OECD Economic Outlook,* December 2020. http://www.oecd.org/economic-outlook/december-2020/. Accessed: 4 March.

OECD and European Observatory on Health Systems and Policies. 2019. *Germany: Country Health Profile 2019. State of Health in the EU.* Brussels: OECD Publishing.

Our World in Data. 2021. Cumulative COVID-19 Tests, Confirmed Cases and Deaths Per Million People. https://ourworldindata.org/grapher/cumulative-deaths-and-cases-covid-19.

Papier, H.J. 2020. Umgang mit der Corona-Pandemie: Verfassungsrechtliche Perspektiven. *Aus Politik und Zeitgeschichte*, 70(35): 7.

Pusch, T. and S. Seifert. 2021. Stabilisierende Wirkungen durch Kurzarbeit. Analysen und Berichte Arbeitsmarkt. *Wirtschaftsdienst*, 2021(2): 99–105.

Reinhart, K., A. von Butler and J. Graf. 2020. Darum ist Deutschlands Gesundheitssystem nur Mittelmaß. https://www.faz.net/aktuell/wissen/medizin-ernaehrung/darum-ist-deutschlands-gesundheitssystem-nur-mittelmass-16786078.html. Accessed: 9 March 2021.

Rhein-Kreis Neuss. 2020. Krisenstab des Kreises unermüdlich im Einsatz Landrat: "Höchstmöglicher Schutz der Bevölkerung ist unsere zentrale Aufgabe".

RKI. 2016. *Wissenschaftliche Grundlagen. Nationaler Pandemieplan. Teil II*. Berlin: Robert Koch-Institut.

RKI. 2020a. Daily Situation Report of the Robert Koch Institute. 31/12/2020 – Updated Status for Germany. https://www.rki.de/DE/Content/InfAZ/N/Neuartiges_Coronavirus/Situationsberichte/Dez_2020/2020-12-31-en.pdf?—blob=publicationFile. Accessed: 2 March 2021.

RKI. 2020b. COVID-19-Fälle nach Meldewoche und Geschlecht sowie Anteile mit für COVID-19 relevanten Symptomen, Anteile Hospitalisierter und Verstorbener. https://www.rki.de/DE/Content/InfAZ/N/Neuartiges_Coronavirus/Daten/Klinische_Aspekte.html. Accessed: 2 March 2021.

RKI. 2020c. Todesfälle nach Sterbedatum.

RKI. 2020d. Daily Situation Report of the Robert Koch Institute 07/10/2020 – Updated Status for Germany. https://www.rki.de/DE/Content/InfAZ/N/Neuartiges_Coronavirus/Situationsberichte/Okt_2020/2020-10-07-en.pdf?—blob=publicationFile. Accessed: 2 March 2021.

RKI. 2020e. Daily Situation Report of the Robert Koch Institute 23/12/2020 – Updated Status for Germany. https://www.rki.de/DE/Content/InfAZ/N/Neuartiges_Coronavirus/Situationsberichte/Dez_2020/2020-12-23-en.pdf?—blob=publicationFile. Accessed: 2 February 2021.

RKI. 2020f. Dezember 2020: Archiv der Situationsberichte des Robert-Koch-Instituts zu COVID-19. https://www.rki.de/DE/Content/InfAZ/N/Neuartiges_Coronavirus/Situationsberichte/Dez_2020/Archiv_Dezember.html. Accessed: 2 Ferbuary 2021.

RKI. 2020g. Vorbereitungen auf Maßnahmen in Deutschland. Version 1.0. Ergänzung zum Nationalen Pandemieplan – COVID-19 – neuartige Coronaviruserkrankung. https://www.rki.de/DE/Content/InfAZ/N/Neuartiges_Coronavirus/Ergaenzung_Pandemieplan_Covid.pdf?—blob=publicationFile. Accessed: 9 March 2021.

Rothgang, H., D. Domhoff, A.C. Friedrich, F. Heinze, B. Preuss, A. Schmidt, K. Seibert, C. Stolle and K. Wolf-Ostermann. 2020. Pflege in Zeiten von Corona: Zentrale Ergebnisse einer deutschlandweiten Querschnittsbefragung vollstationärer Pflegeheime. *Pflege*, 33(5): 265–275.

RTL. 2021. Das denken die Deutschen über die Lockdown-Verlängerung. Forsa-Umfrage: Mehrheit glaubt nicht an den Erfolg der neuen Corona-Maßnahmen.

Schrappe, M., H. Francois-Kettner, M. Gruhl, D. Hart, F. Knieps, P. Manow, H. Pfaff, K. Püschel and G. Glaeske. 2020a. Die Pandemie durch SARS-CoV-2/Covid-19 – der Übergang zur chronischen Phase – Verbesserung der Outcomes in Sicht Stabile Kontrolle: Würde und Humanität wahren Diskursverengung vermeiden: Corona nicht politisieren.

Schrappe, M., H.F. Francois-Kettner, M. Gruhl, D. Hart, F. Knieps, P. Manow, H. Pfaff, K. Püschel and G. Glaeske. 2020b. Die Pandemie durch SARS-CoV-2/CoViD-19 - Zur Notwendigkeit eines Strategiewechsels. www.schrappe.com/ms2/index_htm_files/Thesenpap6_201122_endfass.pdf. Accessed: 31 October 2024.

Schwäbisches Tagblatt. 2021. Thomas Aigner: „Als Ausdruck meines Protestes", 6.1.2021. www.tagblatt.de/Nachrichten/Thomas-Aigner-Als-Ausdruck-meines-Protestes-485149.html, Accessed: 15 March 2021.

Simon, M. 2020. Das ERG-Fallpauschalsystem für Krankenhäuser. Kritische Bestandaufnahme und Eckpunkte für eine Reform der Krankenhausfinanzierung jenseits des DRG-Systems. Working Paper Forschungsförderung der Hans-Böckler-Stiftung. Nr. 196.

Staatskanzlei des Landes Nordrhein-Westfalen. 2021. Expertenrat Corona. Ministerpräsident Armin Laschet beruft „Expertenrat Corona". https://www.land.nrw/de/expertenrat-corona. Accessed: 2 Ferbuary 2021.

Ständige Impfkommission, Deutscher Ethikrat, Nationale Akademie der Wissenschaften and Leopoldina. 2020. Wie soll der Zugang zu einem COVID-19-Impfstoff geregelt werden? Positionspapier einer gemeinsamen Arbeitsgruppe, Berlin, 9. November 2020.

Statista. 2020a. Anzahl durchgeführter Tests für das Coronavirus (COVID-19) in Deutschland nach Kalenderwoche. https://de.statista.com/statistik/daten/studie/1107749/umfrage/labortest-fuer-das-coronavirus-covid-19-in-deutschland/. Accessed: 1 March 2021. Accessed: 2 March 2021.

Statista. 2020b. Todesfälle mit Coronavirus (COVID-19) in Deutschland nach Alter und Geschlecht. https://de.statista.com/statistik/daten/studie/1104173/umfrage/todesfaelle-aufgrund-des-coronavirus-in-deutschland-nach-geschlecht/. Accessed: 2 March 2021.

Statista. 2020c. Share of Hospitals in Germany in 2018, by Sponsorship and State. https://www.statista.com/statistics/578451/hospital-share-germany-by-sponsorship-state/. Accessed: 4 March 2021.

Streeck, W. 2021. Welchen Wissenschaftlern folgen wir in der Pandemie? https://www.faz.net/aktuell/feuilleton/debatten/corona-beitrag-der-soziologie-zur-bewaeltigung-der-krise-17138966.html. Accessed: 2 March 2021.

Süddeutsche Zeitung. 2020. Amtsarzt legt sich mit dem Freistaat an, 4.11.2020. www.sueddeutsche.de/bayern/aichach-amtsarzt-puerner-kritik-versetzung-1.5104412, Accessed: 15 March 2021.

Thielbörger, P. and B. Behlert. 2020. COVID-19 und das Grundgesetz: Neue Gedanken vor dem Hintergrund neuer Gesetze. https://verfassungsblog.de/covid-19-und-das-grundgesetz-neue-gedanken-vor-dem-hintergrund-neuer-gesetze/. Accessed: 2 March 2021.

Thüringer Allgemeine. 2021. Bayerischer Verwaltungsgerichtshof widerspricht Corona-Urteil des Amtsgerichts Weimar. https://www.thueringer-allgemeine.de/

leben/recht-justiz/bayerischer-verwaltungsgerichtshof-widerspricht-dem-corona-urteil-des-amtsgerichts-weimar-id231408135.html. Accessed: 2 March 2021.

Van Dooren, W. and M. Noordegraf. 2020. Staging Science: Authoritativeness and Fragility of Models and Measurement in the COVID-19 Crisis. *Public Administration Review*, 80(4): 610–615.

Vereinigung der kommunalen Arbeitgeberverbände. 2020. Bedeutung kommunaler Krankenhäuser.

Wagschal, U., S. Jäckle, A. Hildebrandt and E.M. Trüdinger. 2020. Ausgewählte Ergebnisse einer Bevölkerungsumfrage zu den Auswirkungen des Corona-Virus. www.politikpanel.uni-freiburg.de/docs/Auswertung_PPD_Corona_Umfrage_Mai2020.pdf. Accessed: 31 October 2024.

WELT. 2020a. In Deutschland wurden fast eine Million Operationen abgesagt, 29.5.2020. https://www.welt.de/wirtschaft/article208557665/Wegen-Corona-In-Deutschland-wurden-908-000-OPs-aufgeschoben.html. Accessed: 16 March 2021.

WELT. 2020b. 21 Prozent der „Querdenker" wählten die Grünen, 4.12.2020. https://www.welt.de/politik/deutschland/article221812060/Corona-21-Prozent-der-Querdenker-waehlten-die-Gruenen.html. Accessed: 2 Ferbuary 2021.

WELT. 2020c. Die Pandemie ist kein Geschehen mehr, das man mit Beschränkungen ausbremsen könnte, 19.11.2020. https://www.welt.de/politik/deutschland/plus220506980/Kritik-an-Corona-Politik-Die-Pandemie-kein-Geschehen-das-man-mit-Beschraenkungen-ausbremsen-koennte.html. Accessed: 2 March 2021.

Wikipedia. 2021. Proteste in Deutschland während der COVID-19-Pandemie. https://de.wikipedia.org/wiki/Proteste_in_Deutschland_w%C3%A4hrend_der_COVID-19-Pandemie. Accessed: 9 March 2021.

Wissenschaftlicher Beirat Corona Landesregierung Thüringen. 2020. Impulspapier 5: Pandemiemanagement in Schulen und Kindertageseinrichtungen, 27 September 2020.

ZDF. 2020. Buyx zur Corona-Warn-App. Ethikrat: Weniger Datenschutz wäre vertretbar, 29.10.2020.

Pertinent Laws and Regulations

Drittes Gesetz zum Schutz der Bevölkerung bei einer epidemischen Lage von nationaler Tragweite (Drittes Bevölkerungsschutzgesetz), 18. November 2020, BGBl. Teil I Nr. 52, 18. November 2020, S. 2397.

German-Language Weblinks

AGI. Arbeitsgemeinschaft Influenza. influenza.rki.de

DIVI. Deutsche Interdisziplinäre Vereinigung für Intensiv- und Notfallmedizin. www.divi.de.

Expertenrat Corona, NRW. www.land.nrw/de/expertenrat-corona

Grippe-web. grippeweb.rki.de

Leopoldina. Nationale Akademie der Wissenschaften. www.leopoldina.org/leopoldina-home/.

NRZ. Nationales Referenzzentrum für Influenzaviren. www.rki.de/DE/Content/Infekt/NRZ/Influenza/influenza_node.html.

Wissenschaftlicher Beirat Corona-Management Landesregierung Thüringen. https://thueringen.de/regierung/wissenschaftlicher-beirat. Accessed: 31 October 2024.

3 Sweden's Responses to COVID-19

Carl Dahlström and Johannes Lindvall

3.1 Introduction

When the new coronavirus SARS-CoV-2 began to spread across Europe in early 2020, Sweden adopted public-health policies that were markedly different from those of most other Western European states. Sweden's government, parliament, and public-health authorities refrained from the sorts of coercive policies that other countries put in place and did little to restrict the freedom of movement or the freedom of assembly. Preschools, elementary schools, and lower-secondary schools remained open throughout the spring, as did most restaurants and shops. Instead of resorting to coercion, Swedish authorities issued voluntary recommendations that were meant to limit the spread of the virus by persuading citizens to reduce their social interactions and protect themselves and others from the disease.

A few months later, in the autumn of 2020, Sweden, like most of Western Europe, was hit by a second wave of the COVID-19 epidemic, which proved to be even deadlier than the first. During this period, Sweden's government, parliament, and public health authorities put in place policies that were more restrictive, and that made the Swedish approach to the COVID-19 crisis more similar to that of other countries. By January 2021, the parliament had adopted new legislation that authorized the government to impose new restrictions on shopping centers and other businesses, and children in lower secondary schools were taught in their homes in many parts of the country.

This chapter examines Sweden's public-health policies in the twelve-month period between January 2020, when Swedish authorities took the first steps to prepare the country for the new epidemic, and December 2020, when Sweden found itself in the middle of the epidemic's second wave and new, more restrictive policies were being prepared and enacted (Dahlström and Lindvall 2021). We begin with a brief overview of the spread of the new coronavirus in Sweden, examining the number of known infected, the number of fatalities, and the pressures on the health

DOI: 10.4324/9781003362760-3

care system. In the section that follows, we describe the public-health policies Sweden put in place in 2020. We then turn to an analysis of the social and political factors that explain Sweden's distinctive approach to public-health policy during the first phase of the COVID-19 pandemic.

3.2   The COVID-19 Epidemic in Sweden

On January 16, 2020, the Public Health Agency of Sweden published the first news about COVID-19 on its website. The agency informed the public about the discovery of a new coronavirus in Wuhan, China, but assessed the risk of the disease spreading to Sweden as "very low". On January 31, however, the first COVID-19 case was detected in Sweden. In February, the agency informed the Swedish public of new COVID-19 outbreaks in South Korea, Iran, and Italy. At the end of the month, on February 25, the Public Health Agency changed its assessment of the risk of more cases in Sweden to "high," but the risk of community transmission of the disease within Sweden was still seen as "low". The next day, the second Swedish COVID-19 case was confirmed, and in the following days, further cases were reported. In the beginning of March, the agency changed its risk assessment again. It now suggested that there was a "very high" risk of more cases and a "moderate" risk of community transmission within Sweden. On March 10, finally, the risk assessment for community transmission of the new coronavirus within Sweden was raised to the highest level, "very high".

Since the rate of testing has varied greatly over time – with many more tests being performed in the autumn than in the spring – it is difficult to compare the infection rates during different phases of the COVID-19 crisis in Sweden. One must keep this in mind when considering Figure 3.1, which shows how many new coronavirus infections were reported to the Public Health Agency of Sweden in that year, beginning with the first case and ending on December 31, 2020: the figure underestimates the number of infected in the spring, since so few tests were performed then compared with the autumn (see Figure 3.2, which plots the number of tests that were performed per week between late January and the end of December). Nevertheless, the figure shows clearly that there were two distinct waves of the epidemic, one beginning in late March and the other beginning in the middle of October. The two waves are even more clearly visible in Figure 3.3, which describes the number of new COVID-19 patients that were admitted to Swedish intensive care units per day during 2020, and in Figure 3.4, which describes the number of individuals who died with COVID-19 each day.[1] Taken together, these figures show that the virus spread quickly in the month of March 2020, resulting in high morbidity and high mortality at the end of March and in April; the infection rates and the death rates

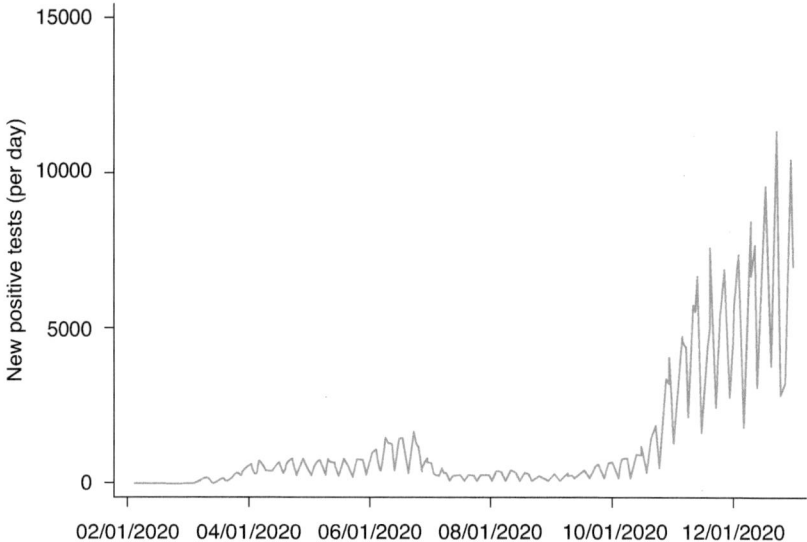

Figure 3.1 New COVID-19 cases reported to the authorities (per day).

Source: Adapted from Folkhälsomyndigheten, accessed 26 January 2021

Note: The figure does not accurately describe the actual number of infected since the rate of testing has changed greatly over the period examined.

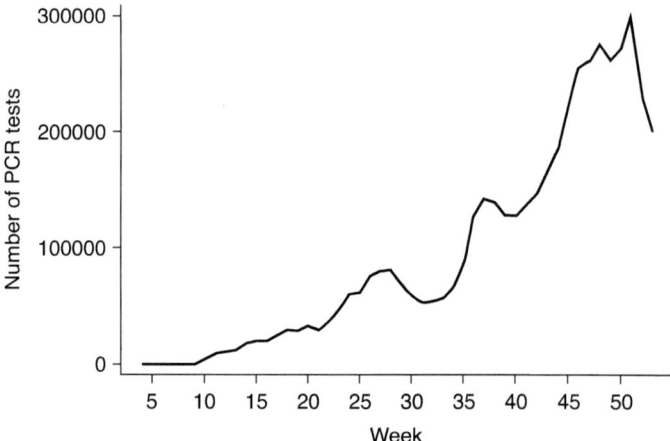

Figure 3.2 COVID-19 tests per week, January to December 2020.

Source: Adapted from Folkhälsomyndigheten, e-mail message 11 January 2021

Note: The data are incomplete since not all laboratories report figures to the Public Health Agency of Sweden, Folkhälsomyndigheten.

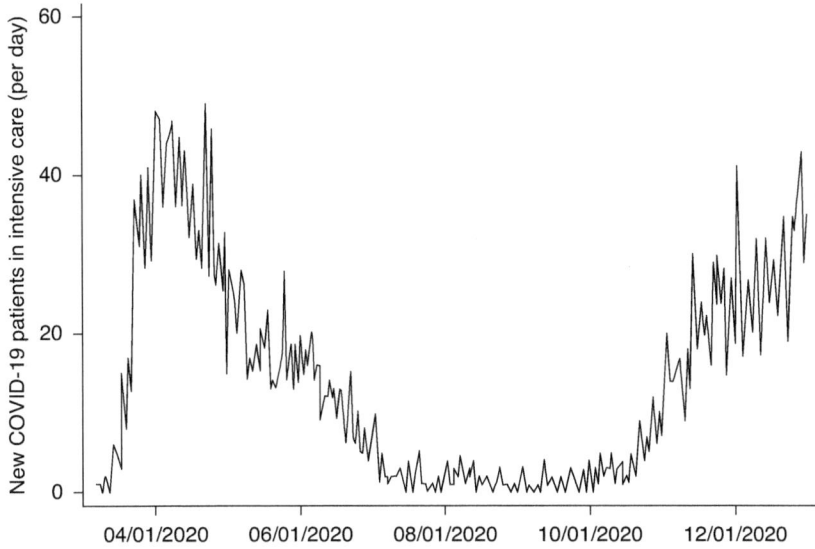

Figure 3.3 New patients with COVID-19 in intensive care (per day).

Source: Adapted from Folkhälsomyndigheten, accessed 26 January 2021

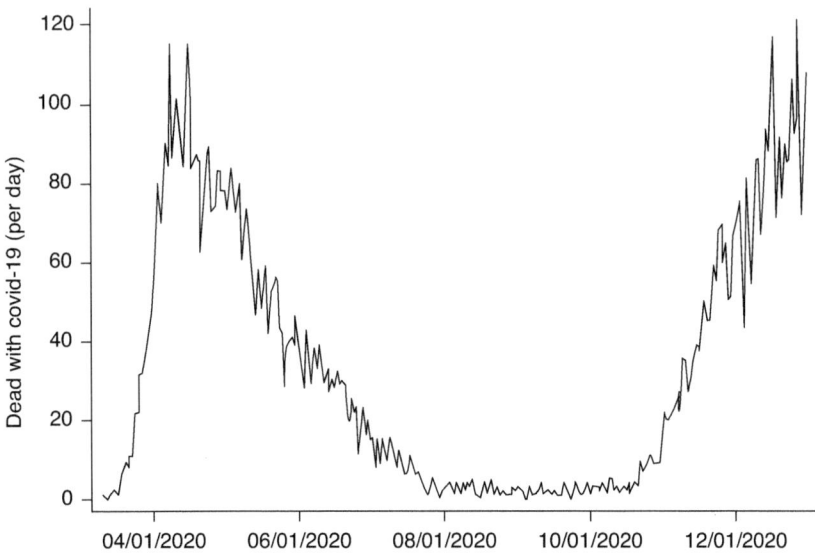

Figure 3.4 Dead with COVID-19 (per day).

Source: Adapted from Folkhälsomyndigheten, accessed 26 January 2021

then fell slowly but surely during the spring, summer, and early autumn of 2020, until the rate of infection picked up again in the middle of October, resulting once more in high morbidity and high mortality in November and December. By the end of 2020, more than 10,000 individuals had died with COVID-19. Since Sweden has a population of just over 10 million, this meant that the total number of deaths exceeded 0.1% of Sweden's population.

The death rate in Sweden was significantly higher both in the spring and in the autumn of 2020 than in Sweden's closest neighbors, Denmark, Finland, and Norway. Starting in the spring and summer of 2020, these differences between the death rate in Sweden and the death rates in the neighboring countries were at the center of a major political debate within Sweden. This political debate was preceded by an intense debate among doctors and public-health experts, where some scholars at Swedish universities were very critical of the Public Health Agency of Sweden and of the methods it relied on. The critics wanted the government and the state authorities to put in place more coercive and stringent policies to halt the spread of the new coronavirus (Carlsson et al. 2020).

As we will discuss in more detail in the next section, it is instructive to distinguish between four phases of the COVID-19 epidemic in 2020: a phase with no (detected) community transmission between January and mid-March, a phase with high community transmission from mid-March until early June, a phase with low community transmission between early June and the middle of October, and, finally, a phase with high community transmission from late October through December. We will now proceed to examine the policies Sweden's government, parliament, and public authorities put in place during these different phases of the pandemic.[2]

3.3   Public-Health Policies in Sweden During the COVID-19 Pandemic

Sweden's epidemic-control policy during the COVID-19 crisis was markedly different from that of other Western European countries. With a few important exceptions, Sweden's government, parliament, and administrative authorities have refrained from introducing coercive policy measures that interfere with the lives of individuals and the activities of private-sector companies and other organizations. The Public Health Agency of Sweden emphasized early on during the crisis that their policy for epidemic control was based on voluntarism and on the idea that a well-informed and motivated public can and will take responsible decisions. In the view of the agency, a policy based on voluntarism is generally more effective than coercive measures (The Public Health Agency of Sweden 2020). The Swedish epidemic-control policy is therefore based on recommendations and general advice from the relevant authorities.[3] It is also primarily such recommendations and general advice that have affected people's lives during the COVID-19 epidemic, not strict rules and regulations.

As we have already mentioned, Swedish crisis management during the COVID-19 epidemic in 2020 can be divided into four different phases: (1) a phase with no (detected) community transmission, from January to mid-March; (2) a phase with high community transmission, from mid-March until early June; (3) a phase with low community transmission, from early June to late October; (4) and a phase with high community transmission, from late October through December.[4]

From January to mid-March, the goal of Swedish public-health policy was to identify all cases of COVID-19 in Sweden. COVID-19 cases were identified by testing individuals who showed symptoms after traveling in areas with documented outbreaks of the disease and people who had been in contact with individuals with confirmed COVID-19. However, there was no quarantine of individuals who had been in areas with documented community transmission of COVID-19. People who returned from affected areas were instead asked to pay attention to symptoms themselves, contact the health care advice platform 1177 Vårdguiden for further assessment and stay in their homes if they had symptoms. The strategy was based on the assumption that individuals without symptoms were not infectious and that there was no community transmission of COVID-19 in Sweden. Until mid-March, preparations were also made for the possibility that more drastic measures might be required. In early February, COVID-19 was added to the list of dangerous diseases in the Swedish Communicable Diseases Act, which made it possible for the coercive measures that the law allows to be used in COVID-19 cases.[5] The Public Health Agency of Sweden turned to the government with this proposal on January 31, 2020, and the government took the decision at a special meeting of the cabinet on February 1. In the beginning of March, travel restrictions were also introduced for certain countries. On March 10, the Public Health Agency of Sweden announced that they saw signs of community transmission of the COVID-19 infection in the Stockholm and Västra Götaland regions and that there was now a "very high" risk of an outbreak with endemic community transmission of the disease within Sweden. Two days later, public gatherings were limited to a maximum of 500 people.

On 13 March, the day after restrictions on public gatherings were introduced, the Public Health Agency of Sweden announced that the epidemic-control policy had entered a new phase. From mid-March – when infection rates in Sweden were already very high – the government, the Public Health Agency of Sweden and the National Board of Health and Welfare (Socialstyrelsen) took a number of new decisions and issued recommendations and general advice that had a strong impact on people's lives as well as on the activities of private companies and other organizations. In the report "Folkhälsomyndighetens föreskrifter och allmänna råd om allas ansvar att förhindra smitta av covid-19 m.m." from the Public Health Agency of Sweden, there were for example several pieces of general advice that severely limited the activities of agencies, companies, municipalities, regions, associations, and religious organizations. The general advice included restrictions on the number of people on the premises to avoid crowds, the suspension of physical meetings, calls to work from home, and to refrain from social events and travel.[6] Moreover, universities, university colleges, and upper secondary schools (gymnasier) were advised to introduce online teaching, and there were more restrictions on public gatherings (a maximum of 50 people) and on restaurants, bars, and cafés. It is from this point that one could reasonably speak of a "lockdown" of Swedish society, although most of the measures that were taken remained voluntary (Ludvigsson 2020).

With a declining number of new patients and falling numbers of deaths with COVID-19 (Figures 3.3 and 3.4), some of the restrictions were eased during the summer and in the first half of the autumn of 2020. In this period, we saw the third phase of the Swedish policy response. The recommendation of online teaching for upper secondary schools, for example, was lifted in June, and though things didn't quite go back to normal, most students and university students started the autumn semester on-site in their schools. The recommendation against non-necessary travel was also lifted in June. Moreover, the authorities withdrew the recommendation that people over the age of 70 should avoid social gatherings, as well as the ban on visits to all nursing homes in the country, in the autumn of 2020.

The Public Health Agency prepared for autumn with locally concentrated outbursts of COVID-19, with testing, tracing, monitoring, and communication as the main measures taken against such local transmission (individual responsibility, social distancing, and hand hygiene were, however, always the backbone of the Swedish strategy). In line with this type of reasoning, the agency opened up the possibility of making stricter recommendations locally during a limited time. When the cases started increasing in October (see Figures 3.1, 3.3, and 3.4), the Public Health Agency of Sweden, in collaboration with regional-level authorities, started implementing this strategy, first in Uppsala on October 20, then in Skåne on October 27, followed by Stockholm, Västra Götaland, and Östergötland on October 29. Within just over a week in late October 2020, the most populated areas in Sweden were again covered by strict recommendations, sometimes even stricter than during the spring.

These regional actions took the Swedish policy response into its fourth phase. The government and the authorities responded to the high and increasing transmission of the virus that causes COVID-19 with more restrictions, also on the national level. In the beginning of December, the Public Health Agency again recommended online teaching for upper secondary schools (gymnasium), and in mid-December the agency made recommendations restricting traveling, social contacts outside the household, sports, shopping, and social contacts with elderly people. In November and December, new and stricter recommendations and regulations for restaurants, bars, and cafés were implemented. For example, the Public Health Agency of Sweden advised against seating more than four guests per table, and the government issued an ordinance banning alcohol after a certain hour (at first, alcohol was not allowed in restaurants, bars, and cafés between 10 pm and 11 am, later the rule was changed to 8 pm–11 am). In the autumn of 2020, the government, its agencies and the regions also prepared for vaccinations against COVID-19 to start in January of 2021. This process started already in late August but intensified later in the autumn.

Since the Swedish authorities emphasized voluntarism throughout all four phases of the COVID-19 crisis, it is important to know if the general public was aware of and followed the recommendations and advice of the authorities. The Swedish Civil Contingencies Agency conducted surveys from 21 March onward to assess behavioral changes among the general public. During the first half of 2020, virtually all respondents (99%) stated that they had changed their behavior in some way. For example, the vast majority stated that they followed the Public Health Agency's advice to wash their hands more thoroughly (86%) and to keep a greater distance from others (85%) (Esaiasson et al. 2020). After 20 August 2020, the Swedish Civil Contingencies Agency also used a new survey item to assess whether the general public had enough information to comply with recommendations. The vast majority of the respondents answered that they were knowledgeable enough. In August and September, about 80% answered that they were well-informed about how to behave in public and private gatherings. About 70% said the same thing concerning testing and vaccinations, and about 60% stated they knew enough to make informed choices in their working lives, in educational contexts, and when they used public transportation (Kantar Sifo 2020a, 2020b). During the fourth phase of the crisis, when specific local and regional actions were taken, the Swedish Civil Contingencies Agency asked respondents if they had enough information about local restrictions and recommendations, and 86% answered that they were fairly or very well-informed (Kantar Sifo 2021). Finally, the Swedish company Telia has made available aggregate cell phone data on traveling patterns within Sweden, and the data show a decline of 20% of daily trips within Sweden. Taken together, these pieces of evidence suggest that the Swedish general public was aware of and followed recommendations and advice from the authorities, but it is difficult to determine what effects these behavioral changes had, and how much effect more stringent rules would have had in comparison.

It is also worth mentioning a few things that didn't happen in Sweden in 2020. Preschools and primary schools did not close, nor did lower secondary schools (although they were closed in January 2021 in many parts of the country). No general recommendations regarding face masks on public transport or in public places were issued. And although both the Ministry for Foreign Affairs and the Public Health Agency of Sweden issued travel advice recommending Swedes to limit travel, no bans on traveling within the country, or on leaving the country, were introduced. In addition, neither health checks nor quarantine were required when entering Sweden, and no policy of confinement was implemented.

Meanwhile, the Swedish parliament and the Swedish government have taken a number of steps to mitigate the economic damage that is caused by the COVID-19 epidemic (Finanspolitiska rådet 2020). The single most costly measure was the new support program for "short-term work" that was introduced in the spring of 2020. Through a government decree and then a new law that applied retroactively from mid-March 2020, it became possible for companies during the COVID crisis to apply for funding for short-term leave for their staff amounting to up to 60% of working hours, a percentage that was later increased to 80% during the months of May, June, and July. Although firms have had the possibility to lay off their staff temporarily, with funding from the government, unemployment has increased. Both the average benefit level in the unemployment insurance system and the cap on high benefits have been raised, and it has become easier for individual employees to qualify for unemployment insurance. Meanwhile, the qualifying day in the health insurance system – a rule that says there is no sick pay for the first day away from work – has been removed. One reason for that rule change was that the government wanted to give employees incentives to stay at home if they had mild symptoms of illness. In addition, the government and the parliament have taken a number of steps to protect Swedish companies directly from the consequences of the economic downturn. The second most costly new measure in 2020, after the short-term work program, was a form of direct support to Swedish companies, which was based on the estimated reductions in their turnover. The third most costly measure was a temporary reduction in social security contributions (which are paid by employers in Sweden). The government has also temporarily taken over the responsibility for sick pay, which is normally paid by the employer in the beginning of a period of illness for an employee.

3.4　Explaining Sweden's Response to the COVID-19 Crisis

In this section, we will discuss the social and political context in which Sweden's distinctive public-health policies during the COVID-19 crisis were adopted and implemented. We concentrate on those characteristics of the Swedish political system that other scholars and political commentators in Sweden and abroad have pointed to when they have sought to explain the choices Sweden's government, parliament, and public-health authorities made during the pandemic.

3.4.1 Experts and Politicians

One important difference between Sweden's approach to the COVID-19 pandemic and that of other comparable countries in Western Europe is that, at least in the beginning of the crisis, many of the operative decisions were made by experts and bureaucrats in public agencies, not by elected political leaders in the government and in parliament. The willingness of Sweden's political leadership to delegate public-health policymaking to administrative authorities – particularly in the beginning of the crisis – has been highlighted by Andersson and Aylott (2020), among others, and it was quite clear to anyone who followed Swedish politics in the spring of 2020: the Swedish government trusted the judgment of the public-health authorities and waited for advice from the bureaucracy before introducing new legislation or government decrees (Andersson and Aylott 2020).

For foreign observers, the relationship between the government and the bureaucracy in Sweden may seem peculiar. It is, for example, different from the relationship between the government and the bureaucracy in Sweden's neighbors Denmark, Norway, and Germany. The Swedish Government Offices, which comprise all ministries, are small and have limited investigative resources compared with government ministries in these other neighboring countries. Swedish administrative authorities also enjoy more operational independence than public agencies in most other democracies, and their independence is protected by the constitution (Ahlbäck Öberg and Wockelberg 2016 and Pierre 2004). In 2020, the Government Offices consisted of the Prime Minister's Office, the Office for Administrative Affairs, and 11 ministries. The Prime Minister's Office is headed by the Prime Minister, and each ministry is headed by a minister. Numerous agencies, such as the Public Health Agency, the National Board of Health and Welfare and the Swedish Civil Contingencies Agency (Myndigheten för samhällsskydd och beredskap), sort under each ministry. In January 2020, there were a total of 341 such agencies. Swedish agencies are quite different from each other, and they include everything from relatively small committees with narrow and specific remits to county administrative boards, large administrative agencies, and universities (Dahlström and Holmgren 2019). In 2020, there were approximately 229,000 annual full-time equivalents employed at these authorities, which can be compared with the approximately 4,600 people that are employed within the Government Offices (i.e., at the ministries themselves). The majority of the resources of the administrative state are thus allocated to the public agencies (The Government Office 2019, The Swedish Agency for Public Management 2020).

According to Swedish administrative law and traditions, bureaucratic agencies make independent assessments that are based on the best available knowledge and the government listens to the experts at the agencies. In international comparison, what is perhaps the most striking is that Swedish ministers are prohibited by the constitution, the Instrument of Government, from giving instructions to agencies in individual cases (Chapter 12, Section 2). A commission of inquiry, Styrutredningen, summarized the Swedish administrative model as follows: "On the one hand, politicians decide and the administration executes, on the other hand, the administration must talk back with a clear voice" (SOU 2007:75, p. 13).

But bureaucratic agencies in Sweden can nevertheless be controlled indirectly, through legislation, executive orders, and written directives. The government's most important formal control instruments are the instructions that authorize each agency's operations, budgets, and yearly spending decisions. For each agency, the government writes a formal instruction that describes the agency's mission and organization. The government is free to change these instructions. The government can also change the budgets of individual agencies, even if it is the Swedish parliament that decides on the state budget. In the yearly spending instructions, written in connection with the budget, the government also gives detailed instructions to each agency on how the funds are to be used. In these spending instructions and in other government decisions, special assignments can be given to an agency (e.g., to increase testing, or coordinate the purchase of protective equipment). Moreover, the government can steer agencies by appointing heads of agencies, although it is constrained by the Instrument of Government's provisions on meritocratic recruitment (Chapter 12, Section 5), and Swedish agency heads have employment contracts with strong employment security for a fixed term. In addition to these formal control instruments, there are informal contacts between the Government Offices and the agencies (Jacobsson 1984, Niemann 2013). These informal contacts are an important part of the governance structure. Ministers and officials at the Government Offices are not prohibited from having informal contacts with agencies under their own ministry for the purpose of obtaining information or achieving certain results – as long as this does not affect decisions in individual cases, which would be a violation of constitutional law. Such informal contacts are made often, and they enhance the ability of the government to steer public authorities, even in a situation such as the COVID-19 crisis (Jacobsson and Sundström 2016, Pierre 2020).

The constitutionally protected independence of administrative agencies means specifically that the parliament or the government may not "decide how an administrative agency should decide in a particular case concerning the exercise of authority vis-à-vis an individual or a municipality or concerning the application of law" (Chapter 12, Section 2). But as we've just discussed, this doesn't mean that the government cannot control public agencies at all: it has several instruments that they can use to this end. It would therefore have been entirely possible for the government and the parliament to adopt policies that were more similar to those adopted in other democracies, even if the public health authorities favored a voluntarist approach. Most importantly, and as we will discuss in more detail below, it would have been constitutionally possible for the parliament to enact new laws, and it would have been legally possible for the government to introduce more far-reaching coercive policies within current legislation since the parliament authorized the government to do so via temporary enabling legislation. The Corona Commission—a government commission of inquiry that was put in place to investigate how Sweden handled the COVID-19 epidemic—reached the same conclusion and argued that the government not only could but also should have taken charge over crisis management in the spring of 2020 (SOU 2022:10 Volume 2).

But even if a more direct political approach would have been legally allowed, Sweden's long tradition of administrative autonomy nevertheless helps to explain the distinctive Swedish response to COVID-19. Since the Swedish government usually lets administrative agencies act autonomously within the framework of existing legislation and regulations, the prevailing views within the public health authorities, especially in the Public Health Agency, did much to shape policy in 2020.

3.4.2   Planning for a Pandemic

Since many of the operative decisions during the COVID-19 pandemic were made by experts and bureaucrats in public agencies, particularly the Public Health Agency, it is important to consider the contingency plans that the Public Health Agency had drawn up for a possible global outbreak of a new infectious disease. In 2019—just before the outbreak of the COVID-19 epidemic—the Public Health Agency published a report called "Pandemic Preparedness," which described the agency's views on appropriate policy during a pandemic (especially an influenza pandemic) and the demands such an event would place on Swedish society. According to that report, the main goals of Swedish policy during a pandemic should be both to "minimize mortality and morbidity in the population" and to "minimize other negative consequences for the individual and society." The report emphasizes in particular the importance of "trying to reduce the spread of infection and delaying the course of the pandemic" so that "the curve is flattened" to reduce "the burden on the healthcare system and society" and to increase "preparation time" before a vaccine becomes available. Social distancing is listed as one possible measure that can be used to achieve these goals. The idea of curbing the spread of a disease in order to "flatten the curve" was thus an integral part of Swedish policy.[7]

But already before the crisis, one notes a certain skepticism on the part of the Public Health Agency concerning the appropriateness of far-reaching "non-medical" measures during a pandemic. On the one hand, the 2019 report emphasizes that in the early stages of a pandemic, there are few opportunities to limit the spread of infection and care for the sick medically, which means that the only "measures that exist to reduce a pandemic's impact on society are so-called non-medical measures," including "hand hygiene, coughing and sneezing etiquette, voluntary isolation in case of illness, avoiding public gatherings and public events, and closing schools." On the other hand, the report emphasizes that the scholarly literature doesn't show conclusively that such policies work. Among other things, the report cites a WHO study suggesting that the evidence for the effectiveness of non-medical measures is low. In addition, the report emphasizes that non-medical measures "may have a negative impact on the functionality of society," so the political response to a pandemic must be "balanced." The Public Health Agency's assessment in 2019 was that the suitability of non-medical measures depended on "the severity, spread and societal context of a pandemic."

When the Public Health Agency and the Swedish government explained the premises of Sweden's COVID-19 strategy in the spring of 2020, they typically referred to this balancing act, taking into account both the expected effect of restrictive measures on the spread of infection and the broader social and economic costs associated with lockdowns. The decision to keep elementary, primary, and lower secondary schools open was justified in two ways, for example. On the one hand, the government emphasized that the spread of infection among children was low. On the other hand, the government noted that the social costs would be high if schools were closed, especially since the healthcare system would suffer if many employees were forced to stay home to take care of small children. In June, Sweden's state epidemiologist, Anders Tegnell, said on the radio that in the beginning of the COVID-19 epidemic, he had assumed that other countries would do much as Sweden did, since he believed that Sweden's strategy was consistent with the prevailing ideas in the international public-health community. These prevailing views within the public-health bureaucracy, combined with the deference that the government in Sweden typically extends to bureaucratic expertise, help to explain the Swedish policy response.

With regard to organizational and administrative issues during a pandemic, the Public Health Agency distinguished in its planning before the COVID-19 crisis between the roles played by international organizations, the government, state authorities, the regions, and the municipalities. Judging from the 2019 report, the assumption was that the government would have a limited role, namely to "ensure access to vaccines and anti-virals," to decide whether a disease should be "classified as dangerous" for the purposes of the provisions of the Communicable Diseases Act, and to decide on an "antiviral storage strategy." The Public Health Agency itself was assumed to have many different tasks, including the coordination of pandemic preparedness at the national level. The National Board of Health and Welfare was expected to oversee and coordinate emergency health care measures regionally and locally and issue regulations on the use of pharmaceuticals. The Swedish Civil Contingencies Agency was expected to coordinate various actors at the national level and to monitor the impact of a pandemic on society as a whole. Municipalities, regions, and regional infection-control physicians were expected to have a number of more operational tasks.

The Swedish approach to COVID-19 was thus in most respects consistent with the ideas that informed prior planning for a pandemic outbreak of a new communicable disease. In other words, what needs to be explained concerning Sweden's distinctive approach is not a change in policy, but the fact that Swedish public authorities—as well as the government and parliament—did not change policies, even if other countries did.

Toward the end of 2020, in what we have referred to as the fourth phase of the Swedish policy response to COVID-19, both the government, parliament, the national public health authorities, and regional decision-makers put in place more restrictions than in the spring, affecting, for instance, lower secondary school students, restaurants and bars, and shops (which were instructed to limit the number of customers they admitted and to take other precautions). It is difficult to determine whether the change in policy came at the initiative of the government or whether the views of the government, the national public health authorities, and local decision-makers co-evolved, but it seems clear that the consequence of this reorientation was to bring Swedish COVID-19 policies closer to the Western European mainstream.

3.4.3 Laws and Lawmaking

One proximate cause of Sweden's choice to refrain from introducing new coercive measures in 2020—in addition to the prevailing views within the public-health bureaucracy and the deference that is usually afforded to administrative agencies in the Swedish political system—is that existing public-health legislation was based on a voluntarist approach. Moreover, there was little legal basis, at least in the early stages of the pandemic, for a nationwide lockdown, restrictions of the freedom of movement, or other sorts of novel restrictions on private individuals and organizations.

Swedish policies concerning the spread of infectious diseases are primarily governed by the Swedish Communicable Diseases Act. The 2004 Communicable Diseases Act, like previous public-health legislation, affords regional infection-control physicians with far-reaching powers when it comes to local coercive measures, such as quarantine, isolation, and restrictions on travel. But the Communicable Diseases Act is also based on the idea that individual citizens bear a great deal of personal responsibility for what happens during an epidemic. The second chapter of the Act begins, for example, by stating that "Everyone shall, by paying attention and taking reasonable precautions, contribute to preventing the spread of communicable diseases." The emphasis on voluntariness in Sweden's COVID-19 policies in the spring of 2020 was thus nothing new—Swedish legislation in the public health domain has long been based on similar principles (Petersson 2020). It is interesting to note that the provisions of the Communicable Diseases Act on extraordinary disease-control measures at the local and regional levels were not in fact applied during the COVID-19 crisis in 2020: since the government declared early on that COVID-19 is a socially dangerous disease, these more coercive provisions of the Communicable Diseases Act could in principle have been applied, but they were not.

Most of the coercive policies that were adopted and implemented during the COVID-19 epidemic were based on other pieces of legislation, primarily the Public Order Act, which regulates order and safety at public gatherings and public events. Most importantly, a ban on public gatherings and public events with more than 50 participants was announced in the spring of 2020. The fact that the Public Order Act is only applicable at public gatherings and public events is an important part of the explanation for the often-noted discrepancy between how different domains of Swedish society were affected by the restrictions that were introduced during the COVID-19 epidemic. For example, more than 50 people could gather in a shop but not at a theater or at a sports event (Wenander 2020). There were also a few that were introduced during the COVID-19 epidemic that were based on laws other than the Public Order Act. For example, in late March, a national ban on visits to elderly-care homes was announced, which was in turn based on a provision of the Social Services Act. Entirely new legislation was also adopted in the spring of 2020, including a new law on temporary infection-control measures at restaurants. But most of the new laws that were adopted during this period dealt with the economic and social fallout of the COVID-19 epidemic, not with preventing the spread of the infection. For example, amendments were introduced in the Swedish Companies Act and in other laws on organizations and associations that made it possible to conduct meetings in a safe manner. Some of the economic policy measures that were introduced during the crisis also resulted in new legislation.

It would be wrong to explain Sweden's distinctive policies during the COVID-19 pandemic with the absence of legislation that authorized the government and the public health authorities to introduce more coercive and stringent measures. It would have been entirely possible for the government to introduce new legislation that provided a legal basis for such a strategy. Indeed, the rapid adoption of legislation that allowed private companies and other organizations to adapt to the pandemic demonstrates that the capacity for immediate political action existed. Perhaps even more importantly, in April 2020, the parliament passed a new law that temporarily gave the cabinet the authority to adopt more drastic policies by government decree in connection with the COVID-19 epidemic. To be more specific, a temporary addition was made to Chapter 9 of the Communicable Diseases Act, which applied until July 2020 and which enabled the Government to:

> issue special regulations on the relationship between individuals and the government that place demands for individuals or otherwise relate to interventions in their personal or financial circumstances, if it is necessary to prevent the spread of the virus that causes COVID-19 and it is not possible to wait for the Riksdag's approval.

The measures that the government was authorized to implement included "temporary closures of shopping centers," "temporary closures of social and cultural meeting places, such as bars, nightclubs, restaurants, cafeterias, gyms and sports facilities, libraries, museums and public meeting places" and "temporary closures or other restrictions of … ports, airports, or bus stations or railway stations." But even if this temporary law existed, the government did not take the opportunity that it afforded to put in place more restrictive disease-control measures in 2020 (Jonsson Cornell 2020). In the beginning of 2021, however, during the fourth phase of the pandemic, the Swedish parliament adopted a similar law, which again authorized the government to regulate private companies and other organizations, and this time the government did put in place more stringent rules.

The work of parliament continued uninterrupted during 2020. On March 16, 2020, the group leaders of Sweden's eight parliamentary parties entered into an agreement on reducing the number of parliamentarians who participated in the votes in parliament, the Riksdag, to 55, in order to "ensure that the Riksdag can fulfill its tasks even in the event of a large number of members of the Riksdag being prevented from participating in the work of the Riksdag." It is worth noting that this institutional change had the form of a voluntary agreement among the group leaders of the parliamentary parties; it was thus not a question of a formal change in the parliament's rules or in other laws. This is not unusual, however, for there are other important rules about parliamentary procedure in Sweden that have the form of agreements among the parties (notably the rules for adjusting the number of voting members when some members are absent). With the new informal rules in place, the parliament remained operational and was highly active throughout 2020, as is evident from our review of the legislative measures that were taken to reduce the spread of infection and the economic policy measures that were taken to mitigate the economic effects of the crisis.

In the beginning of the COVID-19 epidemic, political decision-making was fairly consensual, as we discussed earlier, but the level of conflict increased gradually in the spring of 2020 as it became clear that the death toll in Sweden was much higher than in neighboring countries. The parties on the right have criticized the center-left government for pursuing an overly cautious policy, and they have called for an expansion of more systematic testing and, in the case of the populist-far-right Sweden Democrats, school closings. In the televised party leader debate on 7 June 2020, the differences among the parties were already considerable. The Christian Democrat leader Ebba Busch said, for example, that the Social Democratic-led government had "deliberately allowed the infection to spread." The leader of the Sweden Democrats, Jimmie Åkesson, referred back to the consensual political style in Swedish politics earlier in the spring and declared that the opposition parties must now confront the government on its public health policies.[8]

3.4.4   Constitutional Considerations

On the basis of the arguments we made in the previous section, we conclude that the government could have adopted more stringent measures if it had wanted to do so. Since a temporary law authorizing the government to take more drastic measures was adopted in April 2020, it seems highly likely that the government would have been able to win the Riksdag's support for a different approach. Some observers, such as the economist Lars Jonung (2020), have argued, however, that Sweden's policies during the COVID-19 epidemic are best explained by provisions of the Swedish constitution—the 1974 Instrument of Government—that make it difficult for both the government and parliament to enact laws that suspend individual rights. Jonung refers, among other things, to the protection of civil liberties and rights in Chapter 2 of the Instrument of Government, the principle of municipal self-government, and the independence of Sweden's administrative agencies, which we have already discussed.

Our view is that this interpretation of the Swedish constitution goes too far. When it comes to the protection of civil liberties in Chapter 2 of the Instrument of Government, we begin by noting that the freedom of assembly, which is otherwise highly protected, may be restricted if the purpose is to "counteract an epidemic" (Chapter 2, Section 8). Jonung states that this exception only applies to the freedom of assembly and not, for example, the right to move freely within Sweden. However, the protection of the right of free movement is not absolute either. Like many other freedoms, the freedom of movement may be restricted (Chapter 2, Section 20) if the purpose is "acceptable in a democratic society" and as long as the restrictions do not go "beyond what is necessary with regard to the purpose that has caused them" (Chapter 2, Section 21). It is true that a qualified majority is required to adopt laws that restrict people's freedoms right away—and not with a twelve-month delay—but it seems likely that a big majority in parliament would have been supportive of new, restrictive laws, for in April, as we have noted, the parliament did support a far-reaching, albeit temporary, law authorizing the government to take measures designed to limit the spread of COVID-19. When it comes to municipal self-government, the Instrument of Government allows the parliament to adopt laws that assign new tasks to municipalities, or regulate their services, as long as the restrictions of self-government do not go "beyond what is necessary" (Chapter 14, Section 3).

3.4.5   *The Operational Capacity of Public Authorities and Local Governments*

The political capacity of the government and parliament, which we have discussed in the two previous sections, is one thing. Another related factor that was much discussed in Sweden in 2020 is the operational capacity of the public health authorities and, especially, of regional and local governments. Regional and local governments have played a very important part in the implementation of the national response to COVID-19 since Sweden's regions are responsible for the healthcare system and since the local governments, the municipalities, are responsible for the elder-care sector, which was hit hard by COVID-19. The need to coordinate the response to a pandemic was anticipated in the 2019 report on pandemic preparedness that we cited earlier: it emphasizes that a pandemic requires "collaboration among all actors at all levels" (p. 9). One such structure is the National Pandemic Group, the main task of which is "to promote the coordination of measures planned and implemented to deal with a pandemic"; it includes representatives of the Public Health Agency, the Swedish Civil Contingencies Agency, the Medical Products Agency, the National Board of Health and Welfare, and an organization that represents Sweden's municipalities and regions.

The COVID-19 outbreak was a major challenge for healthcare in Sweden, as in many other countries. The efforts to limit the negative consequences of the pandemic for Swedish healthcare have been focused on reducing the spread of infection, so that the available healthcare capacity is not exceeded, and on increasing capacity in certain areas.[9] The government, the regions, the municipalities, and other authorities have worked to increase the test capacity, the number of hospital- and intensive care units available for COVID-19 patients, and the availability of protective equipment. The Public Health Agency of Sweden and the National Board of Health and Welfare have been responsible for monitoring and coordinating various parts of Sweden's health care system, while the 21 regions and the 290 municipalities have been responsible for implementing new policies within the health care and social care systems during the pandemic.

In mid-March, the Director-General of the World Health Organization, Dr. Tedros Adhanom Ghebreyesus, called on the countries of the world to "test, test, test." Sweden has been able to perform so-called Polymerase Chain Reaction tests (PCR) since January 17, and all university hospitals had the capacity to perform PCR tests from February 28, 2020 (Ludvigsson 2020:11). PCR testing is an established method for identifying an ongoing COVID-19 infection. PCR tests detect the presence of genetic materials from the virus that causes the infection. But the number of PCR tests performed in Sweden was relatively small, due to lack of access to test equipment and because of ambiguities about who was responsible for performing and financing the tests (Ludvigsson 2020:12). In February 2020, fewer than 1,000 individuals were tested. By mid-March, the number had risen to about 10,000 per week. On March 30, the Public Health Agency of Sweden was commissioned by the government to urgently increase the number of tests.[10]

The test capacity has since expanded gradually. The Public Health Agency took measures to increase the analytical capacity of the country's laboratories, with the goal of having a capacity for approximately 150,000 tests per week, a goal that was reached in mid-July. In mid-April, the government and the Public Health Agency announced that 50,000–100,000 tests a week would be carried out. The goal of 50,000 tests during one week was reached in June (week 24). During the autumn of 2020, the capacity continued to increase, and toward the end of the year, almost 300,000 tests were done each week. Figure 3.4 shows the number of individuals who have taken PCR tests in Sweden per week (data from the Public Health Agency). The number of individuals who took PCR tests has varied between 11 (week 4) and just under 300,000 (week 51).

The Public Health Agency has argued that the goals of PCR testing are different during the different phases of a pandemic (The Public Health Agency of Sweden 2020). In the first phase, which Sweden was in until mid-March, the focus was on testing everyone with symptoms and then conducting a thorough infection tracing. After the first phase, priorities were made. The Public Health Agency of Sweden suggested that the most prioritized group are people who have an ongoing illness; the second group is health care staff; the third group is staff in other socially important activities; and the fourth group is everyone else. The Public Health Agency argued further that when the phase of acute community transmission was over, everyone who needed a test could be tested. It should, however, be noted that the Corona Commission has documented that the low number of tests during the spring of 2020 was not a result of strategic planning but of low capacity (SOU 2021:89).

Like many other countries, Sweden experienced a shortage of protective equipment in the early spring of 2020, and during both waves of the epidemic, the capacity of intensive care in Swedish hospitals was put to the test. On March 16, the government commissioned the National Board of Health and Welfare to ensure access to protective equipment and other protective materials, and on March 19, the National Board of Health and Welfare was commissioned to set up a coordination function for intensive care units. According to the Corona Commission, the procurement of protective equipment was, however, not efficiently coordinated by the National Board of Health and Welfare, since their assignment was not clear enough and they lacked the organization and experience of procurement on the world market (SOU 2021:89). Moving on to the coordination of incentive care units, Figure 3.3 shows the number of new intensive care patients per day in Sweden over the year (data from the Public Health Agency, January 26, 2021). There was a sharp increase in the number of patients in intensive care during March and April, and then again from mid-October to the end of the year. Based on information from the National Board of Health and Welfare, between 65 and 70% of the full capacity of Sweden's intensive care units was utilized during the spring. As a national average, capacity utilization never exceeded 75% during the first six months of the year. However, some individual regions were under more pressure (The National Board of Health and Welfare 2020).

The National Board of Health and Welfare cooperates with the Swedish Civil Contingencies Agency and the County Administrative Boards to monitor hospital and intensive care capacity in the regions, as well as the need for medical and protective equipment in the regions and municipalities. The National Board of Health and Welfare has a five-point measure of stress on these systems that ranges from no impact to critical impact.[11] Severe or critical impacts have been reported from a large number of regions for consumables; in other areas, only a few regions have been seriously or critically impacted. Some of Sweden's 290 municipalities also reported that they experienced a serious or critical impact regarding consumables, personnel, home care services, management functions, or the supply of medicines. The strain on the Swedish health care and elderly-care systems was thus great in some parts of the country. The situation was particularly serious in April. The National Board of Health and Welfare wrote in its status report to the Swedish Civil Contingencies Agency on April 16 that the impact within the remit of the National Board of Health and Welfare varied from moderate to critical and that it was expected to increase in the coming weeks. The National Board of Health and Welfare stated that "consequences in two weeks' time include the risk of serious or critical impact in several regions regarding IVA [intensive care] units, protective equipment and medical equipment." The National Board of Health and Welfare also emphasized that there was a risk of "increased impact on municipal health and medical care and social services."

3.4.6   *The Case of Elder Care*

The Swedish elder-care system can be divided into two different types of care: home care and special housing (including residential nursing homes). In Sweden, elder care is the responsibility of the 290 municipalities (which in passing means that it falls under the social services and thus does not primarily belong to health care), but in both home care and special housing there are both public and private providers (Szebehely 2011). In January 2020, 191,910 people over the age of 70 had home care and 79,410 people over the age of 70 lived in special housing. These groups have been very vulnerable. By April 28, 90% of those who had died with COVID-19 were over 70 years old. Half of those individuals lived in special housing while just over a quarter had home care (The National Board of Health and Welfare 2020).

The vulnerable situation of older Swedes has been common knowledge, and measures have been taken to protect those groups, but many observers within Sweden have claimed that not enough was done in this regard. One measure that has already been mentioned was the government's decision on March 30 on a national ban on visits to nursing homes. Other issues that seem to have been important were staff turnover at the nursing homes, protective measures for the staff, and the medical care that was available to residents of the nursing homes. The media has reported major problems when it comes to recruiting personnel and securing protective equipment for both home care and nursing homes (Dagens Nyheter 2020a, 2020b). There have also been media reports claiming that qualified care for fragile elder individuals was not prioritized in certain regions (Dagens Nyheter 2020c, Kurrien 2020). However, these reports have been disputed by the responsible officials (Dagens Nyheter 2020d).

In mid-April, the Government commissioned the Swedish Health and Social Care Inspectorate to investigate how the work against COVID-19 in elder care was conducted in the municipalities. The Swedish Health and

Social Care Inspectorate's reports from late autumn 2020 revealed that there were examples in all regions of infected individuals in nursing homes who did not get individual medical assessments and who were not prioritized for hospital care.

A large evaluation has already been conducted of the measures that were taken to protect individuals within the elder care system from the infection. It is part of a government commission of inquiry into how Sweden handled the COVID-19 epidemic. The Corona Commission published its first report in December 2020, and made several very critical observations concerning the Swedish elder care system in general and the protective measures that were taken by the authorities in particular. The overall conclusion was that the Swedish strategy for protecting old and fragile individuals within the elder care system had failed. The report identified structural weaknesses in Swedish elder care as one of the main explanations of the failure to protect older Swedes. These weaknesses included the organization of the care (too many actors and not enough coordination), the fact that there was too much staff turnover, and shortcomings with respect to the training, the medical skills, and the working environment of the staff within the elder care system. Moreover, when evaluating the specific responses within the elder care during the pandemic, the Commission's conclusion (SOU 2020:80) was that they were often late and insufficient. An international comparison showed that the Swedish response was slower than in the neighboring Nordic countries. According to this report, these delays may have contributed to the high Swedish death toll in Swedish nursing homes (Szebehely 2020).

3.5   Conclusions

The Swedish approach to COVID-19 differed from that of most other comparable democracies in Western Europe, especially in the first phase of the COVID-19 pandemic in the spring of 2020. Rather than putting in place coercive policies that would have restricted the freedom of movement or the freedom of assembly, closing schools, or requiring mask-wearing, the Swedish government and Swedish public authorities chose to issue voluntary recommendations that were meant to limit the spread of the virus by persuading citizens to reduce their social interactions and to protect themselves and others from the new disease.

The Corona Commission—the big government commission of inquiry that was tasked with investigating Sweden's policies during the pandemic (SOU 2022:10 Volume 2)—concluded in its main report in early 2022 that on the whole, this voluntarist approach was sound. But the Corona Commission also criticized the government and the Public Health Agency of Sweden for not taking earlier and more decisive action to prevent the spread of the

SARS-CoV-2 virus in the beginning of the pandemic in the spring of 2020. Judging from the response to the Corona Commission's report, this was a fairly widely accepted view in the aftermath of the pandemic: many observers seemed to agree that the voluntarist approach was well-considered but that more could likely have been done in the first phase of the COVID-19 pandemic to quarantine travelers from Austria and Italy that brought the virus to Sweden in February, protect elder Swedes in nursing homes, and provide adequate testing services. There is less agreement on how best to prepare Sweden for the next pandemic. The Corona Commission recommended far-reaching changes in the crisis-management organization within Sweden's central government offices and in the relationship between the central government offices and the executive agencies, but those ideas have not yet resulted in any concrete proposals regarding administrative reforms.

The main goal of this chapter has been to discuss some of the potential explanations for Sweden's distinctive policy choices in the COVID-19 pandemic that have been suggested in the scholarly literature and in political commentary in Sweden and abroad. We have found little support for some of the explanations that have been suggested, especially the idea that the Swedish government and the Swedish public-health authorities were prevented from responding more aggressively to the COVID-19 crisis because they were bound by prior legislation or by the Swedish constitution. Our view is that the government and the parliament could have put new policies in place if they had wanted to: Sweden's approach was a political choice, not a legal or constitutional necessity. But there are other political explanations that we have not been able to dismiss. We would especially like to mention two interrelated factors that we believe played an important role. The first is that Swedish contingency planning for new global infectious disease such as COVID-19 placed little emphasis on lockdowns, school closures, or other coercive "non-medical" measures since the responsible authorities believed that the social costs were likely to exceed the health benefits of such an approach. The second factor is that Swedish governments typically defer to the expertise of public administrative agencies, as long as those agencies act within their remit, as defined by legislation and the government's general instructions to the bureaucracy.

Notes

1 Note that the information in Figure 3.4 refers to people who were ill with COVID-19 when they died, which does not necessarily mean they died *of* COVID-19.

2 Throughout the pandemic, the official goals of the Swedish epidemic-control policy were to (1) limit the spread of infection in the country; (2) secure resources for health care; (3) limit the impact on socially important activities; (4) mitigate the consequences for citizens and businesses; (5) mitigate people's

concerns, among other things through information, and (6) take the right actions at the right time. See https://www.regeringen.se/regeringens-politik/regeringens-arbete-med-anledning-av-nya-coronaviruset/.

3 The Public Health Agency of Sweden differs between *general advice* and *recommendations*. A general advice is a specification of what the public and various organizations can do to comply with laws, executive orders and regulations. A general advice is not binding in itself but is linked to a binding rule. A recommendation is based on existing knowledge without being linked to binding regulations. For a discussion about this distinction from constitutional and administrative law perspectives, see Wenander (2020).

4 The official goals of the Swedish epidemic control policy have the entire period, according to the government, been to (1) limit the spread of infection in the country; (2) securing resources for health care; (3) limit the impact on socially important activities; (4) mitigate the consequences for citizens and businesses; (5) mitigate people`s concerns, among other things through information, and (6) take the right action at the right time. See https://www.regeringen.se/regeringens-politik/regeringens-arbete-med-anledning-av-nya-coronaviruset/.

5 The ordinance (2020:20) says that the provisions of the Communicable Diseases Act (2004: 168) on generally dangerous and socially dangerous diseases shall be applied to 2019-nCoV infections.

6 "Folkhälsomyndighetens föreskrifter och allmänna råd om allas ansvar att förhindra smitta av Covid-19 m.m."

7 *Pandemiberedskap. Hur vi förbereder oss – ett kunskapsunderlag*. Stockholm: Folkhälsomyndigheten 2019 (19074-1).

8 When it comes to economic policy, as opposed to public-health policies, the political parties have had different views concerning some of the measures taken during the crisis, especially with regard to the timing. For obvious reasons, the government, led by the Social Democrats, has been particularly keen to protect wage earners, for example through changes in unemployment insurance, while the center-right opposition has been more keen to protect business. On the whole, however, economic policymaking during the COVID-19 crisis were consensual. Particularly in the beginning of the epidemic, it was clear that Sweden was moving from a phase of political polarization (which was noticeable during the protracted government formation process of 2018–2019) to a phase where the willingness to compromise was higher. On the 2018–2019 government formation process and the political situation in Sweden after the 2018 election, see Teorell et al. (2020).

9 "Securing resources for health care" is one of the government's goals with their COVID-19 response.

10 "Uppdrag om att skyndsamt utöka antalet tester för covid-19," S2020/02681/FS. On May 8, the government also announced that they had commissioned Harriet Wallberg as test coordinator. She was placed at the Public Health Agency of Sweden. (https://www.regeringen.se/pressmeddelanden/2020/05/harriet-wallberg-ny-testkoordinator-for-coronatester/).

   However, Harriet Wallberg announced that she wanted to end the assignment already after about three weeks (Dagens Nyheter, June 2). In the media it was stated that the reason was that she had not a large enough mandate (Dagens Nyheter, June 3).

11 The five scale steps are: "None," "Moderate," "Significant," "Serious," and "Critical" impact. Information from the National Board of Health and Welfare, e-mail 2020-10-22.

References

Ahlbäck Öberg, Shirin, and Helena Wockelberg. 2016. "The public sector and the courts." In Pierre, Jon (ed.), *The Oxford Handbook of Swedish Politics*. Oxford: Oxford University Press, 130–146.

Andersson, Staffan, and Nicholas Aylott. 2020. "Sweden and Coronavirus: Unexceptional exceptionalism." *Social Sciences* 9(12), 232–249.

Carlsson, Marcus et al. 2020. "Folkhälsomyndigheten har misslyckats – nu måste politikerna gripa in." *Dagens Nyheter*.

Dagens Nyheter. 2020a. *Dagens Nyheter*.

Dagens Nyheter. 2020b. *Dagens Nyheter*.

Dagens Nyheter. 2020c. *Dagens Nyheter*.

Dagens Nyheter. 2020d. *Dagens Nyheter*.

Dahlström, Carl, and Mikael Holmgren. 2019. "The political dynamics of bureaucratic turnover." *British Journal of Political Science* 49(3): 823–836.

Dahlström, Carl, and Johannes Lindvall. 2021. "Sverige og covid-19-krisen." In *Håndteringen af Covid-19 i foråret 2020. Rapport afgivet af den af Folketingets Udvalg for Forretningsordenen nedsatte udredningsgruppe vedr. Håndteringen af Covid-19*. Folketinget, January 2021.

Esaiasson, Peter, Jacob Sohlberg, Marina Ghersetti, and Bengt Johansson. 2020. "How the coronavirus crisis affects citizen trust in institutions and in unknown others: Evidence from 'the Swedish experiment'". *European Journal of Political Research*,60(3), 748–760.

Finanspolitiska rådet. 2020. *Svensk finanspolitik 2020*. Stockholm: Finanspolitiska rådet.

The Government Offices. 2019. *Regeringskansliets årsbok 2019*. Stockholm: Regeringskansliet.

Jacobsson, Bengt. 1984. *Hur styrs förvaltningen? Myt och verklighet kring departementens styrning av ämbetsverken*. Lund: Studentlitteratur.

Jacobsson, Bengt, and Göran Sundström. 2016. "Governing the state." In Pierre, Jon (ed.), *The Oxford Handbook of Swedish Politics*. Oxford: Oxford University Press, 347–361.

Jonsson Cornell, Anna. 2020. "Författningsberedskap i praktiken – en kommentar med anledning av lagen om ändring i smittskyddslagen." *Svensk juristtidning 5–6*.

Jonung, Lars. 2020. "Sweden's constitution decides its COVID-19 exceptionalism." Working Paper 2020:11, Department of Economics, Lund University.

Kantar Sifo. 2020a. Rapport om förtroende, oro och beteende under coronakrisen, 21 mars–24 augusti, Rapport till MSB, 2020-08-24.

Kantar Sifo. 2020b. Rapport om förtroende, oro och beteende under coronakrisen, 21 mars–28 september, Rapport till MSB, 2020-09-28.

Kantar Sifo. 2021. Rapport om förtroende, oro och beteende under coronakrisen. December, Rapport till MSB, 2021-01-10.

Ludvigsson, Jonas. 2020. "The first eight months of Sweden's COVID-19 strategy and the key actions and actors that were involved." *Acta Paediatrica*. Published online on September 20, 2020 Forthcoming.

Niemann, Cajsa. 2013. *Villkorat förtroende: Normer och rollförväntningar i relationen mellan politiker och tjänstemän i Regeringskansliet*. Stockholm: Stockholm University, Department of Political Science.

Petersson, Olof. 2020. "Sverige valde coronastrategi med 2004 års smittskydd-slag." *Dagens Nyheter*, 9 June.

Pierre, Jon. 2004. "Central agencies in Sweden: A report from Utopia." In Pollitt, Christopher and Colin Talbot (eds.), *Unbundled Government*. London: Taylor and Francis, 203–214.

Pierre, Jon. 2020. "Nudges against pandemics: Sweden's COVID-19 containment strategy in perspective." *Policy and Society* 39(3): 478–493.

SOU 2007:75. *Att styra staten – regeringens styrning av sin förvaltning*. Stockholm: Fritzes.

SOU 2020:80. Äldreomsorgen under pandemin. Stockholm: Norstedts Juridik.

SOU 2021:89. *Sverige under pandemin. Volym 1. Smittspridning och smittskydd.* Stockholm: Elanders Sverige AB.

SOU 2022:10. *Sverige under pandemin. Volym 1. Samhällets, företagens och enskildas ekonomi.* Stockholm: Elanders Sverige AB.

SOU 2022:10. *Sverige under pandemin. Volym 2. Förutsättningar, vägval och utvärdering.* Stockholm: Elanders Sverige AB.

The Swedish Agency for Public Management. 2020. Statsförvaltningen i korthet. Stockholm: Statskontoret.

Szebehely, Marta. 2011. "Insatser för äldre och funktionshindrade i privat regi. In Hartman, Laura (ed.), *Konkurrensens konsekvenser. Vad händer med svensk välfärd?* Stockholm: SNS, 215–257.

Szebehely, Marta. 2020. Internationella erfarenheter av covid-19 i äldreboenden. *Report to the Corona Commission* (SOU 2020:80).

Teorell, Jan, Hanna Bäck, Johan Hellström, and Johannes Lindvall. 2020. *134 dagar*. Gothenburg: Makadam Förlag.

Wenander, Henrik. 2020. "Sweden: Non-binding rules against the pandemic – formalism, pragmatism and legal realism." Unpublished manuscript, Lund University.

4 Finland's Responses to COVID-19

Uneven, Fairly Effective, and Craving to Return to Normal

Pertti Ahonen

4.1 Theoretical Background and Research Material

The responses to the COVID-19 pandemic have been approached from the perspectives of numerous academic disciplines. Medical epidemiologists have foregrounded what their specialty stresses and the recommendations that their research results indicate; constitutional law experts, joined by political scientists, have warned us about threats to people's freedoms and liberties; international relations scholars have pinpointed excesses in declaring the pandemic a threat an analogy to a military attack by a hostile power; economists have pinpointed the economic and fiscal consequences of the pandemic and measures to soften these consequences; sociologists and education scholars have focused on the threats of the pandemic to equity and inclusion; and public management scholars have suggested increases to the powers of public authorities to take more rapid, more comprehensive, and more efficient action.

Given the multiplicity of perspectives, any consideration of the responses to the COVID-19 pandemic is by necessity a compromise. However, this chapter does have a theoretical background in critical considerations by political scientists, constitutional law scholars, and international relations scholars concerned with the adverse effects of pandemic governance on civil liberties and freedoms, the recommendable extent of normal adversary politics, and possibilities to keep the public authorities in check (e.g., De Leo 2020; Merkel 2020; Moisio 2020; Nunes 2020; Petrov 2020; VDem 2020; Greer et al. 2021; Karyotis et al. 2021; Kirk and McDonald 2021; Scheinin 2021; Elander et al. 2021; Erickson et al. 2022; Larsson 2022). The research question can be formulated as follows: How to assess the Finnish responses to the COVID-19 pandemic with special reference to nurturing civil freedoms and liberties, the normal functioning of sufficiently adversary democratic politics, and avoiding the aggrandizement of the public authorities?

DOI: 10.4324/9781003362760-4

In a country with a steady rule of law and deep-ingrained political democracy, large amounts of research material become available once a threat like the COVID-19 pandemic has struck. The bulk of the primary research material is comprised of texts of Finnish official legislation and preparatory and evaluative government reports. Secondary material has also been available, including published results of academic research on the pandemic. A third source comprises interviews carried out for this chapter or, although primarily feeding into other studies, utilized in this study. The interview results could only be used to orient this chapter. This limitation was cemented by the promise made to all interviewees that their names would not be connected to the opinions or assessments presented in this chapter.

4.2   Empirical Background

Unlike some other OECD countries, in Finland the political government of the country rather than the central or any other branch of public administration has led the fight against the COVID-19 pandemic. Since December 2019 until October 2022, and until the March 2023 parliamentary elections, Finland had a left-and-center majority government coalition of five parties and a right-and-center opposition of four parties. Parliament, the government and its ministers, the ministries and certain agencies under the ministries played key roles during the pandemic. The Finnish Institute for Health and Welfare (THL) under the Ministry of Social Affairs and Health comprised the foremost expert agency on pandemics, though it had no power to order restrictions (Communicable Diseases Act 1227/2016, Art. 7). In decision-making concerning the combat against the pandemic, a division of labor prevailed (Table 4.1).

In Finland the constitutionally self-governing municipalities were responsible for health care during the COVID-19 pandemic from 2020 until the end of 2022 (THL 2019; Kuntaliitto 2020). To provide for hospital care, each municipality had to belong to one of the statutory federations of municipalities, each managing a hospital district with either one of the university hospitals (in 2022, five in number) or one of the central hospitals (in 2022, 16 in number). Three alternative ways were used to provide primary health care (THL 2019): 74 municipalities had a health center and clinics of their own; 160 municipalities were members of the 33 municipal health care center federations; and 61 municipalities were members of the schemes around 26 municipalities that bore the foremost responsibility for a health center and its clinics, whereas the other 35 municipalities cooperated with the 26 municipalities. It is only at the beginning of 2023 that a long-planned major reform will take effect. Then

Table 4.1 Decision-making in Finland in combat against COVID-19

	Government (Prime Minister and Ministers)	A government ministry or two or more ministries together	Finnish institute for health and Welfare (THL)	A municipality or a health care association of municipalities	A doctor in public health care responsible for contagious diseases	Regional state administrative agency	Others (e.g., other government agencies, employers, or private associations)
Binding decisions							
Restrictions on crossing borders	X						
Restrictions on restaurants, etc.	X						
Closing public spaces		X		X			X
Exceptional educational arrangements		X		X			X
Closing schools, etc.				X		X	
Prohibiting or restricting gatherings				X		X	
Closing private businesses				X		X	
Quarantine					X		
Restricting number of passengers in transportation							X
Recommendations							
Distance work		X		X			
Wearing masks			X	X			
Visits to wards			X	X			
Restricting private gatherings						X	

Source: Finnish Government (2021).

the Finnish municipalities and their hospital and health center federations will lose their functions once the new self-governing health care regions start their operations (Eduskunta 2022), and bear the charge of health care related to the later stages of the COVID-19 pandemic.

4.3   Observable Outcomes in Finland's Combat Against COVID-19

For a Nordic country, let alone in comparison with many other countries, Finland had a reasonably low COVID-19 mortality (Table 4.2) between 2020 and July 2022 (for a focused study on COVID-19 responses in the Nordic countries, see Christensen et al. 2023). A comparison of the first 12-month COVID-19 period in Finland with later developments in this country suggests two different pandemic dynamics with morbidity increasing several times over but also with mortality collapsing in relation to morbidity (Table 4.2). Besides the change of the prevailing virus variant, intervening variables comprise the expanding vaccination coverage and, especially later on, the degrees of immunity achieved by people who had had COVID-19 (THL 2022a). Generally, the characteristics of Finland's

Table 4.2 COVID-19 in Nordic comparison and in Finland

	By 23 October 2020	*By 23 February 2021*	*By 31 July 2022*	*(By 15 December 2023)*
	Deaths caused by COVID-19, per million of population Sweden, Denmark, Finland, and Norway			
Sweden	559	1,223	1,831	2,418
Denmark	118	398	1,116	1,502
Finland	62	143	990	1,961
Norway	51	112	675	1,055
	Cumulative relative COVID-19 morbidity and mortality/morbidity ratio; Finland			
Cumulative morbidity (COVID-19 cases), per million of population, %	0.30%	1.12%	21.67%	26.79%
Mortality/morbidity (cases/deaths) ratio, %	2.06%	1.27%	0.45%	0.72%

Sources: Confirmed Coronavirus Cases in Finland 2020–2021, screenshot 23 July 2021; THL 2022b, screenshot 23 July 2022; Our World in Data 2023; amended; if data from the day indicated has been unavailable, data from the earliest previous available date has been used.

response to COVID-19 correspond to the global empirical predictors of good outcomes (Greer et al. 2021).

The summary of developments with COVID-19 in Finland from early 2020 until 30 September 2022 confirms the above conclusions (Table 4.3). COVID-19 indeed has appeared as if two different diseases, first with a high mortality to morbidity ratio followed by a ratio that scarcely diverges from common influenza epidemics. The spread of vaccinations since late 2020 has also exerted a definitive influence. The burden of COVID-19 upon Finland's health care has generally been bearable contrary to the negative expectations early on during the pandemic.

4.4   Government Policies

4.4.1   Extreme Measures: Two States of Exception

According to Finland's Preparedness Act of 2011, the President of the Republic and the government may jointly conclude that a contingency such as a pandemic requires government state-of-exception decrees (Preparedness Act 1552/2011). These decrees must be sent to Parliament, which will decide whether the decrees will come into force for the period intended, a shorter period, or not at all, and in full or only in part. During the pandemic, Finland had two states of exception, one in spring 2020 and the other in spring 2021.

The Finnish government first passed extraordinary decrees between 17 March and 15 June 2020 (Eduskunta 2020), and a state of exception prevailed like in many other countries (De Leo 2020; Merkel 2020; Petrov 2020). From 17 March to 13 April 2020, state-of-exception arrangements in health care were activated; from 18 March to 13 May 2020, all schools were closed; between 27 March and 16 April 2020 there was a lockdown in Helsinki and in the surrounding region, and from 4 April to 31 May 2020 all restaurants were closed (Eduskunta 2020). The lockdown was "policized," with police patrols preventing traveling between the lockdown areas and other parts of the country, except for force majeure reasons such as work or health. The lockdown was also "militarized": conscripts and commanding officers helped the police to maintain the lockdown in its external borders.

On 1 March 2021, the President and the government again jointly drew the conclusion that a state of exception was necessary (Eduskunta 2020). On 5 March 2021, the government passed four extraordinary decrees, sent these to Parliament for critical consideration, and received Parliament's consent (Valtioneuvosto 2021a). The decrees were to empower the Ministry of Social Affairs and Health and the Regional State Administrative

Table 4.3 Summary of COVID-19 in Finland from January 2020 to 30 September 2022

Incidents	Explanation
First signs of COVID-19	
Wuhan, China	In the Finnish news on 25 January 2020 (Satakunnan Kansa 2020).
First case in Finland	28 January 2020 (Helsingin Sanomat 2020a)
Government preparedness	The first time in a government meeting agenda on 26 February 2020 (Helsingin Sanomat 2020b).
1 March to 15 June 2020	
Expansion	From early March to early April 2020.
Confirmation	First, limited testing capacity.
Peak of deaths	From 4 to 20 April 2020; absolute peak 19 deaths, 20 April 2020.
Testing	5,000/day maximum.
Concentration	Helsinki and the surrounding region, and minor concentrations elsewhere.
Summary	7,300 infections, 800 in general hospital care, 220 in intensive care, 330 deaths.
16 June to 31 August 2020	
Expansion	None.
Confirmation	Increasing testing capacity.
Testing	Maximally 5,600/day in July, maximally 17,000/day in August.
Summary	1,200 infections, few hospitalizations in general or intensive care, 20 deaths.
1 September to 31 December 2020	
Expansion	At the turn of September and October 306 cases/day maximum; since late November until mid-December, 600 cases/day maximum.
Confirmation	Up to 26,000 tests/day; in addition to antigen testing.
Peak of deaths	14 December 2020, 11 deaths.
Testing	From late November to late December 2020, a few days with over 23,000 tests.
Abatement	A plateau from mid-October to mid-November, maximally 289 infections/day.
Concentration	Somewhat more evenly distributed over the country than the first wave.

(Continued)

Table 4.3 (Continued)

Incidents	Explanation
Summary	29,304 infections, 800 in general hospital care, 100 in intensive care, 219 deaths.
Vaccinations	Started 27 December 2020.
From 1 January 2021 to 15 March 2021	
Summary	30,730 infections, 252 deaths, 1,091,134 tests. On 15 March 2021, 217 people in general hospital care, 47 in intensive care.
Vaccinations	680,818 vaccinations; 594,804 first vaccinations; 86,014 second vaccinations.
From 16 March 2021 to 30 September 2022	
Summary	1,225,606 infections, 5,180 deaths, 7,380,860 tests. On 15 March 2021, 217 people in general hospital care, 47 in intensive care.
Vaccinations	12,147,856 vaccinations; 3,841,145 first vaccinations; 4,257,034 second vaccinations, 919,159 fourth vaccinations.

Source: Confirmed Coronavirus Cases in Finland (2020–2021); Situation Update on Coronavirus (2020–2021); THL (2022c).

Agencies to issue orders to actors of public and private sector health care; to enable municipalities to postpone non-urgent health care; to concentrate communication on COVID-19 to the Communication Department of the Prime Minister's Office; and to empower the government chaired by the Prime Minister to resolve disagreements related to COVID-19 between public authorities. The decrees were to be valid from 11 March until 30 April 2021.

Constitutional law experts criticized the 2020 state of exception for excessively restricting constitutional rights and liberties (Helsingin Sanomat 2020c; Moisio 2020), not unlike other countries (Leo 2020; Merkel 2020; Petrov 2020). Later, constitutional experts asked if Art. 23 of the Finnish Constitution (Constitution 731/1999) on basic rights and liberties in situations of emergency could be activated to pass temporary legal norms for the expected duration of a pandemic rather than activating the Preparedness Act (Scheinin 2021). Indeed, the suggestion is included in one of the policies.

During the first state of exception the political opposition stayed calm, suggesting that the pandemic was heavily "securitized" (Nunes 2020; Kirk and McDonald 2021; Larsson 2022), that is, it was understood to represent such an extreme threat that normal adversary and deliberative politics were temporarily set aside. The March 2021 state of exception received the support of all government and opposition parties with the exception of the Finns party on the extreme political right (on this aspect of extreme-right populist parties, see Steuer 2022). In addition, during the pandemic, the Finnish government proposed and Parliament accepted numerous temporary and permanent amendments to the Communicable Diseases Act and other acts to enable stronger measures (Communicable Diseases Act 1227/2016; THL 2020–2022a, b).

4.4.2   *The Finnish Government Hybrid Strategy, Restrictions, Recommendations, and Contact Tracing*

Since the Finnish government's decision-in-principle of 6 May 2020, a hybrid strategy of test-trace-isolate-care became the main policy tool to combat the COVID-19 pandemic (Valtioneuvosto 2020–2022). The government monitored the strategy in three ways (THL 2020–2022b): publishing weekly or bi-weekly a monitoring report on the strategy proper, a report on epidemiological monitoring, and a summary of restrictions and recommendations. The implementation of the hybrid strategy was connected with the phase of the pandemic in different parts of the country (THL 2020–2022a). At the baseline phase, morbidity was low and the proportion of endemic infections was small. The acceleration phase had a regional incidence of 10–15 weekly cases/100,000 people and no more than 25 bi-weekly cases/100,000. Over 1% of tests were positive, and occasional local and regional chains of infection evolved. Sources of infection could usually be traced, and hospital capacity generally sufficed. In the community transmission phase, infections spread regionally or more widely with a weekly incidence exceeding 15 cases/100,000 and a bi-weekly incidence exceeding 25–50 cases/100,000. The daily case growth rate exceeded 10%, more than 2% of tests were positive, and less than half of the infection sources could be traced. The need for hospital care including intensive care grew quickly.

On 26 January 2021, the Finnish government amended its action plan for implementing its COVID-19 hybrid strategy (Valtioneuvosto 2021b). Added to the notion of "phase," indicating the seriousness of the pandemic, was the notion of "tier," signifying the character of the anti-pandemic measures (Table 4.4).

As recommended by constitutional law experts with reference to Art. 23 of the Finnish Constitution, the government proposed to Parliament a temporary 8 to 28 March 2021 amendment to the Communicable Diseases Act (1227/2016). The amendment, which Parliament accepted, enabled the full closure of restaurants and comparable services in regions other than those with low COVID-19 incidence (Eduskunta 2021).

Table 4.4 Phases and tiers related to the COVID-19 pandemic in Finland

		Phases of the pandemic *COVID-19 situation in Finland's regions as monitored by indicators*		
Tiers of prevention measures *with transition to a higher tier if anticipated that the measures so far will not suffice*		Baseline phase	Acceleration phase	Community transmission phase
Tier 1	Epidemic continues, measures fully implemented in areas in the community transmission phase	Restrictions in place according to guidelines	Restrictions in place according to guidelines	Restrictions in place according to guidelines
Tier 2	Threat of the epidemic spreading throughout the country	Measure for the community transmission phase in place throughout the country of specific parts of it		
Tier 3	Epidemic poses a direct threat to the carrying capacity of the health care system or to the health of the population	Emergency conditions; necessary restrictions on movement in addition to the above restrictions		

Source: Adapted from the official source Valtioneuvosto (2021b); note the official term "epidemic" instead of "pandemic."

After the start of the pandemic, foreign traveling to Finland was restricted until the lifting of all travel limitations in spring 2022. As in the spring 2020 state of exception, on 12 October 2020 a temporary end was made to crossing borders without border controls between Finland and the other Schengen treaty countries. To avoid violating the EU Schengen Treaty, on 23 November 2020 health security measures were substituted for border controls (Valtioneuvosto 2020a), although the European Commission later declared that these measures did not resolve the issue.

Besides restrictions, Finnish authorities made numerous recommendations during the pandemic (see, e.g., Valtioneuvosto 2020b, c; Finnish Government 2021). Examples can be given of both the restrictions and the recommendations (Table 4.5). Since 1 March 2022, all restrictions mentioned in the table were lifted.

With the abatement of the pandemic, a major amendment to the hybrid strategy was made in February 2022 (Finnish Government 2022).

Table 4.5 Examples of restrictions, recommendations and health care measures in Finland, mid-March 2021

	Restrictions	Recommendations	Health care measures
Baseline (five hospital districts)	• No more than 20 or 50 people in public gatherings, museums, and youth and indoor sports • Government country-wide restrictions concerning restaurants (limited opening hours, partial use of seating capacity)	• Use masks if any infections during the last two weeks • Keep distances and observe coughing, sneezing and hand hygiene • Use the COVID-19 tracing application • Public sector employees should work from home • Avoid gatherings of more than 10–20 people	• Information campaigns • Preparedness maintenance by means of health care procurement • Creation and maintenance of testing capacity
Acceleration phase (eight hospital districts)	• Limited use of public libraries • 20 people maximum in public gatherings, museums, and youth and indoor sports • Government country-wide restrictions concerning restaurants	• Baseline recommendations apply except where made stricter • All employees do distance work if possible • No private gatherings with more than ten participants • Municipal decisions on distance learning in all education except kindergartens and elementary and junior secondary education • No sports activities for over 20-year-olds • Due care in sports activities for less than 21-year-olds • No traveling to areas in the community transmission phase • No traveling to countries with entry restrictions from Finland	• Increasing testing capacity • Information campaigns • Undelayed testing • Focusing upon incidents of high exposure risk • Readiness to introduce quarantine in cases of mass exposure

(Continued)

Table 4.5 (Continued)

	Restrictions	Recommendations	Health care measures
Community transmission phase (eight hospital districts)	• No inside or outside public gatherings or, alternatively, no such gatherings with over ten participants • Municipal closings of other than the most essential services; yet, possibly, limited use of public libraries • Municipal decisions on distance learning except in kindergartens and elementary and, possibly, junior secondary education • Possibly, prohibitions to visit other than psychiatric, palliative and maternity wards • Government country-wide restrictions concerning restaurants	• In some districts, no private gatherings with over six to ten participants; in other districts, no such gatherings • Due care with high-risk groups • Private providers recommended to close their sports and recreational services	• Preparedness to use available stocks of health care material • Preparedness for substantial increases in health care capacity

Source: See the main text

The amended strategy aimed toward stabilizing society and keeping it as open as possible; supporting post-pandemic crisis management and reconstruction; and adjusting to the global COVID-19 pandemic situation. However, the strategy also acknowledged the possibility of new variants of the virus again causing a serious disease that vaccinations could not substantially alleviate.

The Finnish Institute for Health and Welfare commissioned the contact-tracing application Koronavilkku from a private ICT company and published this application in August 2020 (THL 2020b). Koronavilkku was supposed to help people estimate if they had been exposed to the virus and share their positive test result anonymously. Despite high initial hopes the application failed to become the major tool it was supposed to be. This was especially so since the rationale of contact tracing collapsed when a milder variant of COVID-19 proliferated at the same time as the number of infections skyrocketed.

4.5 Questions of Economic and Expertise Capacity in the Finnish Fight Against COVID-19

4.5.1 *Economics and Public Finance*

The negative GDP impact of the pandemic in Finland was lower than the EU average (European Commission 2020; Valtiovarainministeriö 2020), estimated at 2.8% in 2020 (Tilastokeskus 2021), whereas 2021 and 2022 again became economic growth years. Finnish gross government debt increased substantially, but the rise was more moderate than the EU average. However, while before the pandemic Finland satisfied the EU fiscal policy rules on public sector deficit and public debt, Finland was one of those countries for which the EU waivers of its rules were essential.

From among the three constituents of Finland's public finances, the statutory pension funds were hardly affected. Municipal finances fared reasonably well because of the extraordinary government subsidies, whereas state finances were hard hit (Table 4.6). Indeed, state finances will feel the impact of COVID-19 for a long time to come.

Besides direct government contributions in the annual budget, the Finnish government is a substantial guarantor for businesses, including export industries such as shipbuilding (Kostiainen et al. 2020). During 2020, the ceiling of guarantees and other protection measures that the Finnish government-owned expert credit company Finnvera was allowed to award rose from 134 to 161 billion euros, or 19% (HE 2020, Y97–Y98). It is useful to compare these magnitudes to those of the annual total sums of the state budget in Table 4.6.

Table 4.6 Aspects of the Finnish state budget, 2020–2022 (Selected items with substantial changes due to the COVID-19 pandemic are marked in bold)

Budget Selected items	2020 initial budget decided upon by Parliament	2020 final budget with amendments	2020 final budget/2020 initial budget	Government Budget proposal for 2021	Final budget for 2021 with amendments	Budget for 2022 with amendments until March 2022
	Millions of euros		Per cent	Millions of euros		
Revenue items						
11. Taxes, etc.	47,093	**41,952**	**–10.9%**	45,186	46,553	48,678
15. Borrowing in net terms	2,061	**19,748**	**858.2%**	10,904	12,192	7,633
Total	57,551	68,750	19.5%	64,196	67,839	65,540
Expenditures						
23. Prime Minister's Office	219	219	0%	222	184	223
26. Ministry of the Interior	1,520	1,709	12.4%	1,568	1,788	1,586
26.20 Frontier Guard	267	**429**	**60.6%**	277	476	276
28. Ministry of Finance	18,493	20,721	12.0%	19,478	19,921	21,581
28.90. Supporting municipalities	9,367	**11,447**	**22.2%**	10,077	10,090	10,662
32. Ministry of Economic Affairs and Employment	2,863	6,305	120.2%	3,829	4,545	3,743
32.40. Special funding to business	122	**1,354**	**1,009.8%**	599	1,239	513

33. Ministry of Social Affairs and Health	14,780	17,815	20.5%	17,603	17,974	16,024
33.03.87. Founding a vaccination research company	–	–	–	–	8	0
33.20. Unemployment benefits	2,234	3,644	63.1%	2,815	2,807	2,615
33.60 Municipal social and health care	301	529	75.7%	2,052	2,116	525
33.60.38. Subsidy for COVID-19 costs	–	206	Infinite	1,660	1,615	0
33.70. Promoting health and welfare	37	910	2,361.5%	38	319	133
33.70.20. Acquiring vaccines	31	244	687.1%	31	312	102
33.70.22. Control of epidemics	1	660	7,240.0%	1	0.5	25
36. Interest on state debt	873	911	4.3%	765	771	528
Total	57,552	68,750	19.4%	64,196	67,839	65,540

Source: Valtiovarainministeriö (2022).

To alleviate the effects of the pandemic, the Finnish government made substantial subsidies available to businesses (Table 4.6, item. 32.40.), allowed by the temporary EU lifting of its competitive market rules. Moreover, unemployment benefits were made temporarily available to one-person enterprises, and temporary exceptions were introduced into legislation on bankruptcies (Konkurssilaki 120/2004) and distraint (Ulosottokaari 705/2007).

When considering the Finnish fiscal policies during the pandemic, one is led to the contrafactual consideration of what did not happen, although it was not ruled out in principle. Despite that, the annual increases in the total of Finnish government budgets had typically been only in the range of 1–2%, the increase exceeding 19% from 2019 to 2020 did not bring about intense political debate let alone a political crisis. As indicated above, the "securitization" of the COVID-19 pandemic, that is, experiencing it as nothing more than an existential risk with deadly proportions for Finland, was fully or almost complete. Neither the political opposition comprised political parties of the ideological right nor the traditionally fiscally conservative Center from among the parties of the government coalition dared to rock the boat too vigorously.

4.5.2   Government-Commissioned Studies

Large numbers of special studies related to COVID-19 have been published in Finland, either prepared by government ministries or agencies or commissioned by them, and numerous scholarly studies without government commission were also prepared and came out. However, it is no less relevant to consider what failed to occur in Finland.

In the three other larger Nordic countries, Sweden, Denmark, and Norway, major studies prepared by investigative ad hoc government commissions or for the national Parliament came out (Christensen and Lægreid 2023). This did not happen in Finland. One might ask what were the reasons for this difference. Did the fact that Finland had a majority government, unlike the three other countries run by minority governments, exert an influence? Did this lessen the Finnish urge to launch a major, comprehensive investigation?

4.6   Public Opinion on COVID-19 in Finland

As far as the formation of public opinion was concerned, COVID-19 was at its most critical at the earlier stages of the pandemic up until the time that vaccinations became common. According to one poll, males, young people, people outside the capital city region, and supporters of the Finns party expressed the highest aversion toward wearing masks (Table 4.7).

Another masks poll, whose results are not reported in the table, indicated an equilibrium between accepting and rejecting compulsory mask wearing (Helsingin Sanomat 2020g), with the highest acceptance among older people, and the lowest acceptance among the Finns and the Greens among Finnish political parties. Women, young people, people away from the capital city region, and supporters of the Finns and the Greens were the least willing to take the COVID-19 vaccination (Table 4.7). Males, the youngest and the oldest people, residents in Helsinki and the surrounding region, Social Democrats, Greens and supporters of the Left Alliance were the strongest supporters of the EU COVID-19 rescue package toward its member states (Table 4.7). Companies accepted the government's general measures to combat the pandemic, but were critical toward government measures to alleviate the accompanying economic crisis (Table 4.8).'

4.7   Discussion and Conclusions

The research question to answer was formulated as follows: How to assess the Finnish responses to the COVID-19 pandemic with special reference to nurturing civil freedoms and liberties, the normal functioning of sufficiently adversary democratic politics, and avoiding the aggrandizement of the public authorities? The research question has its theoretical background in critical considerations by scholars concerned with the adverse effects of pandemic governance upon civil liberties and freedoms. normal amounts of political dissensus, and the avoidance of the aggrandizement of public authorities (De Leo 2020; Merkel 2020; Moisio 2020; Petrov 2020; VDem 2020; Greer et al. 2021; Karyotis et al. 2021; Kirk and McDonald 2021; Scheinin 2021; Elander et al. 2021; Erickson et al. 2022; Larsson 2022).

As indicated (Table 4.2; Table 4.3; see also WHO 2022), COVID-19 morbidity was low in Finland as long as virus variants causing a serious disease were predominant and the mortality-to-morbidity ratio was high. The Finnish government reacted with a state of exception from March 17 to 15 June 2020, which, in retrospect, was seen to have been exaggerated where most regions of the country were concerned (Deloitte 2021). The government's main policy tool came to be a "hybrid strategy" of testing-tracing-isolation-care pinned to the phase of the pandemic – baseline, acceleration, and community transmission – in different parts of the country (see the main text). After the later serious aggravation of the pandemic, the president and the government issued a joint statement on the need for another state of exception on 1 March 2021. According to one assessment covering only the early stages of the pandemic, Finland together with such other countries as Germany and New Zealand has been one of the few

Table 4.7 Attitudes related to COVID-19 in Finland

Per cent (%)

	Do you use a mask against COVID-19 where recommended?			Will you take the COVID-19 vaccination once available? December 2020/February 2021			Is it beneficial for Finland to participate in the EU COVID-19 recovery package for the member states?		
	Yes	Don't know	No	Yes	Don't know	No	Yes	Don't know	No
In the total population and by gender									
All respondents	73	7	19	56/75	23/12	22/13	38	24	38
Female	79	6	15	48/74	28/13	25/12	36	18	46
Male	68	8	24	63/76	18/11	19/13	40	30	30
By age groups									
−30 years of age	68	9	22	41/67	23/13	37/20	–	–	–
31–39	64	9	27	39/61	33/25	28/13	–	–	–
40–49	69	9	22	51/67	27/15	21/17	–	–	–
50–59	71	5	24	61/77	22/8	17/14	–	–	–
60–69	81	6	13	72/87	18/7	10/6	–	–	–
70 or above	89	5	6	83/91	14/5	4/4	–	–	–
18–25	–			–			48	19	34
26–35	–			–			41	19	40
36–45	–			–			43	23	34
46–55	–			–			30	23	48
56–65	–			–			30	32	38
66–	–			–			46	27	28

			By place of residence					
Capital city region	81	6	13	–	–	–	–	–	–
other cities or towns	72	8	20	–	–	–	–	–	–
other, dense population	71	7	22	–	–	–	–	–	–
other, sparse population	68	9	23	–	–	–	–	–	–
Helsinki and its region	–	–	–	60/76	22/13	18/17	47	21	32
other Southern Finland	–	–	–	56/76	23/9	21/15	36	24	40
West Finland	–	–	–	49/72	24/14	27/13	–	–	–
Finland-in-between	–	–	–	–	–	–	31	26	43
East and North Finland	–	–	–	57/76	22/12	21/11	–	–	–
East Finland	–	–	–	–	–	–	31	31	38
North Finland	–	–	–	–	–	–	37	20	43
			By political parties					
Social Democratic Party	77	8	15	71/88	15/5	14/7	55	28	17
Coalition	81	2	16	71/92	16/5	12/3	40	22	39
Finns	58	9	34	38/56	22/15	40/13	3	2	95
Center	74	10	16	69/87	12/4	19/9	51	13	36
Green league	86	4	11	58/80	17/8	24/11	74	21	5
LEFT alliance	89	4	7	59/78	25/17	16/5	70	20	10

Source: Helsingin Sanomat (2020d, e, f); Haavisto (2020).

Table 4.8 Company opinions related to COVID-19

		4 May 2020	8 October 2020	1 December 2020
		Per cent		
Success in combating the pandemic	Very well	7.1	4.2	12.8
	Rather well	61.9	51.7	65.2
	don't know	8.3	9.7	9.0
	Rather badly	18.9	28.0	10.9
	Very badly	3.7	6.4	2.2
Success in combating the pandemic-related economic crisis	Very well	2.3	1.4	1,5
	Rather well	30.6	20.8	25.9
	Don't know	15.0	11.2	17.2
	Rather badly	38.7	45.4	42.9
	Very badly	13.4	12.2	12.4

Source: STT Info 2020, modified.

countries without violations of democratic and constitutional standards in introducing COVID-19 emergency measures (VDem 2020).

Measures carried out by the Finnish government to combat the pandemic were many. They included legal amendments for the stronger temporary or permanent empowerment of public authorities; budget allocations to cover the direct costs of the pandemic and to alleviate some of the losses to businesses; increasing government borrowing; increasing government guarantees to export industries; and making temporary exceptions to business legislation. After preparations (PMO 2020), the first vaccinations were administered on 27 December 2020, and vaccination activity expanded until the calculated coverage exceeded 99% of the target population (Table 4.2). However, in actual practice the coverage was not this high as there was a contingent of denialists and others who refused to take the vaccination, and there were people who somehow succeeded taking considerable numbers of vaccinations.

The results of this chapter indicate COVID-19-related fault lines (Scambler 2020) between strategically important and vulnerable and other sectors of the economy; between better-off and worse-off socio-economic strata; and between right-wing populist, mainstream, and progressive political party platforms. The results also suggest that while the politicization of the pandemic that introduces authoritarian governance is undesirable (Merkel 2020; Moisio 2020; Petrov 2020), politicization that maintains common adversary and deliberative politics and contributes to social (Van den Broeck 2020) or political (Uldam and Askanius 2020) innovation would be welcome. The Finnish strategy to combat the pandemic was one of majority parliamentarism within strict constitutional constraints. While authoritarian pandemic governance was avoided in Finland, one can claim to detect a temporary visible increase in the powers of the government including the Prime Minister.

One can look for lessons learned during the Finnish governance of the COVID-19 pandemic. One may argue that useful learning transferable to other policy fields has been limited except for preparedness for other versions of the same virus or other sufficiently comparable major epidemics and pandemics. Moreover, the little transferability that possibly existed was wiped out by and large by Russia's unprovoked attack upon Ukraine on 24 February 2022 and its consequences, such as skyrocketing energy prices and accelerating inflation. Note also that Finland has a land border of 1,300 kilometers with Russia. However, it is not ruled out that during the pandemic valuable general learning accumulated on the precariousness of civil liberties and freedoms, healthily adversary democratic politics, and the challenges to avoid the aggrandizement of public authorities.

Having this chapter published in an edited monograph comprised of a number of country studies should support the contextualization of the results of the constituent studies and the drawing of general conclusions (on this, see Migone 2020; Greer et al. 2021). For instance, we know too little about the chains of influence that lead from anti-pandemic policies and other influences to the outcomes including COVID-19 morbidity and COVID-19 mortality. Nor do we have enough comparative research on the conditions of maintaining civil freedoms and liberties, normal adversary politics and obedient public authorities, despite serious threats and crises as well as suggested ways to cope with them.

Acknowledgments

Kalsi, Tapani, MD, Jyväskylä, Finland, for comments on an early version of this text.

Sarapuu, Külli, Associate Professor, Dr., for comments on a related paper by Pertti Ahonen and Susanne Sissonen during a session of the EGPA Permanent Study Group VI on the Governance of Public Sector Organizations, Lisbon, September 6–9, 2022.

Sissonen, Susanna, M.Sc., Head of Biosecurity at the Finnish Institute for Health and Welfare, for good cooperation during her preparation of her doctoral dissertation on pandemics in political science at the University of Helsinki and during the co-authorship of a related paper presented at a session of the above EGPA Permanent Study Group VI on Governance of Public Sector Organizations, Lisbon, September 6–9, 2022.

Interviews

The interviews were carried out on the understanding that the opinions of the interviewees would remain anonymous.

Anonymous recovered COVID-19 patient, 3 January 2021.

Anonymous COVID-19 patient currently with the disease, 23 July 2022. The results of this interview, carried out for another study, were also used to prepare this article.

Hiilamo, Heikki, Professor, University of Helsinki and Finnish Institute for Health and Welfare, 28 December 2020.

Salminen, Mika, Research professor, 2012–2022 Director of Department of Infectious Diseases Surveillance and Control, The Finnish Institute for Health and Welfare, since 1 September 2022 Director of the Department of Public Health and Welfare of the same institute, 14 July, 2022. The results of this interview, carried out for another study, were also used in the writing of this article.

Sane, Jussi, Ph.D., Docent, Senior Consultant, WHO, 12 January 2021. An update interview with Dr. Sane was held on 18 July 2022. The results of this interview were used in this article.

Sissonen, Susanna, M.Sc., Head of Biosecurity, Finnish Institute of Health and Welfare, 17 December 2020.

Tiirinki Hanna, Dr., Expert at the Finnish Institute for Health and Welfare, 21 December 2020.

References

Christensen, Tom, Jensen, Mads Dagnis, Kluth, Michael, Kristinsson, Knut Helgi, Lynggaard, Kennet, Lægreid, Per, Niemikari, Risto, Pierre, Jon, Raunio, Tapio, and Skúlason, Gústaf Adolf. (2023). "The Nordic Governments' Reponses to the Covid-19 Pandemic: A Comparative Study of Variation in Governance Arrangements and Regulatory Instruments." *Regulation & Governance*, 17, no: 3, 658–676 https://doi.org/10.1111/rego.12497.

Christensen, Tom and Lægreid, Per (2023). "Assessing the Crisis Management of the COVID-19 Pandemic – A Study of Inquiry Commission Reports in Norway and Sweden." Policy and Society 42, no 4, 548–563. https://doi.org/10.1093/polsoc/puad020.

Communicable Diseases Act (2016). Act No 1227/2016. *Finnish Ministry of Social Affairs of Health*, Unofficial Translation Without the Latest Amendments. http://www.finlex.fi/en/laki/kaannokset/2016/en20161777.pdf.

Confirmed Coronavirus Cases in Finland (2020–2021). *Constantly Updated.* https://experience.arcgis.com/experience/92e9bb33fac744c9a084381fc35aa3c7.

Constitution (1999). Finnish Legal Act No. 731/1999. *Unofficial Translation by the Ministry of Justice.* https://www.finlex.fi/en/laki/kaannokset/1999/en19990731.pdf.

De Leo, Andreina (2020). "The Italian Approach to the COVID-19 Crisis: A State of Exception Ruled by Technicians." *Amsterdam Law Forum* 12, no. 3: 1–5.

Deloitte (2021). *Selvitys Koronakriisin Aikana Toteutetun Valtioneuvoston Kriisijohtamisen ja Valmiuslain Käyttöönoton Kokemuksista* [A Finnish Government-Commissioned Study on Crisis Management Related to the COVID-19 Pandemic]. https://julkaisut.valtioneuvosto.fi/bitstream/handle/100 24/162677/2021_1_VN_Selvitys.pdf?sequence=1&isAllowed=y.

Eduskunta (2020). *Valmiuslain Käyttöönottaminen Korona-Aikana* [Parliament on Introducing the Preparedness Act]. Not dated; constantly updated. https://www.eduskunta.fi/FI/naineduskuntatoimii/kirjasto/aineistot/kotimainen_oikeus/LATI/Sivut/valmiuslain-kayttoonottaminen-koronavirustilanteessa.aspx.

Eduskunta (2021). *Hallituksen Esitys Eduskunnalle Laiksi Majoitus-ja Ravitsemis- toiminnasta Annetun Lain Väliaikaisesta Muuttamisesta.* HE 22/2021 vp. [Government Proposal No. 22 of 2021 to Parliament on Activating the Preparedness Act]. https://www.eduskunta.fi/FI/vaski/KasittelytiedotValtiopaivaasia/Sivut/HE_22+2021.aspx.

Eduskunta (2022). Miten Löydän Sote-Uudistukseen Liittyvät Eduskunta-Asiakirjat? [Parliament on Documentation on the Social Welfare and Health Care Reform]. Not dated. https://www.eduskunta.fi/FI/naineduskuntatoimii/kirjasto/tietopalvelulta-kysyttya/Sivut/miten-loydan-sote-uudistukseen-liittyvat-eduskunta-asiakirjat.aspx.

Elander, Ingemar, Mikael Granberg, and Stig Montin (2021). "Governance and Planning in a 'Perfect Storm': Securitising Climate Change, Migration and Covid-19 in Sweden." *Progress in Planning*, online 9 November 2021, https://doi.org/10.1016/j.progress.2021.100634.

Erickson, Peter, Marco Kljajic, and Nadav Shelef (2022). "Domestic Military Deployments in Response to COVID-19." *Armed Forces & Society* 48, online 26 March 2022, https://doi.org/10.1177/0095327X211072890.

European Commission (2020). *European Economic Forecast November 2020.* https://ec.europa.eu/info/sites/info/files/economy-finance/ip136_en_2.pdf.

Finnish Government (2021). Restrictions During the Coronavirus Epidemic. https://valtioneuvosto.fi/en/information-on-coronavirus/current-restrictions.

Finnish Government (2022). *Hybrid Strategy to Manage the COVID-19 Pandemic.* https://valtioneuvosto.fi/en/information-on-coronavirus/hybrid-strategy-to-manage-the-covid-19-epidemic.

Greer, Scott L., Elizabeth J. King, Elize Massard da Fonseca, and André Peralta-Santos (Eds.) (2021). *Coronavirus Politics: The Comparative Politics and Policy of COVID-19.* Ann Arbor: University of Michigan Press.

Haavisto, Ilkka (2020). *"Epäilyttävä Paketti" [Report on the Results of a poll by a Business think Tank on Attitudes Related to the COVID-19 Pandemic].* https://www.eva.fi/wp-content/uploads/2020/12/eva-arvio-029.pdf.

HE (2020). Hallituksen Esitys Eduskunnalle Valtion Talousarvioksi Vuodelle 2021 [Government Proposal to Parliament for the 2021 Budget]. 5 October 2020. https://www.eduskunta.fi/FI/vaski/HallituksenEsitys/Documents/HE_146+2020.pdf.

Helsingin Sanomat (2020a). "Tartunta varmistui koronavirukseksi Suomessa" [Article on the First Ascertained COVID-19 Case in Finland]. 28 January 2020. https://www.hs.fi/kotimaa/art-2000006387778.html.

Helsingin Sanomat (2020b). "THL:n Salmisen Mukaan Päättäjiä piti Herätellä Koronauhkaan" [Awakening Decision-makers to COVID-19 Risks]. 22 November 2020. https://www.hs.fi/politiikka/art-2000007627650.html.

Helsingin Sanomat (2020c). "Professori Arvostelee Valmiuslain Perusteluita" [Professor Criticizes the Motivations of Activating the Preparedness Act]. Newspaper article. 17 March, 2020. https://www.hs.fi/politiikka/art-2000006442797.html.

Helsingin Sanomat (2020d). "Maskeja on Alettu Käyttää Enemmän" [More Use of Masks]. Newspaper article. 21 November, 2020. https://www.hs.fi/politiikka/art-2000007630258.html.

Helsingin Sanomat (2020e). "HS-gallup: Suomalaisista 56 Prosenttia Valmis Ottamaan Koronarokotteen". Newspaper Article. [Gallup: 56 Per cent Ready to Take the COVID-19 Vaccine]. 4 December, 2020. https://www.hs.fi/politiikka/art-2000007661632.html.

Helsingin Sanomat (2020f). "Kysymys Maskipakosta Jakaa Suomalaisia" [Finnish People Divided on Compulsory Mask Wearing]. Newspaper Article. 13 December 2020. https://www.hs.fi/politiikka/art-2000007680114.html.2

Helsingin Sanomat (2020g). "Jo 75 Prosenttia Suomalaisista Haluaa Ottaa Koronarokotteen" [As Many as 75 per cent of the Finnish People Ready to Take the COVID-19 Vaccine]. Newspaper Article. 8 February 2021. https://www.hs.fi/politiikka/art-2000007788942.html.

Interview (2020/2021/2022). Any of the Interviews for this article. See the list of Interviews above.

Karyotis, Georgios, John Connolly, Sofia Collignon, and Andrew Judge (2021). "What Drives Support for Social Distancing? Pandemic Politics, Securitization, and Crisis Management in Britain." *European Political Science Review* 13, no. 4: 467–487.

Kirk, Jessica and Matt McDonald (2021). "The Politics of Exceptionalism: Securitization and COVID-19." *Global Studies Quarterly* 1, no 3: 1–12.

Konkurssilaki (2004). Finnish Legal Act No. 120/2004 [Act on Bankruptcy]. https://www.finlex.fi/fi/laki/ajantasa/2004/20040120?search%5Btype%5D=pika&search%5Bpika%5D=konkurssi.

Kostiainen, Juho, Sakari Lehtiö, Sami Napari, and Markku Puumalainen, M. (2020). *Katsaus Valtion Taloudellisiin Vastuisiin ja Riskeihin*, syksy 2020 [A Survey of State Economic Responsibilities and Risks]. Helsinki: Ministry of Finance. https://julkaisut.valtioneuvosto.fi/handle/10024/162546.

Kuntaliitto (2020). *Erikoissairaanhoito* [Hospital Health Care in Finland]. https://www.kuntaliitto.fi/sosiaali-ja-terveysasiat/terveydenhuolto/erikoissairaanhoito.

Larsson, Oscar Leonard (2022). "The Swedish Covid-19 Strategy and Voluntary Compliance: Failed Securitization or Constitutional Security Management." *European Journal of International Security* 7, no 2: 226–247.

Merkel, Wolfgang (2020). "Who Governs in Deep Crises? The Case of Germany." *Democratic Theory* 7, no. 2: 1–11.

Migone, Andrea Riccardo (2020). "The Influence of National Policy Characteristics on COVID-19 Containment Policies: A Comparative Analysis." *Policy Design and Practice* 3, no. 3: 259–276.

Moisio, Sami 2020. "State Power and the COVID-19 Pandemic: The Case of Finland." *Eurasian Geography and Economics* 61, no. 4–5: 598–605.

Nunes, João (2020). "The COVID-19 Pandemic: Securitization, Neoliberal Crisis, and Global Vulnerabilization." *Cadernos de Saúde Pública* 36, no. 5. https://doi.org/10.1590/0102-311X00063120.

Our World in Data (2023). Cumulative Confirmed COVID-19 Deaths, Excess Mortality Per Million People. https://ourworldindata.org/covid-deaths.

Petrov, Jan (2020). "The COVID-10 Emergency in the Age of Executive Aggrandizement: What Role for Legislative and Judicial Checks?" *The Theory and Practice of Legislation* 8, no. 1–2: 71–92.

PMO (2020). "Government Adopts Resolution on Finland's COVID-19 Vaccine Strategy." Prime Minister's Office, Finland. 10 December, 2020. https://vnk.fi/en/-/government-adopts-resolution-on-finland-s-covid-19-vaccine-strategy.

Preparedness Act (2011). Finnish Legal Act No. 1552/2011. Finnish Ministry of Justice, Unofficial English Translation, without the Latest Amendments. https://www.finlex.fi/fi/laki/kaannokset/1991/en19911080_20030696.pdf.

Satakunnan Kansa (2020). "Wuhanin Virus tuli Varmuudella Eurooppaan" [Entry of the Wuhan Virus into Europe Ascertained]. 2 Newspaper article. 5 January 2020. https://www.satakunnankansa.fi/kotimaa/art-2000007027904.html.

Scambler, Graham (2020). "Covid-19 as a 'Breaching Experiment': Exposing the Fractured Society." *Health Sociology Review* 29, no. 2: 140–148.

Scheinin, Martin (2021). "Suomi Tarvitsee nyt Rytminvaihdoksen Kilpailussa Koronavirusta Vastaan" [Finland Needs a Change of Rhythm in Combatting the Coronavirus]. *Perustuslakiblogi.* https://perustuslakiblogi.wordpress.com/2021/01/07/martin-scheinin-suomi-tarvitsee-nyt-rytminvaihdoksen-kilpailussa-koronavirusta-vastaan/.

Situation Update on Coronavirus (2020–2021). Constantly Updated. https://thl.fi/en/web/infectious-diseases-and-vaccinations/what-s-new/coronavirus-covid-19-latest-updates/situation-update-on-coronavirus).

Steuer, Max (2022). "The Extreme Right as a Defender of Human Rights? Parliamentary Debates on COVID-19 Emergency Legislation in Slovakia." *Laws* 11, no. 2, https://doi.org/10.3390/laws11020017.

STT Info (2020). *Kauppakamarikysely* [The Chambers of Commerce Poll]. 3 December 2020. https://www.sttinfo.fi/tiedote/kauppakamarikysely-yritysten-tyytyvaisyys-hallituksen-koronatoimia-kohtaan-kasvanut-alkusyksysta-silti-yli-puolet-yrityksista-antaa-huonon-arvosanan-hallitukselle-talouskriisin-hoidosta?publisherId=25106402&releaseId=69895580.

THL (2019). "Avainlukuja Perusterveydenhuollon Järjestämisestä Suomessa 2013–2019" [Key figures on organizing health care in Finland, 2013–2019]. *Finnish Institute for Health and Welfare.* https://www.julkari.fi/bitstream/handle/10024/138496/URN_ISBN_978-952-343-386-1.pdf?sequence=1&isAllowed=y.

THL (2020–2022a). *Communicable Diseases and Vaccinations.* Constantly updated with web page title Changes. Finnish Institute for Health and Welfare. https://thl.fi/en/web/infectious-diseases-and-vaccinations/what-s-new/coronavirus-covid-19-latest-updates/situation-update-on-coronavirus/the-covid-19-epidemic-regional-situation-recommendations-and-restrictions.

THL (2020–2022b). Koronaviruksen Seuranta [Monitoring the COVID-19]. *Finnish Institute for Health and Welfare.* Constantly updated with web page title changes. https://thl.fi/fi/web/infektiotaudit-ja-rokotukset/ajankohtaista/ajankohtaista-

koronaviruksesta-covid-19/tilannekatsaus-koronaviruksesta/koronav
iruksen-seuranta.

THL (2020b). Koronavilkku Has Been Downloaded More than 2.5 Million
Times. *Finnish Institute for Health and Welfare.* 5 November 2020. https://thl.
fi/en/web/thlfi-en/-/koronavilkku-has-been-downloaded-more-than-2.5-million-
times-widespread-use-increases-the-app-s-effectiveness?redirect=%2Fen%2Fw
eb%2Finfectious-diseases-and-vaccinations%2Fwhat-s-new%2Fcoronavirus-
covid-19-latest-updates.

THL (2022a). Koronaepidemian Vaikutukset Hyvinvointiin, Palveluihin ja Talou-
teen [The Influence of the Corona Epidemic on Welfare, Services, and the Econ-
omy]. Finnish Institute for Health and Welfare. https://www.julkari.fi/bitstream/
handle/10024/140880/Viikko%204-2021%20-%20Koronaepidemian%
20vaikutukset%20hyvinvointiin%20palveluihin%20ja%20talouteen.
pdf?sequence=5.

THL (2022b). Situation Update on Coronavirus. Finnish Institute for Health
and Welfare. https://thl.fi/en/web/infectious-diseases-and-vaccinations/what-s-new/
coronavirus-covid-19-latest-updates/situation-update-on-coronavirus.

Tilastokeskus (2021). *Talouden Tilannekuva* [A Situation Picture of the Econ-
omy]. Finnish Statistics Centre. http://www.stat.fi/ajk/koronavirus/korona
virus-ajankohtaista-tilastotietoa/miten-vaikutukset-nakyvat-tilastoissa/
talouden-tilannekuva.

Uldam, Julie and Tina Askanius (2020). "COVID-10 and Online Activism: A
Momentum for Radical Change?". *E-International Relations.* https://www.e-ir.
info/2020/08/21/covid-19-and-online-climate-activism-a-momentum-for-
radical-change/.

Ulosottokaari (2007). Finnish legal Act No. 705/2007 [Act on Distraint]. https://
www.finlex.fi/fi/laki/smur/2020/20200341.

Valtioneuvosto (2020–2022). Koronakriisin Vaikutukset ja Suunnitelma Epidem-
ian Hallinnan Hybridistrategiaksi [Government Hybrid Strategy to Combat
COVID-19]. The Finnish Government. Constantly updated with webpage title
changes. https://valtioneuvosto.fi/documents/10616/21411573/VN_2020_12.pdf.

Valtioneuvosto (2020a). Entry Restrictions and Health Measures in Place in Finland. The Finnish Government. https://valtioneuvosto.fi/en/entry-restrictions.

Valtioneuvosto (2020b). Rajoitukset ja Suositukset Koronaepidemian Aikana
[Restrictions and Recommendations During the COVID-19 Pandemic]. The Finnish Government. https://valtioneuvosto.fi/tietoa-koronaviruksesta/rajoitukset-ja-
suositukset.

Valtioneuvosto (2020c). Hallitus Linjasi Valtakunnallisista ja Alueellisista Suosituk-
sista Koronaepidemian Leviämisen Estämiseksi [Government Outline of Recommendations Related to the COVID-19 Pandemic]. The Finnish Government. 15
October 2020. https://valtioneuvosto.fi/-/10616/hallitus-linjasi-valtakunnallisista-
ja-alueellisista-suosituksista-koronaepidemian-leviamisen-estamiseksi.

Valtioneuvosto (2021a). Valtioneuvoston Yleisistunto 5.3.2021 VN 21/2021 [The
Government General Session 5 March 2021]. The Finnish Government. https://
valtioneuvosto.fi/paatokset/istunto?sessionId=0b00908f80713bf3.

Valtioneuvosto (2021b). Valtioneuvoston Periaatepäätös COVID 19-epidemian hillinnän hybridistrategian toteuttamisesta annetun toimintasuunnitelman täydennyksestä [Government Decision-in-Principle on Amending the COVID-19 Hybrid Action Plan]. The Finnish Government. 26 January 2021. https://valtioneuvosto.fi/paatokset/paatos?decisionId=0900908f80707714

Valtiovarainministeriö (2020). Economy Will Recover at Pace Set by Coronavirus Epidemic. Finnish Ministry of Finance. https://vm.fi/-/talous-elpyy-koronaepidemian-maaraamassa-tahdissa?languageId=en_US.

Valtiovarainministeriö (2022). Valtion Talousarvioesitykset [Government Proposals for the State Budget]. Finnish Ministry of Finance. Constantly updated. https://budjetti.vm.fi/indox/sisalto.jsp?year=2021&lang=fi&maindoc=/2021/taet/hallituksenEsitys/hallituksenEsitys.xml&opennode=0:1:71:429.

Van den Broeck, Pieter (Ed.) (2020). *Social Innovation in the Face of the COVID-19 Pandemic*. Leuven: KU Leuven. https://esdp-network.net/insist-cahier-4-social-innovation-in-the-face-of-covid-19-pandemic.

VDem (2020). Pandemic Backsliding: Democracy Nine Months into the COVID-19 Pandemic. https://www.v-dem.net/media/filer_public/13/1a/131a6ef5-4602-474 6-a907-8f549a5518b2/v-dem_policybrief-26_201214_v31.pdf.

WHO (2020–2022). WHO Coronavirus Disease (COVID-19) Dashboard. Constantly updated. https://covid19.who.int/?gclid=CjwKCAiAiML-BRAAEiwAu WVggsC6HEQ0iI0N1filOD7AgGwfgRqQU99F6Ev6c2tsLia0fyaOYpvF-jxoCMg8 QAvD_BwE

5 The United States' Responses to COVID-19

Science, Uncertainty, and Partisanship

Louise K. Comfort

5.1 Introduction: An Evolving Risk at Multiple Scales

As the novel coronavirus, SARS-CoV-2, moved silently across the world during the months of 2020, a sobering documentation of losses ranked the United States to be the nation with the highest number of confirmed cases and the highest number of deaths. Two years later, the United States accounted for more than 15.6% of the world's confirmed cases and over 16% of the world's deaths but only 4% of the world's population (Johns Hopkins University Coronavirus Resource Center, September 21, 2022). There is no lack of basic capacity. The United States is the world's largest economy and has a previous record of successful experience in managing infectious disease. It has a premier medical research community, experienced public health managers, and an internationally recognized research institution in the Centers for Disease Control. The grim toll of infections and deaths escalated over the months of 2020 with no clear national policy guiding operations, until two vaccines were approved for distribution in December 2020, offering a change of course in public response to the disease.

What factors could explain the extraordinary trajectory of this lethal disease in a nation that has previously taken a leading role in mitigating public health risks? What resources finally produced a workable strategy for bringing a runaway pandemic under control in early 2021? This chapter will examine three primary factors that contributed both to the initial failures in managing the crisis and the hard-won arrival of vaccines as an effective strategy of containment. The intersection among science, uncertainty, and partisanship exacerbated the challenges confronting public managers at national, state, and local operational levels in coping with the crisis, altering established policy and practice in unanticipated ways.

5.2 Science and the Role of Expertise

The first challenge confronting public managers was to determine what exactly was causing the sudden surge in illnesses and deaths, first identified

DOI: 10.4324/9781003362760-5

in Wuhan, China, but that quickly escalated to become a global pandemic. On December 31, 2019, the cause was identified as a novel virus, but the symptoms were difficult to diagnose and distinguish from lesser ailments. Further, the novel virus had markedly different effects on people, ranging from mild symptoms to death. Scientists and medical experts had little knowledge of this virus and were literally discovering the mechanisms of transmission and possible treatments by direct observation of cases in real time. Weeks of delay in determining the characteristics of the disease allowed the virus to spread, unchecked, through populations via multiple modes of travel within and between countries in the early months of 2020. Standard public health methods of testing, tracing, and isolating cases of infected persons were implemented, but these methods proved inadequate to control the spread. Every minute of delay led to further infections which multiplied again.

Once community transmission was confirmed, there was no vaccine, no known treatment, no means of control other than stopping transmission through physical measures of distancing from other people, deep cleaning all surfaces, and wearing masks. This confirmation shifted the problem of potential infection to a different level, requiring a social response rather than medical. The methods of science require slow, systematic, rigorous testing and documentation of results, acknowledging the limits of knowledge. Different experts proposed alternative explanations, generating substantial controversy over the role of expertise and the insistence of various persons who claimed expertise, but had no evidence to uphold their radical recommendations. This situation fostered an uneasy climate of anxiety and uncertainty over the extent of the threat and actions to counter it, given the unknown characteristics of the virus.

5.2.1   Uncertainty in Policy and Practice in the U.S.

In the absence of a clear, scientific characterization of the virus, credible evidence, and a widely accepted strategy to reduce the risk, there was a broad reliance on heuristics and biases for decision making at the national level in the United States, rather than science (Kahneman, Slovic, and Tversky, 2013). The biases were evident in decisions made by national policy makers, as some accepted single cases of infection as "representative" of a larger group. Others would take whatever case was "available" as the basis for judgment, either for or against a certain practice. Still others would "anchor" their judgment on an early experience and use that experience as the justification for a much wider set of activities that had no basis in fact. Since there was no national policy, different states in the U.S. and different counties and cities within states struggled to define policies that fit their local understanding of the risk. The result was a wide variance in performance across the country, allowing the virus to spread at exponential rates.

As people tried valiantly to follow different guidelines, the shifting policies led to confusion and division in the society. The inability to control the spreading virus destabilized performance in every aspect of public life: business, education, culture, and sports. Businesses asked employees to work from home; others, unable to do so, closed. Applications for unemployment assistance skyrocketed, as workers were furloughed or eventually dismissed. Schools moved classes largely to online instruction, creating a special hardship for students without access to the internet. Museums closed and sought innovative ways of giving virtual "tours" to keep clients interested and to raise modest revenue for the arts. Even sports teams canceled their games when outbreaks occurred during training sessions, despite extensive preparations to minimize exposure, disrupted schedules, and led to contagion. The economic impact of the lockdowns led to a dramatic decline in GDP for 2020 (Casselman, 2020).

The disproportionate impact of economic losses fell hardest on those with low incomes, on minorities, and people of color. Often working in low-paying jobs with high exposure to the virus, but little access to health care, blacks and Hispanics were consistently over-represented in the numbers of infections and deaths. The inequalities in power and authority between low-income groups, minorities, and the dominant decision-making groups were laid bare by the pandemic. Cascading crises of race, police brutality, social inequality, economic losses, wildfire, floods, hurricanes, and COVID-19 exacerbated the level of social anxiety.

5.2.2   *Partisanship*

The year, 2020, marked the quadrennial presidential election that presents an opportunity for change in national leadership. The incumbent president, deeply unpopular with the majority of the population but protected by an intensely loyal base of supporters and a small coterie of officials who, if not sufficiently loyal, were readily dismissed, sought re-election by any means. The incumbent president took a sharply partisan view of the public health risk, downplaying the threat of COVID-19 as a minor, temporary event, refusing to wear a mask, branding the rise in cases as a partisan issue, and delaying federal resources to governors in Democratic states. Republican governors largely followed the president's lead, until the rampant spread of the virus in their own states required different actions. Democratic governors largely followed the science and built alliances among their states to share resources and to establish common protocols for travel and trade. Mayors of large cities made their own decisions, often conflicting with their respective state governors. The nation was deeply divided, pitting coastal states with densely populated urban regions against inland states with sparsely populated rural areas. To some, change in national leadership was urgent. To others, anxious and defiant at new restrictions imposed to thwart an unseen virus, the president's false promises offered a preferable alternate reality, no matter the lack of evidence. The resulting patchwork of policies failed to stop transmission of the virus across the nation.

5.3   The United States as a Complex, Adaptive System

The interaction of science, uncertainty, and partisanship, as outlined above, affirms the characterization of the United States as a complex, adaptive system. These three factors, operating under the intense pressure of a sudden, unexpectedly severe, public health crisis, created negative feedback loops that seriously damaged the performance of public agencies in coping with COVID-19 across all levels of government: federal, state, county, and municipal. The established programs for disaster management in the U.S. were forged in response to natural and technological hazards (FEMA, 2006), and since 2001, terrorist attacks, operating under the Department of Homeland Security and the Federal Emergency Management Agency.

Public health crises, instead, were managed by the Department of Health and Human Services, with the lead agency designated as the Centers for Disease Control. Both major agencies had undergone changes in personnel, with secretaries appointed by a president insistent on loyalty to his agenda. The Department of Homeland Security, for example, had seven different secretaries in four years, two confirmed by the Senate and five as acting directors who did not go through a Senate confirmation process (*The Economist*, 2020). The Department of Health and Human Services had three secretaries within a four-year presidential term (HHS, 2017, 2018, 2021). The high rate of turnover in leadership positions in key federal agencies with designated responsibilities for managing extreme events underscored the inability to forge a national policy to meet a once-in-a-century health crisis.

The lack of a national policy to respond to the size, scale, and urgency of the public health threat from COVID-19 meant that 50 different states recognized the risk at 50 different stages and times. The complexity of this response was exacerbated by the federal administrative structure of the U.S. which created multiple points of decision, presumably intended to check excessively authoritarian policies. As the virus spread at different rates across the country, interdependent systems of trade, transportation, education, and health care slowed, at enormous cost to the functioning society. The situation created significant strain on the performance of the overall system, as negative interactions among interdependent systems led to conflict and distrust. This inquiry into the evolution of the U.S. response to COVID-19 draws on three interrelated streams of research to set the problem in the context of administrative theory: (1) complex adaptive systems, (2) collective cognition and action, and (3) complex time.

5.3.1 Complex Adaptive Systems

The theoretical framework of complex adaptive systems of systems (CASoS) provides a systematic approach to identifying the interdependencies and uncertainties that characterize the occurrence of extreme events (Glass et al., 2011; Carlson et al., 2014; Comfort, 2019). CASoS reflects the interconnectedness among the physical, technical, ecological, social, and economic systems that characterize a dynamic society. The challenge is to identify the interdependent conditions that lead to crises and to model the types of actions (or inactions) that escalate destructive forces that initiate a cascade of crises, as well as the organizations and institutions that could reverse the flow of negative energy to achieve positive interactions among human actors, technology, and ecological conditions.

In the social world, information serves as the catalyst that activates change among people and organizations. Bridging the natural and social worlds are hazards such as infectious diseases, wildfires, hurricanes, and floods. Understanding hazards as a transition in forms of energy from the natural to the social world (-Smith and Morowitz, 2016) allows the human community at risk to identify, redesign, and reorder its actions and resources to adapt to a novel threat in more timely, constructive ways. The process of self-organizing criticality, as defined by Bak (1996), is driven by information in both the natural and social worlds.

5.3.2 Collective Cognition

The gap between cognition and action has posed a long-standing dilemma in public affairs. Officials inform people regarding risk and provide detailed instructions regarding the reduction of risk; individuals listen, understand intellectually what actions would reduce risk, but fail to act in the context of obvious risk. This lack of action despite public warning is repeated again and again in reference to known hazards like earthquakes, floods, and wildfire. If risk reduction is understood as a learning process, the first step is cognition, or that flash of comprehension that frames a risk situation for action (Comfort, 2007). It derives from both social and cultural conditions.

Importantly, for shared risk, or risk that affects the whole community, cognition includes empathy, or the capacity to understand the impact of one's actions, or inactions on others. This understanding of risk is shared with others through communication to mobilize collective action to reduce risk for the benefit of the whole community (Comfort et al., 2020). Acting collectively, the community at risk can coordinate a range of separate, but interrelated activities to achieve the shared goal of bringing the risk under control. Developing collective cognition is especially critical in reference to novel or infrequent risks. Cognition initiates a learning process among actors but depends upon the available communication processes to circulate information through the community. The extent of learning depends upon the time available for action and the rate of change in conditions that generate risk; it is further confounded by the conditions of complex time.

5.3.3   Complex Time

Underlying the conceptual framework of complex adaptive systems is a conceptual measure of time that acknowledges varying sets of activities occurring in different physical locations at different rates of change (Krakauer, 2020). This measure of time differs from the classic concept of time as a unidirectional, asymmetrical "arrow" that moves only forward, never back (Layzer, 1975; Coveney and Highfield, 1992). Although activities in different locations proceed ever forward and do not go back, the "arrows" move at different rates, and time is perceived as adaptive (Krakauer, 2020). This difference in performance among the sub-systems creates a strain on the macro system that requires internal adaptation among the sub-systems for the macro system to continue to function productively.

The concept of complex time enables analysts to identify a set of events as interconnected via a common, underlying dimension of information flow that reveals a shared goal. Complex time anticipates that successive events in a system under strain are likely to generate either further disruption of existing response actions or activation of new patterns of adaptation within the larger macro system. To the extent that disparate activities relate to the same shared goal, complex time allows the analysis of concurrent processes of learning within the macro system that evolve toward coherent behavior. To the extent that disparate activities reflect different goals, the processes of communication and learning in the sub-systems fracture and strain the overall performance of the macro system. Under strain, the weakened system is vulnerable to cascading crises.

5.4   Main Trends of Observable Outcomes in the United States

The primary trend in COVID-19 infections has been a rolling wave across all 50 states, with peaks increasing and decreasing at different times in different states, reflecting the lack of coherence in policies and practice, and leading to a sobering toll in lives and lost opportunities for the entire country. Figure 5.1, shows the profile of infections and broad outline of

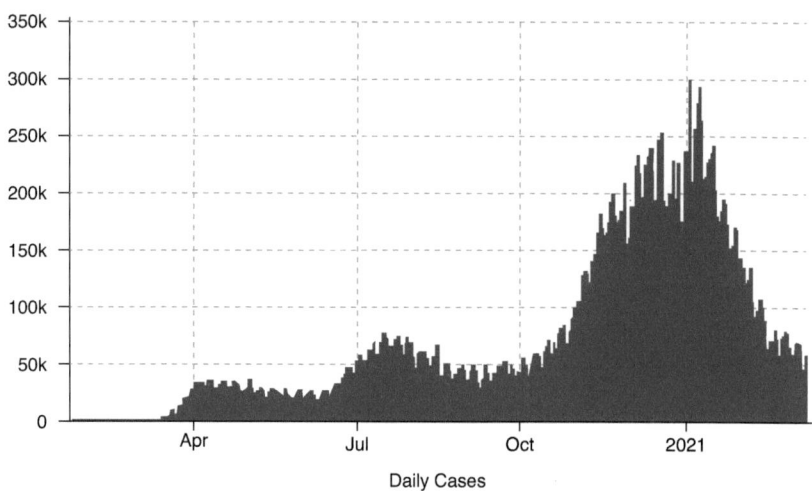

Figure 5.1 Cumulative profile, United States, confirmed cases of COVID-19 infections by month, January 2020 to March 2021.

Source: Adapted from JHU Coronavirus Resource Center, 3-10-2021.

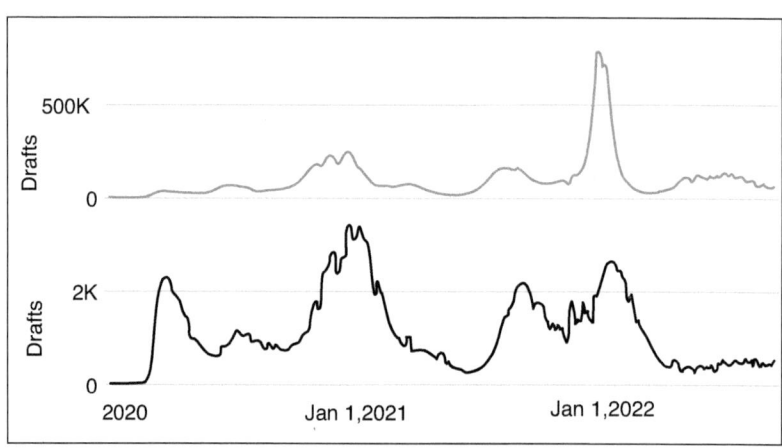

Figure 5.2 Cumulative profile, United States, confirmed cases of COVID-19 infections, deaths, March 2000 to September 2022.

Source: Adapted from JHU Coronavirus Resource Center, 9-25-2022 (cases and deaths data from JHU CSSE; testing and vaccine data from JHU CCI; and hospitalization data from the U.S. Department of Health and Human Services).

the progression of the disease in the U.S. over fourteen-plus months, January 1, 2020, to March 10, 2021. Figure 5.2, shows the cumulative profile of infections and deaths from COVID-19 from January 1, 2020, through January 1, 2023, more than 36 months, that document the continuing range of the pandemic.

Figure 5.2 shows the sharp spike in cases and deaths following the Omicron virus surge in January 2021 and the marked drop in both cases and deaths as the vaccination drive is implemented with full backing of the Administration in March, 2021.

5.4.1   Rapid Escalation of Infections

The World Health Organization (WHO) reported the discovery of a novel coronavirus infection in Wuhan, China on December 31, 2019 (WHO Situation Reports, 2020). Figure 5.1 shows that few infections were reported in the U.S. during the months of January and February 2020, with cases beginning to rise during March and leading to a rapid escalation to nearly 50,000 cases in April, 2020. The increase in infections in March led to a series of nonpharmaceutical measures to curb infection rates adopted by different states at different times that slowed the spread slightly in June, but the number of cases spiked again after the July 4th national holiday. The number of cases dipped slightly in August and early September but began to spike again in late September/October as some states allowed reopening measures, but others did not. The continuing escalation of cases across the country revealed dramatic increases in November and December with the Thanksgiving and Christmas/New Year's holidays. These spikes drove the number of cases to more than double that of India, the country with the next highest number of cases, 11,262,707 and 158,063 deaths, as reported on the JHU Coronavirus Resource site, but with four times the population at 1.37 billion people in comparison to 330 million in the United States.

The U.S. earned the unenviable status of having the highest numbers of reported infections and deaths in the world, with these numbers only beginning to drop in late January 2021. As of March 13, 2021, the total number of confirmed cases stood at 29,384,489 and the total number of deaths at 533,671, reported by the Johns Hopkins University Coronavirus Resource Center. Figure 5.1 shows the number of infections and deaths reaching an extraordinary peak of nearly 300,000 new cases reported per day in early January 2021 but declining markedly to just over 50,000 new infections per day by mid-March 2021.

Figure 5.2 documents the continuation of the pandemic in the United States throughout 2021, 2022, and early 2023, as new variants emerged and circulated quickly through the population, sickening largely unvaccinated people, many of whom fell seriously ill and died. Regrettably, confirmed cases rose to 103,802,702 and the death count rose 1,123,836 as reported on March 10, 2023, by the JHU Coronavirus Resource Center, even though 81.5% of the population had received at least one dose of a vaccine. Although there was wide variation among the 50 states, these data show that social connections and ideological beliefs of people in different parts of the country likely influenced their actions negatively toward taking protective measures against the virus.

How did this jagged trajectory evolve in the United States, and what factors continued the progression of new cases month after month, even as more information about the structure of the virus and its modes of attachment to humans became more widely known? What factors finally contributed to the decline in new cases beginning in late January 2021, but led to the increase in cases in 2022 as new variants emerged? This inquiry explores the evolution of this national profile through dynamic interactions among different actors in complex time.

5.4.2   Overall Assessment of the United States' Response to COVID-19

Searching for the principal factors to explain the United States' performance in public health policy and management will undoubtedly engage many analysts over a period of many years. There is no easy, simple answer to explain the management strategies that have, in practice, led to over 1,123,836 deaths in 38 months, and disrupted economic, social, and cultural activities across all 50 states. Efforts to combat the virus essentially put the nation "on hold" as public agencies, businesses, medical, educational, and cultural institutions grappled unevenly with policies and procedures to bring the infection under control. From a macro perspective, the intersection of science, uncertainty, and political partisanship created a dysfunctional process of decision making at the national scale, leaving management of response operations to sub-national levels of government that enacted scattered and disparate policies.

5.4.3   Comparison of the United States' Response to Selected other Countries

To put the U.S. response in global perspective, it is useful to compare the trends in the U.S. with a select set of nations that were coping with the threat of COVID-19 at the same time. Table 5.1 shows a comparison of numbers of infections and deaths against their respective populations for six selected nations by their ranking among 192 United Nations' member states, as of March 2021.

Table 5.1 Selected nations ranked by number of confirmed cases and deaths from COVID-19, with population figures, March 2021

United States in comparison to selected countries				
Global pandemic	*Confirmed cases: 119,958,400*		*Deaths: 2,644,428*	
Country	*Rank*	*Cases*	*Deaths*	*Population*
United States	1	29,096,048	527,699	330,227,055
India	2	11,262,707	158,063	1,380,004,385
Germany	10	2,569,726	75,362	83,970,413
Sweden	29	712,527	13,146	10,142,867
S. Korea	85	95,176	1,667	51,269,185
Australia	115	29,112	909	25,705,034

What were the key factors that led to this outcome for the United States?
Source: Adapted from Johns Hopkins University Coronavirus Research Center, March 13, 2021.

The figures in Table 5.1 show the remarkable discrepancy between the United States and all other nations. Even India, with more than four times the population of the United States, has less than 39% of the reported confirmed cases and less than 30% of the deaths reported for the United States. While accuracy in reporting cases and deaths may vary by nation, these figures show an extraordinary gap in performance between the United States and other nations in managing the same threat.

Remarkably, this ranking among nations shifted substantially in the 18 months from March 2021 to September 2022. Table 5.2, reports the rankings of the same six nations via the Worldometers.info/coronavirus site in terms of confirmed cases and deaths from COVID-19 recorded on September 30, 2022, for the 192 UN member nations. The JHU Resource Center had discontinued publishing rankings but continued to record cases and deaths. In the ensuing 18 months, the number of confirmed cases tripled, and the number of deaths doubled, as the U.S. maintained its unenviable status as the nation with the highest number of confirmed cases and deaths in the world.

India quadrupled its number of confirmed cases and deaths due to COVID-19 but maintained its ranking as second behind the U.S. in terms of cases and deaths. Germany increased its number of confirmed cases more than tenfold but kept the number of deaths to approximately double the previous mark over the 18-month period between March 2021 and September 2022, moving its rank to 5th place among the 192 nations of the world. The next three nations – Sweden, S. Korea, and Australia – dramatically shifted their rankings, with Sweden dropping down to 41st place, but S. Korea climbing to 6th place among nations with confirmed cases and deaths from 85th place, and Australia climbing to 14th place from 115th place in just over 18 months. Clearly the dynamics in place that had

Table 5.2 Selected nations ranked by number of confirmed cases, deaths from COVID-19, with population figures, September 30, 2022

United States in comparison to selected countries

Global pandemic	Confirmed cases	615,061,946	Deaths:	6,536,828

Country	Rank	Cases	Deaths	Population
United States	1	98,248,623	1,084,891	332,403,650
India	2	44,594,487	528,673	1,417,598,208
Germany	5	33,386,229	150,064	84,380,708
Sweden	41	2,588,441	20,194	10,142,867
South Korea	6	24,819,618	28,489	51,367,217
Australia	14	10,240,031	15,221	25,890,773

What key factors led to this outcome for the same set of nations?
Source: Adapted – Data: Johns Hopkins University Coronavirus Research Center, September 30, 2022; Rankings: www.worldometers.info/coronavirus

enabled S. Korea and Australia to keep cases and deaths to low numbers in the first 15 months of the pandemic shifted markedly as the two nations relaxed the stringent requirements that had kept the infection from entering their borders and spreading through their populations as new variants emerged. Despite the availability of vaccines to these six populations, the policies and practices enacted by the respective nations had limited capacity to reduce exposure and illness from the virus.

5.5   Key Phases in the U.S. Response

The data shown in Figure 5.1 indicate five distinct phases in the U.S. response, with the first four phases becoming progressively worse, until finally, the fifth phase reported a decline in new infections and deaths accompanied by the roll-out of three vaccines. A sixth phase addresses briefly the uneven progress made after the vaccines became available, but when new variants emerged to infect largely unvaccinated people.

5.5.1   *Early Discovery and Denial: January 1–February 29, 2020*

The months of January and February 2020 were essentially months of scattered discovery of single cases of COVID-19 in coastal states and largely denial of a major public health threat by the incumbent president. The first case in the United States was reported in Washington State on January 20, 2020, of a man who had recently traveled from Wuhan, China. That case led to efforts to implement classic public health methods of testing, tracing, and isolating infected cases. Public health experts called for a wide program of testing and tracing to monitor the spread of the disease in the country but needed test kits to do so. The Centers for Disease Control sought to develop its own test kits for COVID-19, but in fact failed in the first attempt, losing critical weeks for implementing a widespread testing regime. As an increasing number of confirmed cases were reported in several countries, the World Health Organization declared COVID-19 to be a Public Health Epidemic of International Concern (PHEIC) on January 30, 2020. One day later, President Trump declared a public health emergency for the United States on January 31, 2020, and imposed a ban on travelers entering the country from China.

After initially denying requests from international scientists to learn more about the origin and characteristics of the virus, China hosted a visit of international scientists, including U.S. scientists, to Beijing and Wuhan in mid-February 2020 (WHO, 7 July 2020). The visit, while graciously managed by the Chinese, yielded little new information. In the United States, the number of cases steadily increased from state to state, and governors of multiple states called for federal assistance. In response, President Trump established a National Coronavirus Task Force on February 26, 2020, to be chaired by the Vice President, Mike Pence, not the Director of the Centers for Disease Control, as was previous practice (Doyle, 2020). While some actions were taken during this two-month period, they were scattered and directed more toward building a public relations campaign against the virus than coordinating a rigorous program of stopping the spread of the virus.

5.5.2   *Uneven Recognition of Threat: March 1–May 27, 2020*

By early March 2020, community transmission had been verified in California, Washington, and New York, and calls for testing and tracing were matched by calls for personal protective equipment and ventilators as patients were beginning to fill the hospitals in New York, Chicago, and Seattle. Six counties in the San Francisco Bay Area declared a shutdown of public gatherings, and asked residents to wear masks and observe social distancing rules. The count of confirmed cases increased particularly in coastal states that were entry points for travelers. Assuming that most infections were arriving in the United States from other countries, President Trump imposed a travel ban on European nations on March 11, in addition to his earlier ban on travel from/to China. Noting the increasing rate of infections, President Trump declared a national emergency for COVID-19 on March 13, 2020, invoking the Stafford Act that provided federal funds to be used for emergencies and the National Emergencies Act that provided authority for the use of emergency powers to waive restrictions and allow mobilization of services to meet a national emergency. States began to follow as California declared a state emergency to release state funds for response operations on March 19, 2020.

In effect, most states, not all, implemented lockdown measures. Schools closed and moved instruction – from kindergarten to university classes – online. This created a massive dislocation for education and revealed the stark gap in access to internet connections and electronic devices for children of rural areas and low-income families. Businesses moved operations online, encouraging those who could, to work from home. Again, the lockdown revealed significant disparities between upper income, white-collar workers who could work from home and agricultural workers, restaurant personnel, or delivery workers who could not. This meant that low-income and minority workers were more exposed to the virus, and more susceptible to infection; unemployment rose to 14.7% in April, 2020. The consequences were severe: economic costs, job losses, high numbers of applications for unemployment assistance, and businesses cutting back employees or closing altogether. Against this background of economic loss, the numbers of confirmed cases, hospitalizations, and deaths increased steadily, with the centers of escalating cases moving around the country, from New York to Chicago to Florida.

The most consequential step taken by the federal government in response to the burgeoning challenges of COVID-19 was the passage of a $2.2 trillion relief bill, the CARES Act, that was signed into law by President Trump on March 27, 2020 (S.4459-116th Congress, 2020). This bill provided immediate relief in payment of $600 checks that were sent directly to the bank accounts of people with incomes under $75,000 and extended unemployment assistance and rental assistance to keep people in their homes. The President further announced, on May 15, Operation Warp Speed, a program of public support for pharmaceutical companies and scientists to find a vaccine that would prevent illness and death from COVID-19, with luck, before the end of 2020. Despite these very positive steps, communications from the White House continued the false assurances that the virus would disappear with warmer weather and dubious recommendations for treatment with hydroxychloroquine and bleach.

5.5.3   *Mixed Signals across Jurisdictional Levels: May 28 to October 14, 2020*

The trends in infections, deaths, and operational response varied significantly across the 50 states throughout the summer months of 2020. The Trump Administration did not develop a national policy but essentially shifted the responsibility for managing pandemic actions to the governors of the 50 states. This led to a patchwork of policy responses, with some governors enacting strict mandates for wearing masks, limiting travel, closing public venues, and reducing the size of meetings, followed by cities, counties, and school districts enacting their own policies and practices, and other governors rejecting public health guidelines presumably to protect economic activity. Ironically, the evidence showed that the primary means to protect the economy was to protect public health. Instead, President Trump and his followers viewed requirements to protect public health as an infringement on personal freedom, leading to a partisan interpretation of public health guidelines. The result was a rolling wave of infections across the country as one state's practices to slow the virus was limited by the neighboring state's refusal to do so.

The increasing polarization of views toward public health restrictions was sharply exacerbated by a white police officer's action that deliberately led to the death of a black man in Minneapolis on May 25, 2020. The actions were captured on a cell phone video that went viral after the killing and led to widespread protests against police brutality in city after city across the country. The protest events compounded the concern for COVID-19, and although the protests were outdoors, largely peaceful, and multiracial with participants wearing masks, they served as a flashpoint for far-right militant groups who asserted their own right to bear arms in states that permitted open-carry gun laws. President Trump exacerbated the situation in an election year by sending federal troops to Portland, Oregon ostensibly as a show of law and order, but effectively as an act of intimidation to the protesters. These events created even more unrest and anxiety in a nation already straining under economic and social pressures from exposure to the virus.

Despite CDC guidelines asking people to stay home, many gathered to celebrate the national holiday, July 4th, and the number of cases spiked again in July. These spikes were further exacerbated by a severe set of natural hazards striking different parts of the country – wildfires in the western states of California, Oregon, and Washington; hurricanes in the Gulf Coast states of Texas, Louisiana, and Mississippi, and flooding in the midwestern states of Iowa, Illinois, and Missouri. States, already burdened with expenses related to managing COVID-19, struggled to provide operational response to these extreme hazard events as they were coping with cascading crises, each contributing to cumulative strain on the society. The stock market tumbled; unemployment was rising; trust in government was eroded by partisan rivalry and lack of substantive action to cope with the increasing burden. In the absence of substantive policy at the national level, governors of neighboring states formed alliances to share stocks of personal protective equipment (PPE) and to coordinate policies on testing, tracing of cases, interstate travel, and commerce.

5.5.4   *Rampant Escalation of Cases and Deaths, October 15, 2020 to January 19, 2021*

The months between mid-October 2020 and mid-January 2021, as shown in Figure 5.1, brought the worst escalation of cases and deaths over the entire year of 2020. These months coincided with the tentative decision of some schools and universities to reopen classes on campus, consequent flare-ups of infections, followed by shutting down in-person instruction and closing campuses again. Most critical were the Thanksgiving and Christmas holidays, when people who had been largely staying home for a year, defied CDC guidelines and traveled to be with family and friends whom they had not seen in person for months. Spikes in the numbers of confirmed cases, hospitalizations, and deaths increased exponentially over the numbers from March and April, and each day reported a new breach of the previous day's total of infections and deaths for the nation, with the virus spreading to rural states as well as urban coastal states.

At this point, benefits provided by the CARES Act were due to expire. Most urgent, unemployment assistance under CARES was scheduled to expire on December 31, 2020, bringing further economic hardship for low-income and minority groups. The House had passed a second relief bill, but the Republican majority leader refused to bring the HEROES Act, as it was named, to the Senate floor for a vote. The national Coronavirus Task Force stopped giving briefings, as they had been transformed essentially to campaign rallies for the president. Governors, mayors, health personnel were taking the actions available to them at their respective levels of authority, but the overall approach was mixed, with no consistent action or policy followed across the nation. Throughout these months, the presidential campaign continued, with efforts to dismiss or downplay the pandemic by the incumbent administration (Woodward, 2020), but with the opposing Democratic candidates making a major issue of the failed management of the pandemic and the unnecessary losses in lives and livelihoods as a result (C-SPAN, October 23, 2020).

During this time of runaway escalation in the numbers of confirmed cases, hospitalizations, and deaths, two events fundamentally changed the trajectory of managing the pandemic in the United States. On November 3, 2020, the presidential election produced a record-high turn-out of voters across the country in the midst of the pandemic. The Democratic candidate, Joe Biden, won a resounding majority of the popular vote, and narrow majorities in key swing states to win a sizable majority, 306 to 232, in the electoral college, securing the election. The electoral college is an anachronistic legal mechanism that favors rural states with lesser populations; in 2016, large numbers of voters disenchanted with both candidates stayed home, and narrow majorities in swing states returned a majority of electoral votes for Donald Trump. Given his unexpected victory in 2016, Donald Trump refused to concede his loss to Joe Biden in 2020, and continued a false narrative that he won the election, filing more than 60 lawsuits to challenge the results, but losing virtually every case, including two cases filed before the Supreme Court. Despite Trump's determined efforts to overturn the election, the election results were verified by all 50 states, and Joe Biden was certified the winner of the 2020 election, poised to assume leadership of the country, and importantly, to manage pandemic response operations on January 20, 2021, when he would be formally sworn in as president.

The second major event was transformative in a quiet, profoundly hopeful way. In December 2020, the U.S. Food and Drug Administration authorized two vaccines for emergency use (www.fda.gov), bringing long-awaited access to a pharmaceutical means to halt the spread of the disease. The Pfizer vaccine, shown in trials to be 95% effective against COVID-19, was approved for distribution to the population on December 11, 2020. It was followed one week later, December 18, 2020, by approval for the Moderna vaccine, shown in trials to be 94.1% effective in preventing infection by COVID-19. The two vaccines brought a practical solution to stopping rampant transmission of the virus, but the task of vaccinating at least 270 million people to achieve a state of collective immunity where the virus no longer propagates quickly through the U.S. population of 330 million required a massive, complex mobilization of both transport and personnel for implementation. Complicating the task further was the emergence of new mutations of the virus with still unknown characteristics in transmissibility and severity of infection. The policy task was enormous, even as the solution became clearer in practice. Yet, these two events, taken together, offered the potential for major change in managing the pandemic response in the United States.

5.5.5   *Change in Presidential Leadership; Vaccination Policies, Practice, January 20 to March 30, 2021*

The change in presidential leadership led to a marked change in managing the response to the pandemic, as President Biden had made controlling the pandemic the first priority of his new administration. With two approved vaccines available, the task now turned to producing sufficient vaccine to vaccinate the estimated 80% of the population that would be necessary to stop reproduction of the virus within the United States. This task was not easy. It required a major logistical operation to ship vaccines, which must be kept frozen at sub-zero temperatures until they are ready for use, to every state, county, city, and hamlet in the country. It meant recruiting medical personnel who can give the vaccinations safely to the wide range of demographic groups in the country. It also meant setting priorities for vaccination by greatest need: elderly, essential workers, those with pre-existing medical conditions who are most vulnerable; establishing vaccination sites, and scheduling appointments for people in terms of the priorities set. This task was made more difficult by the lapse in transition planning from the Trump Administration to the Biden Administration, and the discovery that little planning for distribution of vaccines had been done by the previous administration.

With a new strategy of vaccination against COVID-19 available and responsible for the production and distribution of the vaccines, President Biden moved quickly to set a new course of action for the U.S. in terms of managing the pandemic. He developed a rigorous plan to deliver vaccines to all 50 states and territories. To do so, he mobilized the Defense Production Act to produce sufficient vaccine for 300 million people, going beyond the target of 80% of the population needed for "herd immunity." He authorized the use of the National Guard to assist with vaccinations, agreeing to reimburse the states for deploying their National Guard troops for this purpose. He called for volunteers and contributions of space and personnel to carry out this massive effort, indeed, a "whole of nation" response.

The changes in presidential leadership, management strategy, and the scientific discovery of the vaccines reversed the trajectory of failed, uncoordinated management to the threat of COVID-19 in the preceding months of 2020 and placed the United States in a leading position among nations of the world in vaccinating its population. A third, single-dose vaccine, produced by Johnson & Johnson, was approved for distribution on February 28, 2021. As of March 11, 2021, fully 10% of the U.S. population, 33 million, had been fully vaccinated, and another 64 million persons had received at least one dose of the vaccine (Smith-Schoenwalder and Lurye, 2021). The U.S. set a record of vaccinating over 4 million people in one day on March 14, 2021, and the nation was on track to have sufficient vaccine and capacity to vaccinate every person in the United States by the end of May 2021. When asked at a news conference what he would do if the U.S. had surplus vaccines, Biden's response was immediate: "the U.S. would share the vaccines with the rest of the world" (PBS, May 17, 2021).

5.5.6   *Struggle to Bring the Pandemic Under Control, April 2021 to September 2022*

The hopeful and much-anticipated goal of bringing the pandemic under control in the United States by July 4th, 2021, proved too ambitious. Even though vaccines were made widely available without charge, and major efforts were undertaken to set up convenient vaccination sites in ball parks, neighborhood sites, and public distribution centers, a substantial proportion of the population was hesitant to get the vaccination shots. Misinformation about the vaccines circulated through internet platforms, reinforcing an initial reluctance to take the active step of vaccination to ensure protection from the virus. The same three factors that had hampered the initial response to COVID-19 continued to disrupt the public response to the national vaccination program initiated by the Biden Administration in 2021 – questions concerning the validity of the science that produced the vaccines; uncertainty regarding the reliability of the vaccines; and partisanship toward a government-sponsored program of vaccination.

The vaccination campaign had varied rates of success during the year 2021, but as it progressed to the end of August 2022, at least 79% of the U.S. population had received at least one dose of vaccine, while 68% of the population were considered fully vaccinated. The campaign proved largely successful in the coastal states of Washington, Oregon, and California in the West, and in the northeast, Massachusetts, New Hampshire, Vermont, New York, Connecticut, and New Jersey. It achieved moderate success in the Midwest states of Wisconsin, Illinois, and Minnesota, but it met substantial resistance in rural states and the Southeast, where residents clung to the partisan belief that getting vaccinated was a matter of personal choice and viewed the government-sponsored vaccination program as an infringement on their liberty (Galston, Brookings Institution, October 1, 2021). Table 5.3 shows the fractured distribution among the 50 U.S. states and the District of Columbia by percent of population vaccinated as of August 31, 2022.

Despite the availability of vaccines, social constraints inhibited certain groups in the population from accessing them for their own protection. Regrettably, as highly transmissible variants of the Omicron virus and BA.2 emerged, the rapid increase in cases and deaths occurred largely among the unvaccinated (Scharfstein, March 2022).

5.6 Interacting, Dynamic Conditions in Policy and Practice

At least five interacting, dynamic conditions contributed to the sobering record of response operations to COVID-19 in the United States. These conditions reflect the three factors initially laid out in this analysis – science, uncertainty, and partisanship – but the impact of the pandemic altered the social and economic contexts of the nation in lasting ways. Further, the decision processes were constrained by the administrative context of a federal system that assumes the slow process of building consensus over time. Time proved to be a critical factor in the progression of the virus that did not wait for adaptation at different scales of operation. Although identified in the earlier discussion of the phases of response, five conditions shaped the operational context in the United States and are summarized below.

Table 5.3 Comparison of Vaccination Status among 50 U.S. States and DC, August 31, 2022

Percent of U.S. population vaccinated against COVID-19 with at least one dose by state +DC (N=51)

>95%	>90%	>80%	>70%	>60%	>50%	Total, N/%
Connecticut	Maine	California	Alaska	Alabama	Wyoming	
District of Columbia	New Hampshire	Colorado	Arizona	Arkansas		
Massachusetts	New Jersey	Delaware	Illinois	Georgia		
Rhode Island	New Mexico	Florida	Kentucky	Idaho		
Vermont	New York	Hawaii	Minnesota	Indiana		
		Maryland	Nebraska	Iowa		
		North Carolina	Nevada	Kentucky		
		Pennsylvania	Oklahoma	Louisiana		
		Virginia	Oregon	Michigan		
		Washington	South Dakota	Mississippi		
			Texas	Maryland		
			Utah	Montana		
			Wisconsin	North Dakota		
				Ohio		
				South Carolina		
				Tennessee		
				West Virginia		
5 (9.8%)	5 (9.8%)	10 (19.6%)	13 (25.5%)	17 (33.3%)	1 (2%)	51 (100%)

Source: Adapted from USAfacts.org/visualizations/covid-vaccine-tracker-states.

5.6.1 Scientific Context

The novelty of the coronavirus and the uncertainty surrounding its mode of transmission and capacity to infect humans were primary factors in shaping the decision processes in reference to COVID-19. Scientists and medical personnel had little knowledge of the virus when it first emerged. Instead, they discovered its mechanisms of transmission and treatment by direct observation and experience. Conflict existed between scientific standards of evidence and uncertainty regarding the characteristics of the novel virus. The search for established evidence to meet scientific rigor takes time, but the virus was highly transmissible. The gap in time between the date at which the virus was first detected and the date by which practical measures were taken to stop transmission led to an exponential escalation of infections across the world.

In the United States and globally, the Centers for Disease Control (CDC) had a reputation for professional excellence, but the Trump Administration pressured the leadership to downplay the virus and weaken public health guidance to give false assurance to the U.S. public that the virus was under control (Goldstein and Sun, 2020; Woodward, 2020). The president made misleading claims; professional staff at the CDC left the agency in disagreement, and the CDC lost credibility both in the United States and the world. The limits of the scientific method in highly uncertain contexts exacerbated the public's vulnerability to false narratives that were intended to create political certainty where none existed.

5.6.2 Political Context

The pandemic occurred in an election year with a minority president intent on minimizing the virus as harmful to his chances of re-election. There was a virtual absence of leadership to counter COVID-19 at the national level, leaving governors of the 50 states to navigate the situation largely on their own. The result led to conflicting policies and practices among the states, and widespread escalation of infections as people and trade traveled among the states. Further, there was a continuing battle over access to health care; even during the pandemic, the incumbent administration pursued a case before the Supreme Court to limit access to health care at the very time when people needed it most (Pingree, 2020). Missteps in managing the pandemic became a major factor in the electoral defeat of Donald Trump but led to a change in national leadership that placed control of COVID-19 as the first priority for the incoming Biden Administration.

5.6.3 Economic Context

As businesses closed, transportation stalled, schools and universities moved to online instruction, unemployment rose to 14.7% in April and still hovered around 8.4% in August. The cost was and still is enormous. Congress passed, and President Trump signed into law a $2.2 billion program of benefits to cope with COVID-19 called the CARES Act on March 27, 2020, but the initial federal stimulus payments ended in July, and the follow-up HEROES bill, passed by the House, was never placed on the floor of the Senate by the Republican majority leader. During the months of 2020, by any measure, the economy suffered as the pandemic spread across the country. Federal borrowing reached new highs; the stock market was volatile; small business owners had to close. Workers suffered the largest job losses since the Depression of the 1930s. The incoming Biden Administration brought a focused perspective to controlling the virus and used new tools through three approved vaccines to do so. The new Administration signed into law a major American Rescue Plan on March 11, 2021, that provided $1.9 trillion in assistance not only for COVID-19 relief and implementation of vaccinations but also provided much-needed assistance to families with children, addressing some of the most critical gaps in social inequality.

5.6.4 Social Context

The cascade of interdependent effects from COVID-19 fell most heavily on minorities. People of color were most vulnerable to the virus and suffered disproportionately serious consequences and death from infection. People of color often worked in front-line jobs and were more exposed to contagion, yet the first to be laid off as businesses closed. This cumulative economic burden exposed the latent racial inequality in the U.S. economic system that was accentuated by long-standing police brutality against African-Americans in some cities. Brutal acts by the police against blacks, captured on social media, led to massive demonstrations against racial injustice that crossed race, age, income, education, and gender lines across the country through the summer months of 2020. The incumbent president responded with threats, insults, and questionable use of federal forces, further escalating tensions and compounding social and economic losses with the virus threat.

The pandemic exposed long-standing weaknesses and disparities in racial justice, income, access to health care, and police brutality that initiated a cascade of crises that affected low-income people. These crises were exaggerated further by intense natural hazard events: wildfires in California, Oregon, and Washington; hurricanes in Texas and Louisiana; flooding in Illinois and the Carolinas. Measures taken by the incoming Administration to address these long-standing disparities worsened by COVID-19 provided a positive step toward healing the social inequalities laid bare by the pandemic.

5.6.5   *Administrative Context*

The federal administrative structure in the U.S. allows different decision processes across the 50 states and within the 50 states. Absent leadership at the federal level, states and cities were left to manage the public health risk on their own, leading to fragmented policies and escalating transmission of the virus across state, city, and regional lines. Intensely partisan divisions turned a public health threat into a political/cultural war. The federal system of administrative government creates multiple points of decision that make it more difficult to reach consensus in a large, complex society with a population characterized by diverse demographic and ethnographic groups. The underlying assumption is that people will learn and will eventually reach consensus that all can support, but this assumption is valid only when there is candid, factual communication of the current state of operations. The incumbent administration, rather, produced its own set of facts that were repeatedly at odds with reality (Porter, 4 July 2020).

5.7   Cumulative Uncertainty Across Policy Spheres

Each of these five conditions contributed to building a cumulative uncertainty regarding the most appropriate, timely, practical way of coping with the virus. The sobering fact was that peoples' lives were at stake, and any delay in responding to public health requirements worsened the economic consequences. Economic losses exacerbated political tensions that were heightened by severe natural hazards which increased in scale and scope, representing a major threat from climate change largely ignored by the Trump Administration. As the cascading crises increased the pressure for change, the nation shifted, in the November 2020 presidential election, to a tested, experienced political leader who could frame the issues for action with empathy, allowing at least the majority to forge a common strategy.

The incoming Biden Administration focused on a consistent national strategy to bring COVID-19 under control through a program of rapid, mass vaccination backed by the full authority of the federal government. This strategy began the slow, deliberate process of healing a divided nation, but achieving that goal rests on the nation's capacity to learn from serious missteps in coping with a global pandemic. The challenge is to forge more informed, constructive models for coping with future complex global risks that surely will come.

5.8   Designing a Collective Learning Process

The critical question is how will the U.S. correct the massive missteps observed in response to the global threat of COVID-19, and importantly, who will mobilize the change? There are indeed corrective steps in motion, but are they moving in a consistent, coherent direction? The challenge is to integrate a collective learning process that is strong, consistent, constructive and enables the society to learn and adapt to dynamically changing conditions in a timely, informed, socially responsible mode. Returning to the theoretical concepts used to frame this analysis – complex adaptive systems, collective cognition and action, and complex time – these basic concepts have been affirmed through the narrative analysis of the five phases of response operations from January 1, 2020, through March 15, 2021.

5.8.1   *Collective Learning in Complex, Adaptive Systems Under Stress*

Collective learning is not a simple process under normal operating conditions, but it becomes especially challenging when the whole system is under life-threatening stress. There are no shortcuts. It is essential, first, to identify, understand, and assess the operating components of the system before it is possible to forge a reasoned strategy to manage threats to a changing system. Given the size, complexity, and scale of operations in the United States, this is no easy task. It likely exceeds the capacity of current administrative practices that rely on informed consent. The time and effort required to explain, encourage, and coach 330 million people to adopt new behaviors to protect themselves and others, as well as to avoid old behaviors that put themselves and others at risk under present modes of administrative action clearly was not wholly effective, as shown through phases one through four noted above.

What proved effective in scattered instances of unplanned collective action were the symbols and signals of others taking constructive action in informed, positive ways, modeling constructive behavior like wearing masks, keeping six feet apart, and assisting others in need. For example, people did learn to wear masks in most parts of the country, but modeling the practice and engaging them in a shared effort to protect themselves and one another appeared more effective than legal mandates that provoked defiance and anger (Bowen, July 4, 2020).

The models, however, need to be based on sound evidence and current assessment of the state of risk. Current information technologies can be used to great advantage to monitor changing patterns among demographic groups, types of exposure, notifications of exposure, and conditions of vulnerability. Using the full power of information technologies to track cases of infection and the movement of infections within different population groups proved effective in other countries like South Korea and Taiwan. While such methods need to respect privacy concerns and be carefully designed and executed, the data produced could model different strategies to control contagion. Determining who is most at risk, and modeling different modes of transmission among vulnerable groups are critical analytical methods. The devastating impact of COVID-19 on elderly patients in long-term care homes is only one example of losses to be avoided with careful monitoring, reporting, and analysis (Slick and Wu, 2022).

5.8.2   Collective Cognition

Building collective cognition of risk includes the crucial capacity for empathy essential to build social coherence (Fligstein and McAdam, 2012). It is the capacity to understand the conditions that others are experiencing, and to recognize the impact of one's actions – or inactions – on the larger community that creates a sense of commitment to action. This critical factor was missing in national leadership for the months of 2020, and, in practice, was left to governors, mayors of cities, leaders in private and philanthropic organizations to build a commitment to action at their separate levels of responsibility. This task requires clear, timely, evidence-based information that updates the status of operations in a dynamically changing environment. Patterns of public communication that repeatedly denied facts and distorted scientific findings at the national level misled public understanding of the risks of COVID-19 and hampered efforts by public health experts to build collective cognition of the serious threat posed by the virus. Such distortions can only be countered by valid information and openness to inquiry in public discourse. Establishing valid practice in communicating clearly regarding what is known and what is not known and demonstrating the capacity to correct mistakes are essential skills needed to rebuild public trust in government.

5.8.3   Complex Time

The dynamic effects of complex time were verified in undeniable ways by the progression of COVID-19 across the United States, as different states recognized the risk of the novel virus at different times and responded to the threat in varying degrees. Some states, such as California and Illinois, acted quickly to stop transmission by multiple means while others, such as Texas and Arizona, chose to deny the risk, only to impose lockdown measures after the number of cases spiraled upward and their hospitals filled. The concept of complex time shows the compelling influence of the gap between cognition and action that characterized this dynamic period of virus transmission and efforts at control within the U.S. society as a complex system.

Figure 5.3 provides a simple model of the differential rate of cognition and action in response to the virus at different times, and the impact of the variance in rates of change on slowing down the overall response of the whole system. The model shows only the differential rates among the states, but within each state, there were similar differences among the counties and between the cities and the small towns. As the months progressed in 2020, escalating rates of infections, hospitalizations, and deaths ricocheted back and forth among the 50 states, as actions taken by one state affected the rates of exposure and infections in neighboring states, slowing down the capacity of the whole national system to bring the virus under control.

Complex Time

- Classic conception of time: "arrow" of time moves only forward, never back
- In complex adaptive systems, time is perceived differently in different contexts

Control of the virus is a macro-level problem, as different states, counties, and cities have different rates of exposure to risk, different levels of resources and knowledge, and consequently muster different levels of organization and management to cope with the disease. Only by adapting their respective performances on testing, tracing, social distancing, travel, and exchange of goods could the 50 states achieve a nationwide level of control for the country. Such an effort requires national-level leadership and the articulation of a shared goal for the nation, accompanied by the resources and trained personnel to achieve a national standard of reporting and action. Building the capacity for self-organization and risk

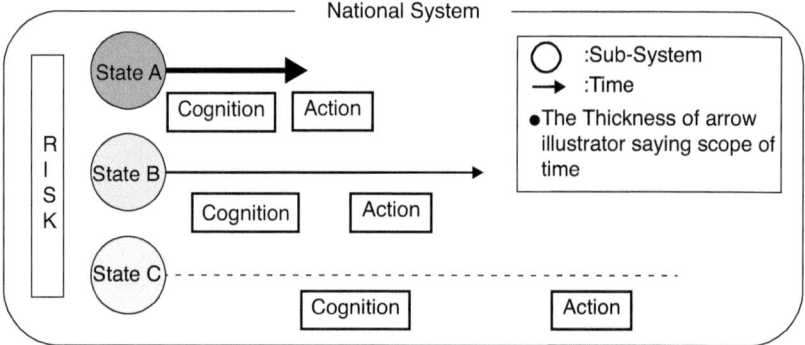

Figure 5.3 Complex time in differential response operations to COVID-19 at the state level.

Source: Adapted from Comfort and Rhodes (2022), p. 8.

management at different scales of operation in a large, complex, dynamic nation requires flexibility, adaptation, and iterative learning under continuing conditions of uncertainty.

5.9 Conclusions

The United States will recover, chastened by its sobering performance during the months of 2020 on the global scale, and heartened by the discovery of vaccines and strong mobilization of vaccine distribution in early 2021. Three areas are likely to be fundamental in moving this recovery forward.

First, the role of science, essential to policy decisions regarding public health, will regain public influence and credibility as new discoveries are supported by governmental agencies practicing their legal responsibilities of inquiry and oversight. The CDC, under new leadership, is resuming its former professional status and again providing rigorous guidance for managing infectious diseases, including COVID-19. Gone are the efforts to mold CDC guidance to fit an incumbent president's preferred position. In authority again are senior scientists who had resisted political pressures to report the actual status of the infections and are establishing the organizational policies and procedures to ensure that such politicization does not happen again. Key priorities include allocation of the financial and professional support needed for the medical and public health research community to explore and anticipate other infectious diseases likely to emerge in the future.

Secondly, the power of information technologies needs to be harnessed to increase the capacity for collective learning at multiple scales of operation. The speed and pervasiveness with which the SARS-CoV-2 virus was transmitted throughout the nation meant that no state, county, city, or small town in the nation escaped exposure. The size and scale of the risk exceeded the capacity of standard administrative processes to manage it, and the tasks of monitoring and modeling alternative strategies to cope with an unknown virus require sophisticated data collection, analysis, and modeling techniques. Building the organizational capacity to collect data on changing performance of multiple systems simultaneously and the disciplinary expertise to analyze the data to anticipate potential strategies of action become an essential investment to reduce emerging risk. These capacities need to be developed at every level – small towns, big cities, county, state, and federal agencies – to enable communities to address large-scale, dynamic threats like infectious diseases.

Thirdly, investing in a national information infrastructure with equal access to all groups is fundamental to support responsible, self-organizing management of risk within the United States in an ever-changing world. People learn, they adapt and change, but to do so, they need the basic infrastructure to search, exchange, store, and update information on the status of their respective communities. Such an information infrastructure is as essential to developing the capacity for societal learning as the inter-state highway system is to commercial trade and economic development. The basic institutions for such a national information infrastructure are already in place, with land-grant universities in all 50 states. The land-grant universities were founded with a public mission to serve the educational and research needs of the residents of each state. Linking these universities together through the power of current information technologies is the next step toward building this capacity at a national scale.

Importantly, achieving the capacity for continuous learning in one coun-try, even a large, complex, dynamic country like the United States, is only one part of the larger global arena. It will be imperative to build on the lessons learned in all countries from this global pandemic (see, e.g., Moon, 2020) and use these insights to develop the capacity for global cooperation and collaboration in addressing major problems like infectious diseases that one country alone cannot solve. Other issues require global attention: climate change, energy use, clean water and the continuing problems of health, education, and welfare for the nearly 7.7 billion people on this planet. Only through developing an interdisciplinary, international pro-gram of continuous learning and adaptation will the global community of nations be able to sustain a healthy, humane world.

References

Bak, P. 1996. *How Nature Works: The Science of Self-Organised Criticality*. New York: Copernicus Press.

Bowen, K. 2020. Protesters Gather at Texas Capitol for "Shed the Mask" Rally. *FOX 7*, Austin. https://www.fox7austin.com/news/protesters-gather-at-texas-capitol-for-shed-the-mask-rally

Carlson, J.M., D.L. Alderson, S.P. Stromberg, D.S. Bassett, E.M. Craparo, F. Guiterrez-Villarreal, and T. Otani. 2014. Measuring and Modeling Behavioral Decision Dynamics in Collective Evacuation. *PLoS One*, 9 (2): e87380.

Casselman, B. 2020. A Collapse that Wiped Out 5 Years of Growth, with No Bounce in Sight. *The New York Times*, July 30. https://www.nytimes.com/2020/07/30/business/economy/q2-gdp-coronavirus-economy.html

C-SPAN. 2020. Joe Biden Remarks on the Pandemic Response. *Campaign 2020*, October 23, 2020. https://www.c-span.org/video/?477287-1/joe-biden-unveils-coronavirus-pandemic-recovery-planComfort, L. K. 2007. Crisis Management in Hindsight: Cognition, Communication, Coordination, and Control. *Public Administration Review*, 67: 189–197.

Comfort, L.K. 2019. *The Dynamics of Risk: Changing Technologies and Collec-tive Action in Seismic Events*. Princeton: Princeton University Press, Studies in Complexity.

Comfort, L.K., N. Kapucu, K. Ko, S. Menoni, and M. Siciliano. 2020. Crisis Decision-Making on a Global Scale: Transition from Cognition to Collective Action under Threat of COVID-19. *Public Administration Review*, 80 (4): 616–622.

Comfort, L.K. and M.L. Rhodes. 2022. Collective Cognition in Complex Systems. In L.K. Comfort and M.L. Rhodes (Eds.), *Global Risk Management: The Role of Collective Cognition in Response to COVID-19*. New York: Routledge Publishing.

Coveney, Peter and Roger Highfield. 1992. *The Arrow of Time: A Voyage through Science to Solve Time's Greatest Mystery*. New York: Ballantine Books.

Doyle, K. 2020. Trump Announces Coronavirus Task Force. *Washington Examiner*, January 30, 2020. https://www.who.int/news/item/07-07-2020-who-experts-to-travel-to-china.

The Economist. 2020. Assessing Donald Trump's use of the Homeland Security department. https://www.economist.com/united-states/2020/09/19/assessing-donald-trumps-use-of-the-homeland-security-department.

FDA (Food and Drug Administration). 2020. Pfizer Vaccine. *Pfizer*, December 11, 2020, USFDA. https://www.fda.gov/emergency-preparedness-and-response/coronavirus-disease-2019-covid-19/moderna-covid-19vaccine#: ~:text=On%20 December%2018%2C%202020%2C%20the,SARS%2DCoV%2D2.

FDA (Food and Drug Administration). 2020. Moderna Vaccine. December 18, 2020. https://www.fda.gov/emergency-preparedness-and-response/coronavirus-disease-2019-covid-19/moderna-covid-19vaccine#:~:text=On%20December% 2018%2C%202020%2C%20the,SARS%2DCoV%2D2.

FEMA (Federal Emergency Management Agency). 2006. https://www.fema.gov/emergency-managers/national-preparedness/frameworks/response

Fligstein, N. and D. McAdam. 2012. *A Theory of Fields*. New York: Oxford University Press.

Galston, William A. 2021. For COVID-19 Vaccinations, Party Affiliation Matters More than Race and Ethnicity. *Brookings Institution Blog*, FixGov. https://www.brookings.edu/blog/fixgov/2021/10/01/for-covid-19-vaccinations-party-affiliation-matters-more-than-race-and-ethnicity/

Glass, R.J., A.L. Ames, T.J. Brown, S.L. Maffitt, W.E. Beyeler, P.D. Finley, T.W. Moore, J. M Linebarger, N.S. Brodsky, S.J. Verzi, A.V. Outkin, and A.A. Zagonel. 2011. *Complex Adaptive Systems of Systems (CASoS) Engineering: Mapping Aspirations to Problem Solutions*. Albuquerque: Sandia National Laboratories. June (SAND 2011-3354C).

Goldstein, A. and L.H. Sun. 2020. Controversial Change in Guidelines about Coronavirus Testing Directed by the White House Coronavirus Task Force. The Washington Post. August 26. https://www.washingtonpost.com/health/cdc-testing-guidelines-coronavirus/2020/08/26/eb653028-e7af-11ea-97e0-94d2e46e 759b_story.html

HHS (US Department of Health and Human Services). 2018, 2017. HHS Leadership. https://www.hhs.gov/about/leadership/index.html. These appointments are also cited in the *New York Times*, Donald Trump's Cabinet is Complete. May 11, 2017; https://www.nytimes.com/interactive/2016/us/politics/donald-trump-administration.html;

Kahneman, D., P. Slovic, and A. Tversky. 2013. *Judgment under Uncertainty: Heuristics and Biases*. Cambridge: Cambridge University Press. (First printing, 1982).

Krakauer, D. 2020. *Complex Time*. Santa Fe: Santa Fe Institute Seminar Series, July 31. https://www.santafe.edu/research/themes/complex-time

Layzer, D. 1975. The Arrow of Time. *Scientific American*, 233 (6): 56–69.

Moon, M.J. 2020. Fighting COVID-19 with Agility, Transparency, and Participation: Wicked Policy Problems and New Governance Challenges. *Public Administration Review. Covid Viewpoint Symposium*, 80 (4): 651–656.

PBS (Public Broadcasting System). 2021. Biden Boosting World Vaccine Sharing Commitment to 80 Million Doses. https://www.pbs.org/newshour/politics/watch-live-biden-delivers-remarks-on-covid-19-response-and-vaccination-program-2.

Pingree, C. 2020. As Trump Administration Seeks to Overturn ACA, Pingree Votes to Protect & Expand Health Care Coverage. *Press Release*, June 29, 2020. https://pingree.house.gov/news/documentsingle.aspx?DocumentID=3427

Porter, Tom. 2020. Trump Lives in 'alternative reality' and Truly Believes His Election-Fraud Claims, Says UK Film-Maker with Him Around Jan. 6. *Insider*, July 4, 2020. https://www.yahoo.com/entertainment/trump-lives-alternative-reality-truly-155156876.html

S.4459-116th Congress: CARES Congressional Oversight Commission Diversity Act of 2020. *www.GovTrack.us.2020*, October 6, 2022. https://www.govtrack.us/congress/bills/116/s4459.

Scharfstein, J. *Here We Go Again: The BA.2 Version of Omicron. Interview, Public Health on Call.* Bloomberg School of Public Health, Johns Hopkins University, Baltimore, MD. March 22, 2022. https://publichealth.jhu.edu/2022/here-we-go-again-the-ba2-version-of-omicron.

Slick, J. and H. Wu. 2022. The Need to Protect the Most Vulnerable: The COVID-19 Crisis in Long-term and Residential Care in Canada. In L.K. Comfort and M.L. Rhodes, (Eds.), *Global Risk Management: The Role of Collective Cognition in Response to COVID-19.* New York: Routledge Publishing. Pp. 182–207.

Smith, E. and H.J. Morowitz. 2016. *The Origin and Nature of Life on Earth: The Emergence of the 4th Geosphere.* Cambridge: Cambridge University Press.

Smith-Schoenwalder, C. and S. Lurye. 2021. Uneven Reporting Raises Doubts About CDC Vaccination Numbers. *US News and World Report.* December 2021. https://www.usnews.com/news/health-news/articles/2021-12-21/uneven-reporting-raises-doubts-about-cdc-vaccination-numbers.

WHO (World Health Organization). 2020. *Situation Reports, 2020,* 7 July 2020. https://www.who.int/emergencies/diseases/novel-coronavirus-2019/situation-reports

Woodward, B. 2020. *Rage.* New York: Simon & Schuster.

6 Aotearoa New Zealand's Responses to COVID-19

Sophie Henderson and Matt Withers

6.1 Introduction

The COVID-19 pandemic has presented an almost unprecedented challenge to public healthcare systems around the world. While the very interconnectedness of the global economy facilitated an initial rate of contagion that outpaced scientific understanding of the disease and policy consensus around effective containment measures, high- and low-income countries alike have since struggled to weigh public health interventions against their political and economic implications. Across the OECD – the group of high-income countries best-resourced to respond to such an emergency – transmission and mortality rates have typically been no better than the world average (Bretschger et al. 2020). Aotearoa, New Zealand (NZ) is, in many ways, the most striking outlier in this respect. Having acted relatively swiftly, decisively, and with a clear prioritization of public health over economic concerns or the preservation of civil liberties, NZ was able to "flatten the curve" of COVID-19 infections during the early stages of the pandemic and thereafter pursue a strategy of elimination that few others have been able to emulate.

In this chapter, we explain NZ's comparatively successful management of the pandemic by examining how distinctive situational and institutional factors combined to produce a policy environment conducive to staunch public health interventions. We preface our analysis with an overview of aspects of NZ's geographic, political and demographic context relevant to the pandemic. We then provide an in-depth assessment of government policy responses during critical phases of the COVID-19 timeline – assessing how key policies were informed, formulated, communicated and implemented – before linking these interventions to an underlying matrix of political, analytical and operational capacities. Importantly, we identify that these capacities (or lack thereof) not only enabled NZ's highly restrictive response but constrained the ability to pursue alternative measures that may have attained similar outcomes with fewer shortcomings.

DOI: 10.4324/9781003362760-6

Finally, we consider some of these shortcomings with respect to ongoing social and economic hardships arising from unilateral border closures, quarantine management and periodic lockdowns.

First, though, it is important to convey NZ's milestones in controlling COVID-19 with reference to caseload data and key events in the chronology of the pandemic (Figure 6.1). The SARS-Cov-2 virus that causes COVID-19 was first reported to the World Health Organization (WHO) on December 31, 2019, following a spate of pneumonia diagnoses with an unknown cause in Wuhan, China. In the weeks that followed, cases began spreading within China and, by January 13, the virus was transmitted internationally for the first time when a confirmed case was reported in Thailand. Wuhan was placed under strict lockdown and on January 30th NZ made its first intervention when it arranged a charter flight to evacuate citizens stranded in the city, who were then placed into quarantine for 14 days (Reuters 2020). No COVID-19 cases were recorded among those repatriated nationals, but on February 3 entry restrictions were enforced for all inbound travel from China, marking the first instance in which border closures were used as an integral component of the government's policy response (Henrickson 2020). Almost a month later, on February 28, NZ recorded its first case of COVID-19 when a resident tested positive after returning from Iran. The first instance of community transmission was recorded shortly thereafter on March 5 and in the two weeks that followed, the local caseload increased to 28.

On March 19 NZ announced the closure of its international borders, effectively barring inbound and outbound travel, to everyone except citizens and residents – a hallmark policy that remains in place as of March 2021 (Roy 2020). After the closure of NZ's borders, imported cases declined dramatically, but community transmission persisted (Robert 2020). An escalating caseload in the week following the border closure resulted in the introduction of a four-level alert system on March 21. These levels correspond with "prepare," "reduce," "restrict," and "eliminate" warnings that are each accompanied by lockdown measures of varying severity (New Zealand Government 2020b). The country was placed at level two at the time of the announcement, but with growing daily cases, it was placed on level three on March 23, before a State of National Emergency declaration on March 25 and the imposition of a four-week level four lockdown on March 26 (New Zealand Government 2020a).

The level four restrictions entailed a stringent nationwide lockdown with complete home confinement of the population outside of essential frontline work and essential personal movement (New Zealand Government 2020b). At the start of the level four restriction period, NZ was experiencing 73 new cases per day; two weeks later, it dropped to 26 daily cases, and after four weeks, it stood at just five daily cases (Figure 6.2).

Date (2020)	Event
February 28	First case of COVID-19 reported in NZ in a resident returning from Iran. Entry restrictions placed on people travelling from Iran.
March 5	First confirmed person-to-person transmission of COVID-19 in NZ.
March 11	WHO declares COVID-19 a pandemic.
March 14	All people entering NZ must self-isolate for 14 days, except arrivals from Pacific Island countries. Cruise ships are banned.
March 19	A total of 28 cases of COVID-19 in NZ, all linked to overseas travel. Borders are closed to everyone except NZ citizens and residents.
March 21	A total of 52 cases confirmed in NZ. A four-level alert system introduced: level 1 (prepare); level 2 (reduce); level 3 (restrict); level 4 (eliminate). The country is placed at level 2.
March 23	NZ placed at level 3 with additional restrictions imposed.
March 25	State of Emergency declared.
March 26	NZ enters level 4, lockdown restrictions initially imposed for 4 weeks.
March 29	First death caused by COVID-19 in NZ.
April 9	A total of 29 new cases of COVID-19 reported. The lowest daily total since 23 March.
April 27	NZ re-enters level 3, with some lockdown restrictions eased.
May 14	NZ enters level 2, with further restrictions eased.
June 9	NZ has no active cases of COVID-19 and enters level 1 for the first time with minimal restrictions in place.
August 11	After more than 100 days of no community transmission of COVID-19 outside managed isolation, a cluster of 4 new cases detected in a single family in Auckland.
August 12	Auckland is placed under level 3. The rest of NZ is placed under level 2.
September 23	Auckland moves to level 2, the rest of NZ moves to level 1 (no restrictions).
October 7	Auckland moves to level 1 (no restrictions).
October 17	PM Jacinda Ardern wins a landslide victory in NZ's general election and credits her government's decisive COVID-19 response for the win.

Figure 6.1 Timeline of the NZ government's response to COVID-19.

Source: Created by the author.

Level four restrictions were extended for five days before transitioning to more moderate level three restrictions for two weeks commencing April 27. By May 4, NZ reported no new cases and entered a phase of controlled de-escalation of lockdown measures as the objective of containment gave way to a more ambitious strategy of complete elimination.

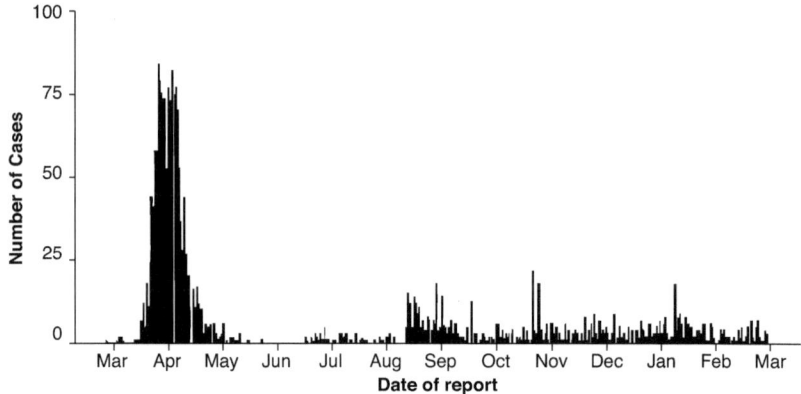

Figure 6.2 Daily confirmed cases.

Source: Adapted from Ministry of Health NZ 2021.

This paradigm shift entailed the continuation of strict border controls, quarantine protocols for repatriated citizens, and further planning to ensure national preparedness for instances of re-escalation. After more than 100 days without any community transmission, such an episode did occur on August 11, when four new cases from an unknown source were detected in Auckland, catalyzing a second outbreak of the virus (New Zealand Government 2020a). Having learned from the first wave of cases, alert level restrictions were rapidly implemented: Auckland was placed at level three on August 12, and the rest of the country on level two. Restrictions for both jurisdictions were then scaled back on September 23, to levels two and one, respectively, before Auckland was also reduced to level one on October 7. With cases again brought under control by quick and decisive intervention, incumbent Prime Minister (PM) Jacinda Ardern went into the NZ general election on October 10 buoyed by public support for her government's handling of the pandemic and won by an outright majority for the first time since 1951 (Shaw 2020).

In the following section, we begin our analysis of NZ's track record of containing the virus by contextualizing, demographic, political and geographic factors that influenced the country's position toward handling a pandemic event of this nature. We then examine specific policy responses in greater detail, delineating between public health and economic policymaking, and critically evaluating these interventions relative to comparably situated countries. In the next section, we link these policymaking decisions to a matrix of underlying capacities – highlighting that NZ's response is largely the outcome of robust political and analytical capacities against a backdrop of operational constraints, particularly with regard to healthcare infrastructure. Finally, and despite the relative merits of NZ's response, we locate continuing challenges associated with the approach, emphasizing the social and economic hardships arising from unilateral border closures and severe lockdown measures.

6.2 Country Profile and Background

Aotearoa NZ is a high-income remote island nation of five million people situated in the Southwest Pacific Ocean. New Zealanders predominantly live in urban areas on the North Island. The city of Auckland is inhabited by approximately one-third of the country's population, while the capital city – Wellington – accounts for a further 500,000 (Stats NZ 2020a). NZ is home to an increasingly diverse and multi-ethnic society. In the latest Census, 70.2% of the population were identified as European, 16.5% were indigenous Māori, 15.5% were Asian, 8.1% were Pacific peoples, 1.5% were Middle Eastern, Latin American or African and 1.2% were of other ethnicity (Stats NZ 2020a).

The NZ economy and labor market were robust going into the COVID-19 lockdown. The economy experienced an annual growth of 2.3% during 2019, while the labor market grew 1.6% in the quarter ending March 2020 (Ministry of Business, Innovation and Employment 2020). NZ has an internationally competitive economy with primary sector exports accounting for NZ$46.4 billion out of a total of NZ$58.3 billion worth of good exports the year ended June 2019 (Ministry for Primary Industries 2019) and contributing to 7% of GDP. NZ is one of the top five dairy exporters globally and these products ranked first among primary exports, closely followed by its other primary exports of meat, wool, forestry, horticulture and seafood, the majority of which are sent to China. Tourism is another highly significant sector for NZ's economy. For the year ending March 2020, the tourism industry directly employed 8.4% of the NZ workforce and delivered NZ$41.9 billion to the country, accounting for 20.1% of foreign exchange earnings and contributing 9.3% to GDP (Stats NZ 2020b). However, international tourism has been the worst hit industry by the pandemic amid NZ's ongoing border closure from March 2020.

NZ has a unitary system of governance characterized by highly centralized policymaking. In the absence of a written constitution to specify power-sharing with lower levels of government, national decision-making power rests predominantly with a political executive drawn from the ranks of the majority party (Bromfield and McConnell 2020). Local government bodies in NZ consist of regional councils and territorial authorities, which are responsible for providing local services and overseeing environmental resource management. NZ enjoys a largely civil political environment with a strong center-left government led by PM Jacinda Ardern. Ardern was first sworn in as NZ's youngest-ever PM in October 2017, although her Labor Party fell short of a majority and was forced to form a coalition with the New Zealand First party. Throughout her first term, Ardern's popularity grew, and she won praise nationally and abroad for her compassionate handling of the Christchurch mosque shootings in March 2019 (which resulted in 51 deaths), and the Whakaari/White Island volcanic eruption in December 2019 (which resulted in 22 deaths). These two crises prepared Ardern to effectively contend with the COVID-19 pandemic, which in turn played a large part in her re-election and landslide victory at the October 2020 parliamentary elections.

NZ is also a gateway to numerous Pacific Island Countries (PICs) and is a major stakeholder in the region's economic development and public health strategy. In particular, Samoa's devastating experience with the influenza pandemic of 1918–1919 (H1N1) established a historical rationale for NZ's response to COVID-19. NZ suffered severely during the second wave of the influenza pandemic with a death toll of approximately 8,000, of which at least 2,160 were Māori, and an overall death rate of 7.8% per thousand (Rice 2020). The fatal course of the pandemic through the Pacific Island nations can be traced to the movements of NZ's regular steamship service to these islands: the Talune. The Talune was allowed to dock in the ports of Samoa rather than remain in quarantine, despite having passengers on board infected with influenza. The NZ Departments of Public Health and Defence failed to notify the Samoan health authorities about the spread of influenza before it was too late. Samoa's subsequent death toll of 8,000 constituted over 22% of the population (Tomkins 1992). Therefore, NZ initially used its pre-existing national Influenza Pandemic Plan, revised in 2017, as a framework for responding to COVID-19 in a manner that would prevent disparities and minimize transit of infection to lower-income PICs.

However, NZ's Influenza Pandemic Plan is based on a mitigation model focused on "flattening the curve" and delaying the epidemic peak to reduce the overall public health impact of an influenza pandemic (Ministry of Health NZ 2017). Once NZ became aware of the differences in the function of the biology and epidemiology between an influenza pandemic and COVID-19, i.e., that COVID-19 has a longer incubation period (median of 5–6 days) than influenza (1–3 days), meaning influenza can spread faster than COVID-19, the country changed direction and refined its plan shortly before the first case arrived on February 28, 2020 (Baker, Wilson, and Anglemyer 2020). In a major departure from pandemic influenza mitigation, NZ adopted an elimination strategy involving the early introduction of strong measures, including strict border control, quarantine, and a full lockdown, all of which are easier to apply for small island nations.

The geographical isolation of NZ has been key in both the timing of the appearance of COVID-19 and the nature of the government's response (Henrickson 2020). NZ's relatively low population density, at 19 per square kilometer, coupled with the country's ability to monitor and secure its clearly defined borders, provided crucial advantages. The secluded location of NZ accounted for its comparatively late exposure to COVID-19, enabling it to observe the pandemic unfold in China, South Korea, and Italy and learn from their early experiences. However, while we examine how NZ was able to eliminate COVID-19 by closing its border and imposing a strict lockdown with an effective communication strategy, we also consider limitations and weaknesses associated with poor management of cases at the border, delayed contact tracing and testing, and an underfunded and ill-equipped public health system.

6.3   New Zealand's Policy Responses to COVID-19

6.3.1   Public Health Response

The NZ government has been closely monitoring the spread of the virus through China and into Thailand, Japan, and South Korea. On January 24, the Ministry of Health set up an incident management team to closely monitor and respond to the international situation and provide public advice and information, although the risk to NZ at this point was assessed as "low" (Ministry of Health NZ 2020a). The government began to charter Air NZ flights to evacuate New Zealanders from affected regions on January 30. New Zealanders returning from China were quarantined for 14 days at a military facility. The WHO (2020b) declared the novel coronavirus outbreak to be a "public health emergency of international concern" on January 30. On February 3, the NZ government placed entry restrictions on foreign nationals traveling from, or transiting through, Mainland China, including Chinese international students. The first official confirmed case of COVID-19 was recorded on February 28 in a NZ resident returning from Iran. The government banned arrivals from Iran that same day, followed by northern Italy and South Korea on March 2 and all cruise ships on March 15. The WHO (2020b) officially declared a pandemic on March 11.v

NZ's efforts to tackle the spread of COVID-19 were orchestrated using an all-of-government approach, predominantly led by the All-of-Government Controller John Ombler, the Ministry of Health, and the National Emergency Management Agency. On March 6, the Emergency Management Agency activated the National Crisis Management Centre (NCMC) to coordinate the national response to COVID-19. The All-of-Government Controller was appointed to lead the NCMC, supported by the

Director-General of Health, the Director of Civil Defence and Emergency Management, the Police Commissioner, and the Ministry of Business, Innovation and Employment. An Operational Command Centre was established within the NCMC to provide operational oversight and day-to-day coordination of response activities across national agencies (National Crisis Management Centre 2020).

By mid-March, it was clear that community transmission was beginning to occur in NZ and the country did not have sufficient testing and contact tracing capacity at this point to contain the virus. NZ's options and preparedness were further constrained by a longstanding lack of public health investment and capability (Gorman and Horn 2020). Early disease modeling indicated that NZ could expect the pandemic to spread widely, overwhelm the health system, and disproportionately burden the indigenous Māori and Pasifika populations who already suffer high health inequalities from pandemic infectious disease (Summers et al. 2020). As a result, when there were 28 active cases, the government made the historic decision to close NZ's borders from midnight on March 19 to anyone who is not an NZ citizen, permanent resident, or their children and partners. Citizens and residents arriving in NZ after this date were required to self-isolate at home for 14 days.

NZ has been widely praised for acting "early" to contain the virus (Jamieson 2020; Henrickson 2020; Robert 2020). However, during the seven days from the WHO declaring a pandemic to NZ's border closure, Gorman and Horn (2020) estimate that approximately 40% of the eventual subtypes of the SARS-CoV-2 virus entered the country, indicating NZ could and should have imposed its border closure earlier before the peak in infections occurred. In contrast, Taiwan began immediate border management measures including initial health screening and exclusion of air passengers as soon as the WHO was informed of the outbreak in Wuhan on December 31, 2019, with more extensive border screening occurring in late January and entry restrictions to non-citizens in early March (Summers et al. 2020). Despite Taiwan's closer proximity to the source of the pandemic and higher population density, its earlier introduction of border control measures likely accounts for a substantially lower case rate of 20.7 per million compared with NZ's 278.0 per million as of August 2020 (Summers et al. 2020).

By March 21, 2020, there were 52 cases in NZ. The Report of the WHO-China Joint Mission on COVID-19 (2020) showed that SARS-CoV-2 was behaving more like severe acute respiratory syndrome than pandemic influenza, in terms of its longer incubation period and transmissibility, suggesting that containment was possible with a sufficiently vigorous response. In light of this and the rising cases in NZ, national leaders decisively moved from their pandemic plan entirely oriented to influenza with limited applicability to other pandemic disease, to a COVID-19-tailored approach focusing on suppressing community spread with a goal of COVID-19 elimination (Jefferies et al. 2020). Despite the detrimental economic impact this approach would have on the agricultural, hospitality, and tourism industries, the government considered that investing in prevention and elimination would be more efficient and cost-effective than having to continuously mitigate an uncontained virus (Jamieson 2020).

Ardern announced the establishment of a four-level alert system on March 21 that could be applied nationwide or to specific areas (New Zealand Government 2020b). Under level one (prepare), COVID-19 is considered to be contained in NZ, but uncontrolled overseas with sporadic imported cases. In response, border entry measures are put in place to minimize the risk of importing COVID-19 cases; intensive testing is undertaken, with rapid contract tracing for any positive case, but no restrictions are imposed on personal movement or gatherings. Under level two (reduce), COVID-19 is still contained in NZ, but limited community transmission could occur with active clusters in more than one region. Therefore, restrictions are tightened on public gatherings with physical distancing of two meters enforced between people in all public venues. The country was placed under alert level two on March 22. The next day, the government issued an Epidemic Notice under section 5 of the Epidemic Preparedness Act 2006 and alert level three (restrict) was announced, meaning multiple cases of community transmission and active clusters are occurring in several regions. Under level three people are instructed to stay-at-home in their "bubble," other than for essential personal movement, and work from home where possible. Public venues must close but certain essential businesses can remain open.

On March 25, a State of National Emergency was declared under section 66 of the Civil Defence Emergency Management Act 2002, activating special legal powers, approximately 12 hours before an announced move to alert level four (lockdown) on March 26 for an initial four-week period. At this level, the entire population must remain in their homes, except for essential reasons such as short periods of exercise, and travel is severely limited. All public gatherings are banned, while non-essential businesses and educational facilities must close. The first COVID-19-related death in NZ was reported on March 2, when confirmed and probable cases had reached 514 (Ministry of Health NZ 2020b). The border closure and sudden move to alert level four came as a surprise to many people, since NZ is a significant tourist destination. There were numerous reports of tourists struggling to leave NZ, as commercial airlines began to cancel flights and drop their routes into NZ (Lock 2020). The government responded by extending the visas of visitors, students, and temporary migrant workers who were unable to leave NZ due to the border closure and international travel restrictions until the end of September 2020 (Collins 2020). This was extended for a further two months under the "COVID-19 short-term visitor visa" to provide more time for visitors and temporary migrants to organize flights home (Moir 2020).

During the lockdown period, the NCMC published a National Action Plan to coordinate the national response during level four, followed by another Action Plan to direct the all-of-government response while transitioning out of lockdown. These Plans were accompanied by a COVID-19 Māori Response Action Plan to establish a strategic framework to address the indigenous health inequities in NZ and protect, prevent and mitigate the impacts of COVID-19 within iwi, hapū, whānau, and Māori communities. The plan facilitated the adoption of culturally appropriate approaches in the design and delivery of services, an increase in outreach services for vulnerable Māori without access to healthcare, and a Māori-focused communication campaign to provide relevant and up-to-date information on protecting their wellbeing during the pandemic (Ministry of Health NZ 2020c).

Following a lack of self-isolation enforcement and several non-compliant returnees, the government announced on April 9 that every person arriving in NZ would have to go into mandatory quarantine/managed isolation for 14 days at an approved facility (repurposed hotels). Each individual is required to have two COVID-19 tests taken on days three and twelve of their time in quarantine. By April 23, the number of cases had increased to 1,451, of whom 1,065 had recovered and 16 had died (Ministry of Health NZ 2020d). Lockdown restrictions in NZ were extended until April 27, 2020, at which point the country moved back to alert level three for two weeks. Several days later, the government announced that some businesses including construction and forestry were permitted to reopen, as well as shopping for essential items under strict regulations governing personal contact. On May 13, the COVID-19 Public Health Response Act 2020 was enacted to provide a bespoke legal framework for managing the public health risks posed by COVID-19. The Act empowers the Minister of Health to issue orders in relation to the movement of people, isolation or quarantine, physical distancing, and provision of information for contact tracing. The country re-entered level two on May 14 shortly after the last known COVID-19 case was identified in the community, which marked the end of identified community spread at that time.

The stringent lockdown was undoubtedly successful in suppressing the incidence of COVID-19 and community transmission, with the daily number of cases dropping below ten by the end of April (Robert 2020). However, it is important to note that countries such as Australia and Taiwan were essentially able to achieve similar disease suppression using a more relaxed, and less economically punitive, strategy with fewer social restrictions because of their superior contact tracing and testing abilities (Gorman and Horn 2020). In particular, Taiwan's well-developed pandemic institutions, with extensive contact tracing abilities through both manual and digital approaches, meant that potential cases could be identified and swiftly isolated without having to impose stringent restrictions on movement in the form of local and national lockdowns (Summers et al. 2020). In contrast, NZ's contact tracing methods did not involve a centralized digital approach involving mobile phone applications and telecommunications data until May 2020, necessitating a national lockdown until the Ministry of Health was able to strengthen its contact tracing and testing capacity (Verrall 2020).

After a slow start, testing kits gradually became available, and testing for COVID-19 went from just 12 tests conducted by March 9 to a daily average of 3,870 tests in April and 4,571 in May (Jamieson 2020). The government introduced the NZ COVID Tracer App on May 20 and encouraged people to download it on their mobile phones in order to scan QR codes displayed by businesses upon entry. In the event of exposure to the virus, the Ministry of Health is then able to contact users who have been in those areas via the Tracer App. On June 9, the government announced a move to alert level one, declaring that there were no more active cases of COVID-19 in NZ, 103 days after the first identified case. As of June 11, NZ had an estimated total of 1,504 cases of COVID-19 and 22 deaths. However, two new cases related to the border were announced on June 16 in two sisters released prematurely from managed isolation to visit a dying parent. Ardern described the incident as an "unacceptable failure of the system" (Graham-McLay 2020).

On August 11, 2020, after 102 days without community transmission of COVID-19 outside of managed isolation, NZ announced that a cluster of four new cases had been detected in a family in South Auckland. The source remains unknown, but work on the genetics of the virus provided the best clue to this being a managed isolation and quarantine facility failure (N. Wilson, Barnard, and Kvalsvig 2020). The response from the government was to immediately reinstate stay-at-home orders at alert level three for several weeks in Auckland, and raise the alert level to two for the rest of the country. The government moved to tighten systems at the border and in isolation facilities, as well as conduct widespread testing. On this occasion, the time between the imposition of restrictions and moving the country back to alert level one on October 8 was 57 days. This outbreak was limited to 179 known cases and three deaths, of which 61% of cases were Pacific peoples and 22% were Maori (N. Wilson, Barnard, and Kvalsvig 2020).

Despite early evidence-based advocacy from public health experts (Kvalsvig et al. 2020) and advice from the WHO, mandatory mass masking to prevent the spread of respiratory infections only became part of the NZ government's approach from August 2020 during the second localized outbreak of community transmission. Unlike the first outbreak, people were required to wear facemasks on public transport and encouraged to wear them in indoor public spaces. Again, this delayed use of face masks stands in contrast to Taiwan's approach, which had a long-established culture of mask use by its public following the SARS epidemic. Summers et al. (2020) note how Taiwan had a proactive policy of supporting production and national distribution of masks to all residents during the pandemic from February 2020 onwards, requiring masks to be worn in confined indoor environments even during periods of no community transmission.

6.3.2   Economic Policy Response

While NZ's elimination strategy has resulted in a low prevalence of COVID-19 compared to most other countries, one significant trade-off from its border closure and lockdown measures is the economic cost. The restrictions placed on activity in the June quarter contributed to the sharpest fall in real GDP on record, with a quarterly decline of 12.2%, causing NZ to experience its first recession since the global financial crisis in 2008. The IMF's (2020) latest World Economic Outlook Update projects the NZ economy to contract by 6.1% in 2020. The return to higher alert levels in August 2020, along with restrictions on international travel, resulted in continued downward pressure on economic growth, mostly concentrated in Auckland. However, the effective containment of COVID-19 and lifting of restrictions enabled most industries to return to normal operations, resulting in the economy bouncing back and GDP growing 14% in the September quarter (Stats NZ 2020c). The long-term effects of the pandemic and closed international borders have had specific and varied impacts at the industry level. Sectors reliant on international arrivals, including hospitality, accommodation, transport, retail, and education, are likely to operate well below capacity for a prolonged period.

The government began to announce and implement a range of economic policies in mid-March, starting with an initial NZ$12.1 billion COVID-19 Economic Response Package. Representing 4% of the country's GDP, the response package was one of the largest in the world on a per capita basis (Robertson 2020a). The package included NZ$5.1 billion in wage subsidies for affected businesses to pay workers up to 80% of their normal wages or salary rather than making staff redundant; NZ$126 million in COVID-19 leave and self-isolation support; NZ$2.8 billion income support package for the most vulnerable, including a permanent NZ$25 per week benefit increase and a doubling of the Winter Energy Payment for 2020; and NZ$100 million redeployment package (Robertson 2020a).

The government also provided targeted support to the aviation sector, including a debt funding agreement with Air New Zealand of up to NZ$900 million, without which the country would be at risk of not having a national airline to continue freight operations and domestic flights.

On May 14, 2020, the government established the COVID-19 Response and Recovery Fund (CRRF), setting aside NZ$50 billion to help rebuild the economy and support recovery from the pandemic. Of this, NZ$4 billion will be used for business support, including an extension of the wage subsidy scheme for businesses with a 50% drop in revenue; NZ$230 million is set to encourage entrepreneurship to kick-start growth; and NZ$900 million is allocated to support the Māori and Pacific community (Robertson 2020b). The government also announced a NZ$400 million Tourism Recovery Package to support tourism operators and drive domestic tourism. The package includes a Strategic Tourism Assets Protection Programme comprising over NZ$230 million in grants and loans for 126 tourism businesses to help protect the jobs of around 3,000 people employed in the industry; NZ$30 million for Māori tourism businesses; NZ$50 million for a Regional Events Fund; and NZ$10 million to help businesses adapt to the new reality by developing digital capability and strategies. In response to the Auckland COVID-19 resurgence in August 2020, the wage subsidy scheme was reintroduced for two weeks, including NZ$585.80 for each employee working 20 hours or more a week and NZ$350 for each employee working less than 20 hours a week. In the event of a future resurgence and alert level escalation, the government has prepared a support payment for businesses that experience a minimum 30% decline in revenue over a 14-day period (New Zealand Treasury 2020). In addition, a short-term absence payment of NZ$350 will be available from mid-February 2021 to help employers support eligible workers to stay home while waiting for a COVID-19 test result.

6.4 New Zealand's Policy Implementation

6.4.1 *Analytical and Political Capacity*

NZ's relatively effective handling of the pandemic and management of community transmission thus far has often been attributed to its geographical good fortune, as a fairly small and remote island nation with clearly monitored borders. While acknowledging these advantages, NZ's effective response is also a result of political choices and strong crisis leadership. The pandemic has tested the leadership and communication abilities of political leaders globally, which has in turn shaped public attitude and compliance with pandemic control measures in each country. Compared to the responses of other countries, the NZ government has excelled in term of its clearly communicated science-led approach. However, its operational capacity faced constraints by a lack of anticipatory policymaking to prepare for a pandemic, weak testing and contact tracing capability, and an underfunded public health system.

From the early phase of the crisis PM Jacinda Ardern prioritized public health, seeking to deliver on her pledge to protect all New Zealanders from the effects of COVID-19. The government's initial focus was to communicate clearly and reassure the public that expert advice had been taken in opting for a particular strategic approach (McGuire et al. 2020). During a post-cabinet press conference on March 16 Ardern stated

> What I want to be really clear on is that there are different models out there around the world that have had different experiences with COVID-19. We do not want to be Italy. We do not want to be those countries who have experienced mass outbreaks . . . What we're going to do is make sure that we take the actions that are required to keep New Zealanders safe, but I'll listen to the evidence and advice around what is the best way to do that.
>
> (Ardern 2020)

Ardern recognized that an evidence-based approach involving specialist expertise, rather than political ideology, was critical to effective policymaking in response to a global pandemic. Epidemiological data and qualified experts, including doctors from within NZ and overseas, were widely sought for commentary in the media and led the national response. In particular, NZ's Director-General of Health Ashley Bloomfield led the near-daily press conferences alongside Ardern. Bloomfield calmly and clearly communicated many complex health issues around COVID-19 to help the public understand how the decisions were being led by science and data. Ardern and Bloomfield have stayed firmly on the same page throughout the crisis, in stark contrast to the strained relationship between President Donald Trump and leading infectious disease expert Anthony Fauci in the United States (Mazey and Richardson 2020).

The government ensured the public remained informed by conducting regular briefings and press conferences on the country's response and progress in tackling the virus. The press conferences were delivered in English and included an NZ sign language interpreter, while translations of COVID-19 materials were made available in Te Reo Māori and 26 other languages. Ardern also engaged in a more personable and informal communication style by participating in a series of Facebook and Instagram Live broadcasts to update the public and directly answer questions about COVID-19. The use of social media platforms was seemingly effective in reaching a wider and younger audience to educate and share detailed information in a more relaxed and approachable manner. According to McGuire et al. (2020), such broadcasts helped to "build a shared experience of COVID-19, supplementing the more institutional role of formal messaging with a human level of authenticity." The government employed clear language and direction to help the public understand their goals and obligations. For example, Ardern introduced an alert level system and asked New Zealanders to stay in their household "bubble" as a way of social distancing. These concepts convey crucial scientific advice and rules in a concise format and quickly became part of New Zealander's everyday vocabulary (S. Wilson 2020).

Once lockdown measures were in place, the government began to emphasize the importance of national unity and social solidarity. In particular, Ardern appealed for individuals to be kind and compassionate, and framed combating the pandemic as "our response" and the work of a "unified team of 5 million" (S. Wilson 2020). The government adopted the campaign slogan "Unite Against COVID-19" as NZ's overarching mission, in order to persuade New Zealanders to bind together to "slow the spread and put NZ in the best position for recovery" (National Crisis Management Centre 2020). Such rhetoric helped to garner community support while working as an effective mobilizing device to ensure public acceptance and adherence to a number of burdensome pandemic-control measures. By fostering a sense of shared purpose and national unity, the discourse quickly shifted to eliminating the virus rather than simply managing or suppressing cases (Mazey and Richardson 2020). During a Facebook Live Broadcast on April 20,, 2020, Ardern reaffirmed this approach:

> Success doesn't mean zero COVID-19 cases. It means zero tolerance for cases, which means as soon as we know we have a case, we go in straight away, we're testing around that person, we're isolating them, we contact trace, and we find out all the people who may have been in contact with them while they could have passed it on. That's how we keep stamping out COVID cases whenever they come up.
>
> (Basu 2020)

This personable and transparent style of communication also worked to build trust in the government and its handling of the pandemic. On account of NZ's unitary system of government, Ardern has not had to compete for political authority nor contend with the policymaking implications and political divergences typically associated with devolved or federal systems (Mazey and Richardson 2020). This stands in contrast to leaders in the United States, Australia, and the United Kingdom, who have often had to negotiate national COVID-19 policy responses with subnational elected leaders. In NZ, there is a strong central government and limited local government, although local councils applied bans to public gatherings, theaters, libraries, and other facilities at the same time as the central government called for such measures. Thus, there was significant cross-party support for the Ardern-led response and minimal intergovernmental conflict, which translated into swift action and high levels of public confidence in the government. Ardern's response to the pandemic was rewarded with a landslide re-election on October 17, 2020, allowing the Labor party to govern alone.

An international poll undertaken by Colmar Brunton (2020a) in early April, when the country had moved into a full national lockdown, showed that 88% of respondents believed they could "trust the NZ government to make the right decisions on COVID-19." Comparatively, this is far above the 59% average trust in government polled across the G7 countries. More broadly, the poll revealed how the public's trust in the NZ government to deal successfully with national problems has soared from 59% pre-crisis to 86% at the end of April. However, the latest poll conducted by Colmar Brunton (2020b) in June 2020 showed signs that public trust in government is waning, dropping from 86% to 77%. An increasing number of New Zealanders – 18% in April to 29% in June – are claiming that the government has focused too much on health and not enough on the economy. This declining support has been expressed through anti-lockdown protests and "freedom marches" across NZ in response to reinstated restrictions after the outbreak of COVID-19 in August 2020 (Bayer 2020).

6.4.2 *Operational Capacity Constraints*

However, while the NZ government adopted a clear communication strategy and collaborated with experts to effectively eliminate COVID-19, the pandemic has exposed major shortcomings in its operational capacity. Unlike Taiwan, Singapore, and South Korea's broader experience of pandemics including severe acute respiratory syndrome (SARS) and Middle East respiratory syndrome (MERS), NZ's response was reliant on its influenza pandemic plan, and it had failed to learn the same lessons as its Asian neighbors to prepare for COVID-19. Taiwan's responsiveness to pandemic diseases is embedded in its national institutions with a dedicated Centre for Disease Control established in 1990. Following the SARS epidemic, Taiwan carried out extensive planning and established a National Health Command Centre (NHCC) in 2004, dedicated to responding to large outbreaks of emerging communicable diseases while acting as the operational command point for direct communications among central, regional and local authorities (Wang, Ng, and Brook 2020). The NHCC unified a central command system that includes the Central Epidemic Command Centre, the Biological Pathogen Disaster Command Centre, and the Central

Medical Emergency Operations Centre. This prior preparation led to the rapid implementation of control measures to respond to COVID-19 in January 2020, such as entry restrictions, health screening before passengers could deplane, systematic quarantine, contact tracing, and cluster control without needing the strict national lockdown used in NZ (Summers et al. 2020).

Taiwan's readiness stands in contrast to NZ's largely non-existent pandemic infrastructure, including a dedicated public health agency equipped with the skills and resources to prevent and manage pandemics and other public health threats. The Communicable Disease Centre – NZ's equivalent organization to Taiwan's Centre for Disease Control – was closed in 1992. The absence of an established institution to address pandemic infectious disease resulted in slow uptake and implementation of essential digital technologies for disease surveillance. The government's decision to "go hard" by closing NZ's borders and placing the population under strict lockdown was arguably the only feasible option available given its severely limited public health system and weak testing and contact tracing capabilities. NZ's national pandemic preparedness was constrained by limited intensive care unit beds – 4.6 per 100,000 population compared to Australia's 8.9 per 100,000 (Betteridge and Henderson 2020); low numbers of ventilators and extracorporeal membrane oxygenation (ECMO); a shortage of intensivists and public health workers; poorly resourced and performing Public Health Units with consequent effects on supplies of Personal Protective Equipment, surveillance and case-tracking and testing capacity (Gorman and Horn 2020).

NZ's reactive policymaking became particularly apparent through mismanagement of its strict border controls and associated quarantine processes. As international flights resumed post-lockdown and NZ citizens and residents started to return in large numbers, the government had set up mandatory 14-day managed isolation in designated hotels. Officials were instructed to test those in quarantine on days three and twelve of their isolation. However, implementation often failed on the ground with the media uncovering a number of cases involving people being released from quarantine early without prior testing or escaping from the hotels and bypassing lax security measures (Mazey and Richardson 2020). Despite being considerably unprepared for the pandemic, resulting in delays and oversights in its handling of the crisis, the NZ government has generally responded to errors and oversights by learning and correcting them. A review into managed isolation was conducted and significant changes made, including an increase in the number of clinical and non-clinical staff at each facility to ensure health checks and testing are consistently delivered; doubling of on-the-ground NZ Defence Force staff to manage the quarantine process; tightened security for transferring returnees; and more frequent testing of staff at the border, workers in managed isolation facilities and airline crews (Woods 2020). Its contact tracing and testing system is now set up and widely available across the country after the slow start and face mask use is now required on public transport. While there have been a small number of resurgences of COVID-19 in the community since the outbreak in August 2020, the government has moved quickly to contain the virus without resorting to lockdown measures, indicating that the government's restructurings are working effectively.

6.5 Continuing Challenges

Despite the NZ government's demonstrated achievements in stemming foreign and community transmission of COVID-19, reliance on strict border management and lockdown measures have created lasting challenges as ongoing pandemic management cements itself as the "new normal." In this section, we consider the social and economic implications of NZ's strategy, highlighting the potential exacerbation of underlying inequalities experienced by native Māori and Pasifika populations, severe financial losses endured by specific sectors of the economy, and indirect consequences for migrant workers and their families.

6.5.1 Social and Economic Implications

Though NZ is a wealthy and relatively equitable country, with a high Human Development Index (HDI) ranking and moderate levels of income inequality and poverty (OECD 2019), underlying disparities in health and socio-economic outcomes for native Māori and Pacific Islander populations are a persistent source of inequality (Poata-Smith 2013; Chin et al. 2018; Ministry of Health NZ 2018). Relative to European-originating populations – or Pākehā – Māori and Pacific Islander populations have significantly shorter life expectancies, almost triple the rate of unemployment, and double the incidence of childhood poverty (Stats NZ 2020a). NZ's strategy for managing the pandemic has both responded to, and potentially aggravated, these expressions of inequality (Khalil 2020). The prevalence of underlying health problems render Māori and Pacific Islander populations particularly susceptible to infectious disease and evidence suggests these groups carry a far higher risk of mortality from COVID-19 (Steyn et al. 2020). This heightened vulnerability overlaps with discriminatory access to NZ's already underfunded healthcare system (Graham and Masters-Awatere 2020), such that early pandemic modeling and policy analysis identified the importance of pursuing an elimination strategy through stringent border closures and lockdown policies to protect at risk groups (Ministry of Health NZ 2020d). While this response has been applauded for safeguarding Māori and Pacific Islander communities who might otherwise have been severely affected by uncontained community transmission, initial research has indicated that these policies have also "furthered the marginalization of communities at the margins" (Elers et al. 2021, 109). Lockdown measures were seen to be particularly detrimental to these communities, as restrictions on non-essential travel and gatherings disrupted collective cultural practices and disconnected vulnerable individuals from social resources (Elers et al. 2021), while the government's fiscal stimulus measures have prioritized support for the private sector over marginalized communities (Khalil 2020). Māori populations have historically fared disproportionately poorly during economic crises affecting NZ and, indeed, Māori and Pacific Islander unemployment rates are projected to increase more steeply over the course of the pandemic than for other ethnic groups (Ministry of Māori Development 2020).

NZ's broad trade-off between safeguarding public health and permitting the continuation of normal social and economic life has also had repercussions for the wider economy. Perhaps the most obvious drawback to NZ's strict border control policies has been the financial impact for sectors of the economy that rely, directly or indirectly, on international travel. The tourism and hospitality industries have been among the hardest hit by the pandemic, but the unilateral cessation of non-resident international arrivals has also disrupted the flow of seasonal workers and working holiday-makers who comprise a significant portion of NZ's agricultural workforce.

As mentioned in Section 1, NZ's tourism industry accounts for 8.4% of employment and contributes 9.3% of GDP (Stats NZ 2020b). International tourism constitutes a major share of revenue for the industry, approximately 41% for the year ending March 2020 (Stats NZ 2020b). Although increased domestic tourism may partially offset this downturn, anticipated losses are expected to amount to a 3–5% reduction in contribution to GDP and substantial job losses (Smith 2020). The loss of international arrivals has been particularly acute for Air New Zealand, the national carrier and third-largest employer, which initially cut 95% of its flights due to the border closure and domestic lockdown measures (Carroll 2020). It has estimated that its revenue could result in a loss of NZ$5 billion (on a reported operating revenue of NZ$5.8 billion in 2019), and it has already announced plans to make up to 1,460 cabin crew employees redundant as well as 387 pilot redundancies (Carroll 2020). In addition to sector-specific stimulus measures outlined in Section 3, the government has launched services to provide support to businesses and individuals within the sector through information updates, skill development, redeployment, and guidance (Tourism New Zealand 2021). One widely-discussed policy option has been to implement a "travel bubble" permitting trans-Tasman travel between Australia, NZ and select Pacific Island Countries, on the provision that community transmission was sufficiently controlled in participating locales and quarantine measures observed (Hunt 2021). Australia is the largest source of tourist arrivals for NZ (Smith 2020), and with similarly few daily confirmed cases of COVID-19 as of March 2021 (Johns Hopkins University and Medicine 2021), it could present a relatively low-risk opportunity for resuming limited international tourism. As of February 2021, only unidirectional quarantine-free travel involving NZ citizens traveling to Australia has been agreed upon, though the Ardern government maintains plans to introduce bi-directional travel in the coming months (Hunt 2021).

Beyond impacts on the tourism and hospitality industries, strict border restrictions have drastically reduced the availability of migrant labor within the agricultural sector – particularly for horticultural employers reliant on Pacific seasonal workers and working holiday visa holders (Nagar 2020; Bedford 2020). Depending on the time of year, Pacific Islanders participating in the Recognised Seasonal Employer (RSE) scheme and working holiday visa holders can make up over a third of the horticultural labor force (Gämperle 2018). Estimates provided by the NZ Institute for Economic Research indicated that the industry was already experiencing labor shortages, particularly during peak harvesting periods, prior to COVID-19 (Gämperle 2018). With border closures effectively halving the number of RSE workers remaining in NZ and reducing working holiday visa holders to one-seventh of their seasonal average (Bedford 2020), these shortages have been significantly exacerbated (Nagar 2020). The implications for industry and the economy are dire, with employers having to discard crops that cannot be harvested, potentially jeopardizing NZ$9.5 billion worth of produce (Nagar 2020). It has also placed NZ's temporary migrant workers – of whom there were 303,000 in March 2020 – into precarious circumstances, being unable to draw upon the same healthcare, welfare, and employment rights that residents and citizens enjoy, while not necessarily having financial means to support themselves, their families, or to return home (Collins 2020). Moreover, the RSE scheme is promoted as one of New Zealand's flagship development initiatives with Pacific Island Countries; the remittances sent home by seasonal migrant workers are an important source of income for nine participating countries and disruptions to recruitment have spillover effects for those economies (Bedford 2020). As of January 2021, 2,000 RSE workers have been permitted to enter NZ in an exception to border policy, the first such concession since restrictions were introduced (Bedford 2021).

6.5.2   Recent Developments

New Zealand remained at Alert Level 1 until the Delta-variant was detected in Auckland on August 17, 2021, at which time the NZ population was only partially vaccinated. After 16 months of relative freedom, the country was immediately moved into a "hard lockdown," with Auckland remaining under Alert Level 4 for four weeks and Alert Level 3 until December 2021. This period of prolonged lockdown provided the time needed to increase vaccination rates among the most vulnerable groups. This particular outbreak, however, proved too difficult to stamp out using the methods that effectively eliminated previous outbreaks, thus the government indicated its intention to transition away from an elimination strategy to a "minimization and protection strategy" in October 2021 (Baker et al. 2021). In marking this transition, the government officially implemented its new "COVID-19 Protection Framework" in December 2021, the objective of which was to contain the spread of COVID-19 in order to keep hospitalizations as low as possible (NZ Government 2022).

Until January 2022, NZ's strict border controls and elimination strategy meant that the country experienced very low rates of COVID-19 and, therefore, few hospitalizations or deaths due to the virus, allowing time for development and delivery of vaccines before widespread COVID-19 circulation. By the end of 2021, NZ had achieved high vaccination coverage, with over 90% of the eligible population having received two doses of the Pfizer vaccination (Vattiato 2022). However, social cohesion and support for pandemic measures that characterized NZ's early response began to fracture in late 2021. Prolonged restrictions and vaccine mandates prompted distrust in the government and triggered regular anti-vaccine protests, the most notable of which involved the occupation and destruction of parliamentary grounds in Wellington for 23 days (Craymer and Menon 2022). This was accompanied by the highly transmissible Omicron-variant quickly becoming established in the community at the beginning of 2022, alongside the loosening of restrictions amid political pressure. Cases subsequently skyrocketed and a total of 1,797 people died due to COVID-19[1] from January 1 to August 26, 2022. This equates to 34 in every 100,000 New Zealanders having died due to COVID-19 during this time period (Ministry of Health NZ 2022).

6.6 Conclusion: Policy Lessons

By objective measures, NZ has been a world-leader in managing COVID-19 from a public health standpoint. The policy choices underscoring this achievement have necessitated considerable social and economic compromises (outlined above) in response to a combination of situational and institutional factors (described in Sections 2 and 3) that narrow policymaking parameters. In essence, NZ has underlying characteristics that heighten its vulnerability to a pandemic event – notably insufficient healthcare infrastructure and substantial at-risk populations – and others that confer a considerable advantage in managing those risks, including a unitary system of government with high levels of public trust, the presence of strong scientific institutions and epidemiological expertise, and the geographical benefits of being a small and secluded island nation. Against this backdrop, it is perhaps unsurprising that NZ long-pursued a strategy of elimination through border controls and strict lockdown measures to avoid the potentially catastrophic public health outcomes foreshadowed by early pandemic modeling.

In addressing opportunities for policy learning, both for NZ and for comparably situated countries, two questions stand out: (i) what could NZ do to improve its management of COVID-19 and future pandemic events? and (ii) what elements of NZ's policy response might be applicable to other countries?

In addressing the former, it is clear that the greatest shortcoming of NZ's handling of the pandemic was a lack of overall preparedness for a pandemic event stemming from weaknesses in operational capacity. Whereas several East Asian countries with previous exposure to the SARS virus were proactive in handling the pandemic, NZ was very much reactive in its approach (Summers et al. 2020). This is evident in terms of overall healthcare infrastructure, the lack of an updated pandemic response plan, and delays in implementing an effective system of contact tracing. Comparing the availability of intensive care beds per 100,000 people among similarly wealthy island countries, for example, reveals that NZ is significantly below the OECD average (Figure 6.3). Greater investment in public healthcare systems would have placed NZ in a better position to deal with the eventuality of surging cases or widespread community transmission. In lieu of a wholesale transformation of existing facilities, however, the establishment of a dedicated agency to plan and manage a national pandemic response could help mitigate those limitations. Key elements of such a response plan could prioritize faster implementation of border controls and more comprehensive contact tracing methods. Both policies could potentially reduce the need for lockdown measures and therefore ease the social and economic drawbacks of NZ's existing management paradigm. For instance, whereas NZ adopted a "wait and see" approach to border management and relied on WHO recommendations before imposing categorical border closures on March 19, Taiwan's pandemic management protocol informed the decision to close borders immediately, thus limiting the potential for imported cases at the outset and circumventing the need for lockdown measures (Summers et al. 2020). Meanwhile, Australia's management of the pandemic has demonstrated the viability of comprehensive contact tracing to manage moderate levels of community transmission while preserving a significant degree of social and economic activity (Finkel, Jasper, and Weeramanthri 2020). It's plausible that NZ's timely implementation

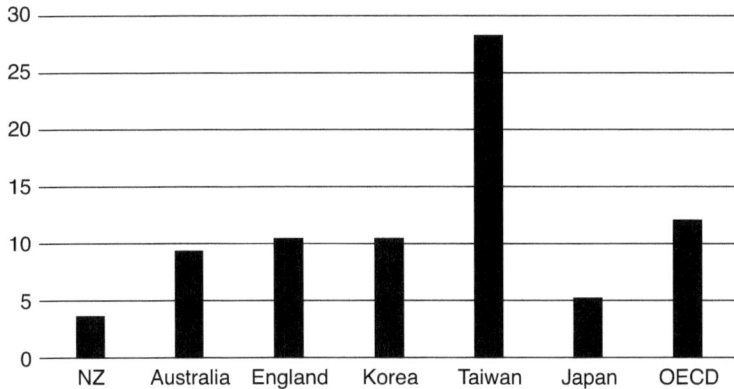

Figure 6.3 ICU beds per 100,000 people.

Source: Adapted from OECD (2020), Phua et al. (2020).

of similar policies could have averted the disruptions caused by level three and level four national lockdowns while achieving similar or better overall public health outcomes.

Despite the potential opportunities for improvement outlined above, NZ's successful management of the pandemic despite an under-resourced healthcare system confers valuable policy lessons for other countries too. Foremost among these is evidence that, particularly for small island countries with limited healthcare capacity, rapid and extensive border closures can be highly efficacious in stemming imported cases of COVID-19 and reducing overall caseload. Island nations that have enforced strict border policies have typically fared better in the management of the pandemic (Lowy Institute 2021), while those that have not taken this approach – such as the United Kingdom (Geddes 2021) – have been comparatively overwhelmed by the pandemic and lost the opportunity to pursue an elimination strategy (Patel and Sridhar 2020). Though preserving economic openness has been cited as a reason to avoid border closures, it is notable that NZ's economy has fared significantly better than those that have maintained open borders but, as a result, have endured "unsustainable lockdown-and-release cycles" (Patel and Sridhar 2020, 1). While NZ did not close its border promptly enough to prevent the need for lockdown measures, its strategy of swift and decisive restrictions – along with a vigilant readiness to extend and reinstate these protocols – has shown that lockdowns can be instrumental in achieving the elimination of the virus. That these measures were adopted and maintained with high levels of public support speaks to the key roles that political leadership, operationalized scientific expertise and clear communication have played in NZ's overall pandemic management

(S. Wilson 2020). To some extent, this may reflect the practical advantages of a unitary system of government that is better able to coordinate a centralized pandemic response, but it also highlights the benefit of administering a response plan having achieved bipartisan support by prioritizing public health ahead of political and economic interests.

Note

1 That is, where COVID-19 was related to the cause of death.

References

Ardern, Jacinda. 2020. Post-Cabinet Press Conference: Monday, 16 March 2020 Press Conference. https://www.beehive.govt.nz/sites/default/files/2020-03/Press%20Conference%2016%20March%202020.pdf.

Baker, Michael G., Amanda Kvalsvig, Sue Crengle, Matire Harwood, Collin Tukuitonga, Bryan Betty, John Bonning, Nick Wilson. 2021. 'The Next Phase in Aotearoa New Zealand's COVID-19 Response: A Tight Suppression Strategy May be the Best Option'. *The New Zealand Medical Journal* 134(1546): 8–16. https://journal.nzma.org.nz/journal-articles/the-next-phase-in-aotearoa-new-zealands-covid-19-response-tight-suppression-may-be-optimal-for-health-equity-and-wellbeing-in-the-months-ahead

Baker, Michael G., Nick Wilson, and Andrew Anglemyer. 2020. 'Successful Elimination of Covid-19 Transmission in New Zealand'. *New England Journal of Medicine* 383(8): e56. https://doi.org/10.1056/NEJMc2025203.

Basu, Arindam. 2020. 'Why Coronavirus Emerges in Clusters, and How New Zealand Plans to Eliminate Outbreaks after Lockdown'. *The Conversation* (blog). 23 April 2020. http://theconversation.com/why-coronavirus-emerges-in-clusters-and-how-new-zealand-plans-to-eliminate-outbreaks-after-lockdown-136942.

Bayer, Kurt. 2020. 'Covid 19 Coronavirus: Hundreds Turn out for Anti-Lockdown Protests'. *NZ Herald*, 5 September 2020, sec. New Zealand. https://www.nzherald.co.nz/nz/covid-19-coronavirus-hundreds-turn-out-for-anti-lockdown-protests/AHE2NJJY3VMTTXLAUHLWIJOODY/.

Bedford, Charlotte. 2020. 'New Zealand's Seasonal Labour Shortage, and How to Solve It.' *DevPolicy Blog*, 7.

Bedford, Charlotte. 2021. 'Pacific Seasonal Workers Return for New Zealand's Summer Harvest.' *DevPolicy Blog*, 5.

Betteridge, Toby, and Seton Henderson. 2020. 'Intensive Care in New Zealand: Time for a National Network' New Zealand Medical Journal 133(1520): 2.

Bretschger, Lucas, Elise Grieg, Paul J. J. Welfens, and Tian Xiong. 2020. 'COVID-19 Infections and Fatalities Developments: Empirical Evidence for OECD Countries and Newly Industrialized Economies'. *International Economics and Economic Policy* 17(4): 801–847. https://doi.org/10.1007/s10368-020-00487-x.

Bromfield, Nicholas, and Allan McConnell. 2020. 'Two Routes to Precarious Success: Australia, New Zealand, COVID-19 and the Politics of Crisis Governance'.

International Review of Administrative Sciences, December, 002085232097246. https://doi.org/10.1177/0020852320972465.

Carroll, Melanie. 2020. 'Coronavirus: Up to 1460 Air NZ Cabin Crew Jobs to Go in Airline's Covid-19 Hit'. *Stuff.Co.Nz*, 9 April 2020, sec. business. https://www.stuff.co.nz/business/industries/120946954/cronavirus-reports-that-1450-air-nz-cabin-crew-jobs-to-go-amid-airlines-covid19-hit.

Chin, Marshall H., Paula T. King, Rhys G. Jones, Bryn Jones, Shanthi N. Ameratunga, Naoko Muramatsu, and Sarah Derrett. 2018. 'Lessons for Achieving Health Equity Comparing Aotearoa/New Zealand and the United States'. *Health Policy* 122(8): 837–853. https://doi.org/10.1016/j.healthpol.2018.05.001.

Collins, Francis L. 2020. 'Caring for 300,000 Temporary Migrants in New Zealand Is a Crucial Missing Link in Our Coronavirus Response'. *The Conversation* (blog). 23 March 2020. http://theconversation.com/caring-for-300-000-temporary-migrants-in-new-zealand-is-a-crucial-missing-link-in-our-coronavirus-response-134152.

Colmar Brunton. 2020a. 'COVID TIMES: Backing New Zealand'. Kantar New Zealand, 24 April 2020, https://www.kantarnewzealand.com/wp-content/uploads/2019/05/COVID-Times-24-April-2020-1.pdf

Colmar Brunton. 2020b. 'COVID TIMES: How COVID-19 Is Changing Us'. Kantar New Zealand, 1 July 2020, https://www.kantarnewzealand.com/wp-content/uploads/2019/05/COVID-Times-3-July-2020.pdf

Craymer, Lucy and Praveen Menon. 2022. 'New Zealand's Parliament Protest Ends with Clashes, Arrests'. *Reuters*. https://www.reuters.com/world/asia-pacific/new-zealand-police-dismantle-tents-tow-vehicles-clear-anti-vaccine-protests-2022-03-01/

Elers, Christine, Pooja Jayan, Phoebe Elers, and Mohan J. Dutta. 2021. 'Negotiating Health Amidst COVID-19 Lockdown in Low-Income Communities in Aotearoa New Zealand'. *Health Communication* 36(1): 109–115. https://doi.org/10.1080/10410236.2020.1848082.

Finkel, Alan, Leigh Jasper, and Tarun Weeramanthri. 2020. *National Contact Tracing Review: A Report for National Cabinet.* Commonwealth of Australia.

Gämperle, Dion. 2018. *Horticulture Labour Supply and Demand: 2018 Update.* Wellington: New Zealand Institute for Economic Research.

Geddes, Linda. 2021. 'Covid: Could Britain Have Been More like New Zealand?' *The Guardian*, 5 February 2021, sec. World news. https://www.theguardian.com/world/2021/feb/05/covid-could-britain-have-been-more-like-new-zealand.

Gorman, Des, and Murray Horn. 2020. 'On New Zealand's Weak, Strong and Muddled Management of a COVID-19 Epidemic'. *Internal Medicine Journal* 50(8): 901–904. https://doi.org/10.1111/imj.14928.

Graham, Rebekah, and Bridgette Masters-Awatere. 2020. 'Experiences of Māori of Aotearoa New Zealand's Public Health System: A Systematic Review of Two Decades of Published Qualitative Research'. *Australian and New Zealand Journal of Public Health* 44(3): 193–200. https://doi.org/10.1111/1753-6405.12971.

Graham-McLay, Charlotte. 2020. 'New Zealand Officials Admit Two Women with Covid-19 Met Friends'. *The Guardian*, 17 June 2020, sec. World News. http://www.theguardian.com/world/2020/jun/17/new-zealand-brings-in-military-after-covid-19-quarantine-fiasco.

Henrickson, Mark. 2020. 'Kiwis and COVID-19: The Aotearoa New Zealand Response to the Global Pandemic'. *The International Journal of Community and Social Development* 2(2): 121–133. https://doi.org/10.1177/25166026 20932558.

Hunt, Elle. 2021. 'New Zealand Stands by "travel Bubble" Plan despite Covid Outbreaks in Australia'. *The Guardian*, 13 January 2021, sec. World news. http://www.theguardian.com/world/2021/jan/13/new-zealand-stands-by-travel-bubble-plan-despite-covid-outbreaks-in-australia.

International Monetary Fund (IMF). 2020. *World Economic Outlook Update*. Washington, DC: International Monetary Fund (IMF).

Jamieson, Thomas. 2020. '"Go Hard, Go Early": Preliminary Lessons From New Zealand's Response to COVID-19'. *The American Review of Public Administration* 50(6–7): 598–605. https://doi.org/10.1177/0275074020941721.

Jefferies, Sarah, Nigel French, Charlotte Gilkison, Giles Graham, Virginia Hope, Jonathan Marshall, Caroline McElnay, et al. 2020. 'COVID-19 in New Zealand and the Impact of the National Response: A Descriptive Epidemiological Study'. *The Lancet Public Health* 5(11): e612–623. https://doi.org/10.1016/S2468-2667(20)30225-5.

Johns Hopkins University and Medicine. 2021. 'Coronavirus Resource Center'. 2021. https://coronavirus.jhu.edu/.

Khalil, Shaimaa. 2020. 'NZ Election: The People Left behind in Ardern's "kind" New Zealand'. *BBC News*, 13 October 2020, sec. Asia. https://www.bbc.com/news/world-asia-54444643.

Kvalsvig, Amanda, Nick Wilson, Ling Chan, Sophie Febery, Sally Roberts, Bryan Betty, and Michael G. Baker. 2020. 'Mass Masking: An Alternative to a Second Lockdown in Aotearoa.' *The New Zealand Medical Journal (Online)* 133(1517): 8–13.

Lock, Harry. 2020. 'Plans to Go Home in Tatters as International Travel Options Crumble Due to Covid-19'. *RNZ*, 24 March 2020, sec. New Zealand. https://www.rnz.co.nz/news/national/412514/plans-to-go-home-in-tatters-as-international-travel-options-crumble-due-to-covid-19.

Lowy Institute. 2021. 'Covid Performance'. *Lowy Institute*. 2021. https://interactives.lowyinstitute.org/features/covid-performance/.

Mazey, Sonia, and Jeremy Richardson. 2020. 'Lesson-Drawing from New Zealand and Covid-19: The Need for Anticipatory Policy Making'. *The Political Quarterly* 91(3): 561–570. https://doi.org/10.1111/1467-923X.12893.

McGuire, David, James E. A. Cunningham, Kae Reynolds, and Gerri Matthews-Smith. 2020. 'Beating the Virus: An Examination of the Crisis Communication Approach Taken by New Zealand Prime Minister Jacinda Ardern during the Covid-19 Pandemic'. *Human Resource Development International* 23(4): 361–379. https://doi.org/10.1080/13678868.2020.1779543.

Ministry for Primary Industries. 2019. *Situation and Outlook for Primary Industries*. Wellington: New Zealand Government.

Ministry of Business, Innovation and Employment. 2020. *Quarterly Labour Market Report*. Wellington: New Zealand Government.

Ministry of Health NZ. 2017. *New Zealand Influenza Pandemic Plan: A Framework for Action*. Wellington: New Zealand Government.

Ministry of Health NZ. 2020a. 'Novel Coronavirus Update – 24th January 2020'. *New Zealand Government*, 24 January 2020. https://www.health.govt.nz/news-media/news-items/novel-coronavirus-update-24th-january-2020.

Ministry of Health NZ. 2020b. 'Sadly, First Death from COVID-19 in New Zealand'. *New Zealand Government*, 29 March 2020. https://www.health.govt.nz/news-media/media-releases/sadly-first-death-covid-19-new-zealand.

Ministry of Health NZ. 2020c. '3 New Cases of COVID-19'. *New Zealand Government*, 23 April 2020. https://www.health.govt.nz/news-media/media-releases/3-new-cases-covid-19.

Ministry of Health NZ. 2020d. *Updated COVID-19 Māori Response Action Plan.* Wellington: New Zealand Government. https://www.health.govt.nz/publication/updated-covid-19-maori-response-action-plan.

Ministry of Health NZ. 2021. 'COVID-19: Current Cases'. *Ministry of Health.* https://www.health.govt.nz/our-work/diseases-and-conditions/covid-19-novel-coronavirus/covid-19-data-and-statistics/covid-19-current-cases.

Ministry of Health NZ. 2022. 'COVID-19 Mortality in Aotearoa New Zealand: Inequities in Risk'. https://www.health.govt.nz/system/files/documents/publications/covid-19_mortality_in_aotearoa_inequities_in_risk_september_2022_29_sept.v2.pdf

Ministry of Health NZ and Ministry of Health. 2018. Achieving Equity in Health Outcomes: Highlights of Important National and International Papers. https://natlib-primo.hosted.exlibrisgroup.com/primo-explore/fulldisplay?docid=NLNZ_ALMA11318167390002836&context=L&vid=NLNZ&search_scope=NLNZ&tab=catalogue&lang=en_US.

Ministry of Māori Development. 2020. *Economic Impact of COVID-19.* Wellington: New Zealand Government.

Moir, Jo. 2020. 'Covid-19 Visa Extensions Allow Visitors, Migrants More Time'. *RNZ*, 4 September 2020, sec. Politics. https://www.rnz.co.nz/news/political/425240/covid-19-visa-extensions-allow-visitors-migrants-more-time.

Nagar, Swati. 2020. 'NZ Needs a Plan to Help Migrant Workers Pick Fruit and Veg, or Prices Will Soar and Farms Go Bust'. *The Conversation* (blog). 25 November 2020. http://theconversation.com/nz-needs-a-plan-to-help-migrant-workers-pick-fruit-and-veg-or-prices-will-soar-and-farms-go-bust-150447.

National Crisis Management Centre. 2020. *COVID19 National Action Plan 3.* Wellington: New Zealand Government. https://covid19.govt.nz/assets/resources/legislation-and-key-documents/COVID19-National-Action-Plan-3-as-of-22-April-extended.pdf.

New Zealand Government. 2020a. 'History of the COVID-19 Alert System'. *Unite against COVID-19.* https://covid19.govt.nz/alert-system/history-of-the-covid-19-alert-system/.

New Zealand Government. 2020b. *New Zealand COVID-19 Alert Levels.* Wellington: New Zealand Government. https://covid19.govt.nz/assets/resources/tables/COVID-19-alert-levels-detailed.pdf.

New Zealand Government. 2022. *History of the COVID-19 Protection Framework (Traffic Lights).* Wellington: New Zealand Government. https://covid19.govt.nz/about-our-covid-19-response/history-of-the-covid-19-protection-framework-traffic-lights/

New Zealand Treasury. 2020. *Government Support for Businesses Recovering from COVID-19*. Wellington: New Zealand Government. https://www.treasury. govt.nz/sites/default/files/2020-12/Govt-support-business-COVID-19-Dec22 2020.pdf.

OECD. 2019. *OECD Economic Surveys: New Zealand 2019*. New Zealand: OECD Economic Surveys, OECD. https://doi.org/10.1787/b0b94dbd-en.

Organisation for Economic Cooperation and Development (OECD). 2020. 'Beyond Containment: Health Systems Responses to COVID-19 in the OECD'. OECD Policy Responses to Coronavirus (COVID-19). OECD. https://doi. org/10.1787/6ab740c0-en.

Patel, Jay, and Devi Sridhar. 2020. 'We Should Learn from the Asia–Pacific Responses to COVID-19'. *The Lancet Regional Health - Western Pacific* 5(December): 100062. https://doi.org/10.1016/j.lanwpc.2020.100062.

Phua, Jason, Mohammad Omar Faruq, Atul P. Kulkarni, Ike Sri Redjeki, Khamsay Detleuxay, Naranpurev Mendsaikhan, Kyi Kyi Sann, et al. 2020. 'Critical Care Bed Capacity in Asian Countries and Regions'. *Critical Care Medicine* 48(5): 654–662. https://doi.org/10.1097/CCM.0000000000004222.

Poata-Smith, Evan Te Ahu. 2013. 'Inequality and Māori'. In *Inequality: A New Zealand Crisis*, edited by Max Rashbrooke, 148–164. Wellington: Bridget Williams Books.

Reuters. 2020. 'New Zealand to Charter Flight to Wuhan to Help Citizens Leave'. *Reuters*, 30 January 2020. https://www.reuters.com/article/us-china-health-newzealand-idUKKBN1ZT09T.

Rice, Geoffrey W. 2020. 'How Reminders of the 1918–19 Pandemic Helped Australia and New Zealand Respond to COVID-19'. *Journal of Global History* 15(3): 421–433. https://doi.org/10.1017/S1740022820000285.

Robert, Alexis. 2020. 'Lessons from New Zealand's COVID-19 Outbreak Response'. *The Lancet Public Health* 5(11): e569–570. https://doi.org/10.1016/S2468-2667(20)30237-1.

Robertson, Grant. 2020a. '$12.1 Billion Support for New Zealanders and Business'. *New Zealand Government*, 17 March 2020. http://www.beehive.govt.nz/release/121-billion-support-new-zealanders-and-business.

Robertson, Grant. 2020b. *Summary of Initiatives in the COVID-19 Response and Recovery Fund (CRRF) Foundational Package*. Wellington: New Zealand Government. https://www.treasury.govt.nz/system/files/2020-05/b20-sum-initiatives-crrf.pdf.

Roy, Eleanor Ainge. 2020. 'New Zealand and Australia Close Borders to Foreigners amid Coronavirus Crisis'. *The Guardian*, 19 March 2020, sec. World News. http://www.theguardian.com/world/2020/mar/19/new-zealand-closes-borders-to-foreigners-amid-coronavirus-crisis.

Shaw, Richard. 2020. 'Jacinda Ardern and Labour Returned in a Landslide'. *The Conversation* (blog). 17 October 2020. https://theconversation.com/jacinda-ardern-and-labour-returned-in-a-landslide-5-experts-on-a-historic-new-zealand-election-148245.

Smith, Mark. 2020. *Economic Note: Impacts of COVID-19 on the NZ Tourism Sector*. Auckland: Auckland Savings Bank.

Stats NZ. 2020a. *2018 Census*. Wellington: New Zealand Government. https://www.stats.govt.nz/information-releases/2018-census-nz-stat-tables.

Stats NZ. 2020b. *Tourism Satellite Account: Year Ended March 2020*. Wellington: New Zealand Government.

Stats NZ. 2020c. 'Quarterly GDP Bounces Back, but COVID Still a Drag on Annual Growth'. *New Zealand Government*, 17 December 2020. https://www.stats.govt.nz/news/quarterly-gdp-bounces-back-but-covid-still-a-drag-on-annual-growth.

Steyn, Nicholas, Rachelle N. Binny, Kate Hannah, Shaun C. Hendy, Alex James, Tahu Kukutai, Audrey Lustig, et al. 2020. 'Estimated Inequities in COVID-19 Infection Fatality Rates by Ethnicity for Aotearoa New Zealand'. Preprint. *Epidemiology*. https://doi.org/10.1101/2020.04.20.20073437.

Summers, Dr Jennifer, Dr Hao-Yuan Cheng, Professor Hsien-Ho Lin, Dr Lucy Telfar Barnard, Dr Amanda Kvalsvig, Professor Nick Wilson, and Professor Michael G Baker. 2020. 'Potential Lessons from the Taiwan and New Zealand Health Responses to the COVID-19 Pandemic'. *The Lancet Regional Health - Western Pacific* 4(November): 100044. https://doi.org/10.1016/j.lanwpc.2020.100044.

Tomkins, Sandra M. 1992. 'The Influenza Epidemic of 1918–19 in Western Samoa'. *The Journal of Pacific History* 27(2): 181–197. https://doi.org/10.1080/00223349208572706.

Tourism New Zealand. 2021. 'Tourism New Zealand's Response to COVID-19'. 18 February 2021. https://www.tourismnewzealand.com/news/tourism-new-zealands-response-to-covid-19/.

Vattiato, Giorgia, Oliver Maclaren, Audrey Lustig, Rachelle N. Binny et al. 2022. 'An Assessment of the Potential Impact of the Omicron Variant of SARS-CoV-2 in Aotearoa New Zealand'. *Infectious Disease Modelling* 7(2): 94–105. https://www.ncbi.nlm.nih.gov/pmc/articles/PMC8993704/

Verrall, Dr Ayesha. 2020. *Rapid Audit of Contact Tracing for Covid-19 in New Zealand*. Wellington: University of Otago.

Wang, C. Jason, Chun Y. Ng, and Robert H. Brook. 2020. 'Response to COVID-19 in Taiwan: Big Data Analytics, New Technology, and Proactive Testing'. *JAMA* 323(14): 1341. https://doi.org/10.1001/jama.2020.3151.

Wilson, Nick, Lucy Telfar Barnard, and Dr Amanda Kvalsvig. 2020. *Potential Health Impacts from the COVID-19 Pandemic for New Zealand If Eradication Fails: Report to the NZ Ministry of Health*. Wellington: University of Otago.

Wilson, Suze. 2020. 'Pandemic Leadership: Lessons from New Zealand's Approach to COVID-19'. *Leadership* 16(3): 279–293. https://doi.org/10.1177/1742715020929151.

Woods, Megan. 2020. 'Government Strengthens Managed Isolation System'. *New Zealand Government*, 28 June 2020. http://www.beehive.govt.nz/release/government-strengthens-managed-isolation-system.

World Health Organisation. 2020a. 'Report of the WHO-China Joint Mission on Coronavirus Disease 2019 (COVID-19)'. https://www.who.int/docs/default-source/coronaviruse/who-china-joint-mission-on-covid-19-final-report.pdf.

World Health Organisation (WHO). 2020b. *Timeline: WHO's COVID-19 Response*. World Health Organisation (WHO). https://www.who.int/emergencies/diseases/novel-coronavirus-2019/interactive-timeline.

7 South Korea's Responses to COVID-19

Kilkon Ko and Yoon Kyoung Cho

7.1 Introduction

When the news about COVID-19 was first heard outside of China in January 2020, few expected it to become a global pandemic. When China suffered heavily from COVID-19 in January and February 2020, most countries did not expect that they would also be pulled into this medical horror. The limited medical information released by China triggered debates on whether the virus spread through direct contact or exposure to aerosolized liquid from the infected before the release of the preliminary China-WHO report on February 26. Uncertainty and a lack of information led to the WHO's late declaration of a global COVID-19 pandemic on March 11, 2020 when it had already proliferated globally. After the official announcement of the pandemic, unprecedented social distancing policies began to be adopted around the globe. Some countries locked down entire cities, and others closed schools and mandated facial mask-wearing.

Unlike other natural disasters, such as earthquakes, floods, hurricanes, or even epidemics such as Severe Acute Respiratory Syndrome (SARS) and Middle East respiratory syndrome-coronavirus (MERS-CoV), COVID-19 rampaged at the global level for a long time. To the best of our knowledge, few disasters have affected the world to this extent and persisted longer than three years. Because of the long-lasting nature of the COVID-19 pandemic, preliminary research done during its early phase has to be revised or updated. In South Korea, concerns about the economic and social impacts of social distancing policies led to their revision (Republic of Korea, 2020). For instance, while the South Korean government introduced stringent social distancing when there were less than 1,000 daily infection cases in 2020, it lifted its outdoor facial mask requirement on April 18, 2022, when there were more than 140,000 daily infection cases.

People's perceived risk of COVID-19 infection and subsequent harm have been significantly changed as well. As of 2022, only a few South Koreans believe that a zero-COVID-19 policy or strong lockdowns are

DOI: 10.4324/9781003362760-7

necessary to control the pandemic. Moreover, countries have had different policy responses. Response efforts were sometimes overwhelmed by environmental pressures, and natural selection is more critical than organizational adaptation, as population ecology theory suggests (Hannan and Freeman, 1977). Many countries adopted similar tests, infection tracking methods, treatments, and social distancing policies, but these efforts produced very different results and were not simply the result of differing administrative resources and capacities.

Organizational adaptation and learning require administrative capacity, which is crucial to successful policy implementation and governance quality (Addison, 2009). Administrative capacity is a multi-layered concept involving many components, including human resources, physical resources, institutional systems, and organizational structures (Ko et al., 2021). Early in the pandemic, many believed that developed countries equipped with qualified medical staff, facilities, and public healthcare systems would have greater administrative capacity to address it than developing countries. However, developed countries responded inadequately (Abbey et al., 2020). The gap between their presumed capacity and actual performance was greater than anticipated. This phenomenon should make us rethink the assumption that successful disaster response is the product of administrative capacity.

This paper adopts an evolutionary perspective, assuming that policy responses are adaptations to new situations. This perspective assumes that the strategies, focuses, and policies of one stage of a disaster will not be relevant or effective in other stages. Agile adaptation to new situations requires flexibility, which is atypical of bureaucracies. Natural selection occurs when organizations fail to adapt to new environments. We will use changes in the infection and fatality rates, available knowledge, statistical information, and related technologies in South Korea to describe the changing environment.

Finally, although dynamic situations require adaptive responses, bureaucratic inertia and resistance to learning frequently cause bureaucracies to fall into the success trap (March 1991). Past experiences are sometimes retrospectively justified as previous successes to learn, but we need to critically review response policies and evaluate our successes and mistakes. The South Korean case is unique in that it included many innovative disease testing, tracking, and treatment methods but not lockdowns, which many countries and international organizations highly valued. This chapter tries to show both positive and negative aspects of the South Korean approach to help develop South Korea's and other countries' disaster response systems.

7.2   COVID-19 Trends and Structural Differences between Stages

Infection rate trends in South Korea clearly show that COVID-19 had different magnitudes and patterns in different stages. The first infection was officially confirmed on January 20, 2020, and the number of new cases rapidly fluctuated over the next few days. However, in retrospect, the severity of the pandemic in 2020 and 2021 seems insignificant compared to that of 2022. The first graph in Figure 7.1 illustrates the number of new infection cases between January 2020 and May 2021. As the graph shows, the number of new infection cases in 2020 and 2021 were relatively small compared to those in 2022. However, when South Korea faced the first wave of the pandemic in February 2020, which originated from massive infections among the Shicheonji religious cult in Daegu, the outbreak invoked the highest alert. Accordingly, the number of newspaper articles on COVID-19 and internet searches for the keyword "COVID-19 (코로나)" were highest in early 2020 and higher than in later waves (Ko et al., 2022). Thousands of Daegu residents voluntarily stayed at home and innumerable doctors and nurses went there to help with the skyrocketing number of patients. As shown in the second graph of Figure 7.1, the first outbreak that started in February 2020 was successfully controlled within a month. The new-case distribution's kurtosis was very high, which meant that the South Korean government controlled the spread of infection within the relatively short time span of around three weeks.

The latter three graphs in Figure 7.1 show the new infection cases in 2020, 2021, and 2022. The graphs use different y-axis scales to show wild fluctuations in the number of new infection cases per year. As the future was unknown in 2020 and 2021, policy responses had to be made based on the relative change in the number of new infection cases. Considering the fact that the COVID-19 transmission mechanism was unknown, medical treatment methods were undeveloped, proper policy tools had not been identified, and vaccine availability was limited in 2020, we cannot retrospectively judge the intense response to the pandemic in 2020 as a policy failure or an overreaction. On the contrary, the South Korean government and people are to be appreciative of their quick reaction to the upsurge in COVID-19 cases, successfully flattening the curve under great uncertainty and with limited information and resources.

The number of new cases significantly dropped by the end of April 2020 and remained stagnant until early August 2020. There were sporadic community outbreaks during this period, but no major ones. Despite the relatively small number of infection cases, many regulatory policies were imposed by the central and local governments during this period. For instance, the Seoul Metropolitan government ordered all bars and nightclubs to close on May 9, 2020, after 40 cases were discovered to be linked to them. However, the government could not provide scientific evidence to justify the prohibition of ordinary business operations based on the small number of infections. Tighter operation restrictions on certain types of businesses in May 2020, when there were well under

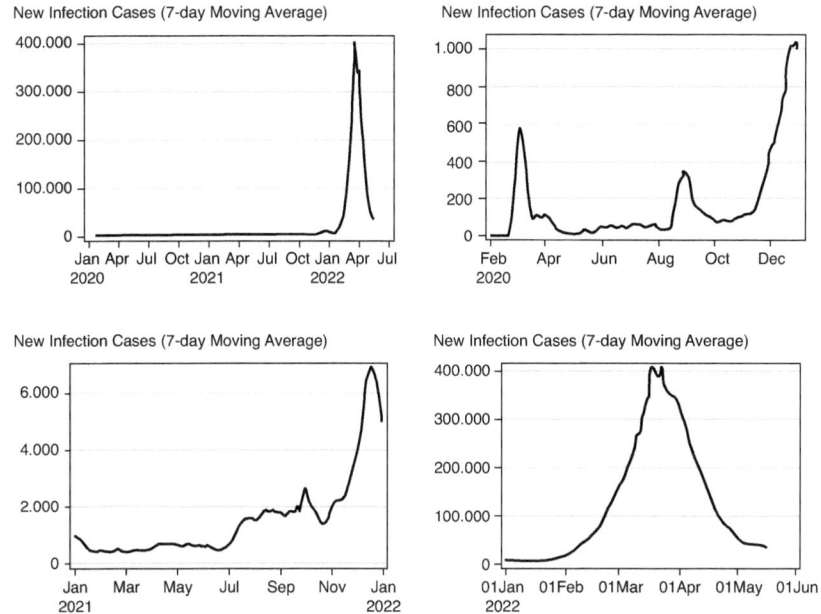

Figure 7.1 New infection cases in South Korea.

Source: Created by authors using Coronavirus Disease 19 (COVID-19) Cases in Korea in Korea Disease Control and Prevention Agency.

100 daily cases, raised questions because most businesses were permitted to operate without restriction during February 2020, when there were significantly more infection cases. However, the mayor of Seoul may have done so to produce the image that he held the decisive and charismatic leadership that many South Koreans prefer despite criticism of policy inconsistency.

In mid-August 2020, in the Seoul metropolitan area, another outbreak occurred that was alleged to have resulted from gatherings in churches and political demonstrations organized by the conservative party. However, in fact, the outbreak was related to community infections originating in health clubs, call centers, etc. During this period, the South Korean government escalated social distancing restrictions from level one to level two. However, as shown in the second graph of Figure 7.1, the highest number of cases in this period was less than the highest number as a result of the Daegu outbreak in February 2020. Despite the absence of strong scientific evidence, the South Korean government strictly prohibited political and religious gatherings. This incurred debate over whether the intent of this policy was to suppress the opposition party.

Compared to previous earlier, more community infections occurred in early November 2020. The social distancing level was elevated as a result, but the number of new cases continued to rapidly increase. At this time, the maximum number of new cases was substantially higher than that of the Daegu outbreak. Moreover, there were more days whose number of new infection cases was over 500, so the infection rate was more persistently high than before. As the infection and death rates rapidly escalated, concerns about hospital facility and medical staff shortages increased as well. Although the South Korean government raised the social distancing level to 2.5, the infection rate did not decrease. From December 2020 to the end of February 2021, the number of daily cases consistently exceeded 200 despite the national government banning gatherings of five or more people and strongly recommending that people not visit family before or after the lunar new year, one of South Korea's major holidays. However, the number of daily infection cases in this period was far smaller than those of Japan, Spain, or the UK, whose populations and economic conditions are comparable to South Korea's. The South Korean government was criticized for being too conservative in refusing to lift the social distancing policy at the cost of people's mobility and business operations.

As the South Korean government expected to start COVID-19 vaccinations in February 2021, the Ministry of Health and Welfare began discussing a new social distancing policy. Although the first vaccination was administered on February 26, a transition plan was deferred until July 12, even after the vaccine supply delay of March 2021 was resolved. Thanks to rapid, widespread vaccinations, severity and mortality rates changed significantly. However, the South Korean government went against public sentiment by keeping rigid social distancing restrictions and continuing to sacrifice the rights of individuals and businesses. A new social distancing plan kept being pushed off due to mass infection cases like in Hongdae in late June 2021 and discoveries of new variants of the coronavirus.

Since July 2021, the surges of new cases, with more than 1,000 per day in early July and more than 3,000 per day in late September, began to change. While the South Korean government stayed hesitant to lift restrictions, it also imposed new policies like limiting the speed of treadmills to 6 km per hour and only allowing music between 100 and 120 bpm in gyms. A lack of scientific evidence supporting the effectiveness of these policies, the unfairness of restrictions differing by business type, and the rigidity of policies relative to countries like the UK and Singapore increased public criticism of governments' responses. The new social distancing policy consisted of four phases, which was simpler than the previous five-phase plan, gave more discretion to local governments, and slightly changed policies about gatherings. However, social distancing restrictions were not lifted entirely until October 2021 because of recurring increases in cases.

However, after more than 70% of the South Korean population was vaccinated in late October, social distancing was finally ended and gradually converted to a back-to-normal, with the Corona policy beginning on November 1, 2021. The gradual back-to-normal policy consisted of three phases whose thresholds were defined according to the vaccination rate and adjusted in response to the appearance of the Omicron variant and the pandemic's resurgence. At last, starting with the end of the outdoor mask mandate on April 18, 2022, other antivirus measures, like quarantining and required PCR testing for international arrivals, were also lifted. Caution is necessary when we interpret the COVID-19 trends in South Korea in 2020. First, we should not overlook the fact that the number of infection cases can be interpreted differently by country. For instance, Spain has a population of 46 million, which is slightly smaller than South Korea's 50 million, so 200 new cases per day in these countries could be considered successful control of the pandemic. However, according to South Korea's three-level social distancing policy, a two-week average of 100 new cases per day was the threshold for raising social distancing restrictions from level 2 to level 3, which was the highest.

Because of the negative social and economic impacts of social distancing, the South Korean government changed the threshold for the social distancing policy from 100 to 800 and the three-level social distancing policy to a five-level policy on November 1, 2020. According to the new policy, 800 new infection cases was the threshold for raising the social distancing level to level 3, the highest level. However, the South Korean government was cautious about actually raising the social distancing level to level 3. Although the week-average new infection cases began to exceed 800 on December 16, 2020, the government did not raise the social distancing policy to level 3. Instead, it announced an administrative order banning mass gatherings in some types of entertainment facilities.

The fatality rate trend shows that the seriousness of COVID-19 has continuously changed. As shown in Figure 7.2, the 30-day, 60-day, and 90-day fatality rates dropped to below 1% in April 2021. This trend persisted in 2022 despite infection cases rising up to 40,000.

The primary concern of COVID-19 policy moved from preventing infection to reducing fatalities after the introduction of the vaccine. When the vaccine was first introduced in December 2020, many people believed that it would significantly reduce the number of infection cases. Also, there appeared to be a significant number of non-symptomatic patients, and the fatality rate was not as severe as was feared. Figure 7.2 shows the fatality rate trend among COVID-19 patients. A notable drop in the fatality rate was associated with increasing vaccination rates and increasing availability of medical services.

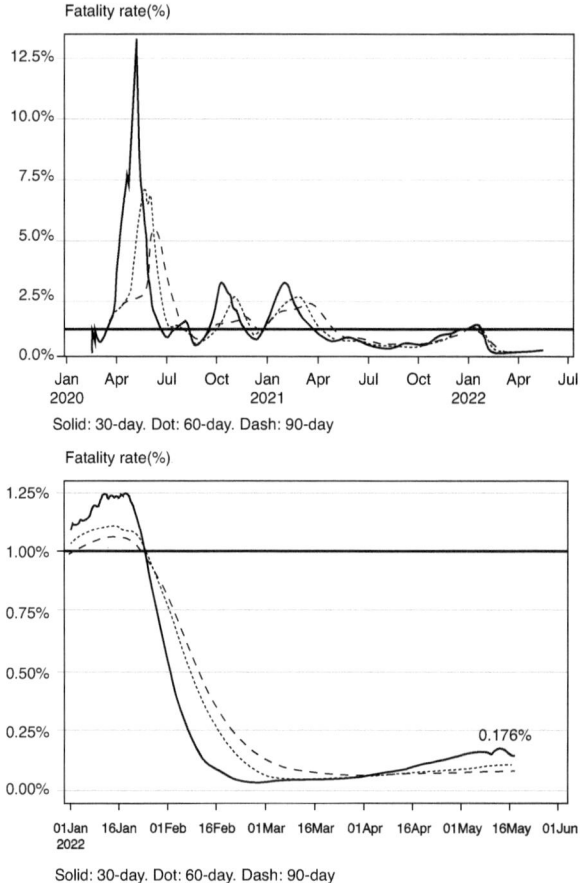

Figure 7.2 Fatality rates in South Korea.

Source: Adapted from Coronavirus Disease 19 (COVID-19) Cases in Korea in Korea Disease Control and Prevention Agency homepage. https://ncov.kdca.go.kr/bdBoardListR.do?brdId=1&brdGubun=11.

As shown in Figure 7.3, South Korea had only 100 intensive care unit (ICU) beds in December 2020, which was not enough. The rapid drop in the fatality rate in early 2021 was mainly attributed to an increase in the availability of medical services, not the vaccination rate, given that it was still below 50% by August 2021.

Comprehensive patient screening was another measure that the South Korean government adopted. As shown in Figure 7.4, the South Korean government performed around 10,000 tests per day, which was very extensive given that there were limited test kits worldwide. In December 2020, the

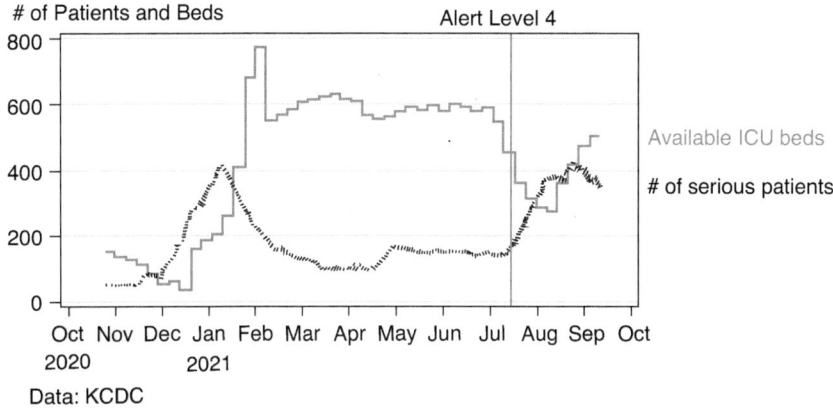

Figure 7.3 Availability of ICU beds for serious patients.

Source: Adapted from KCDC.

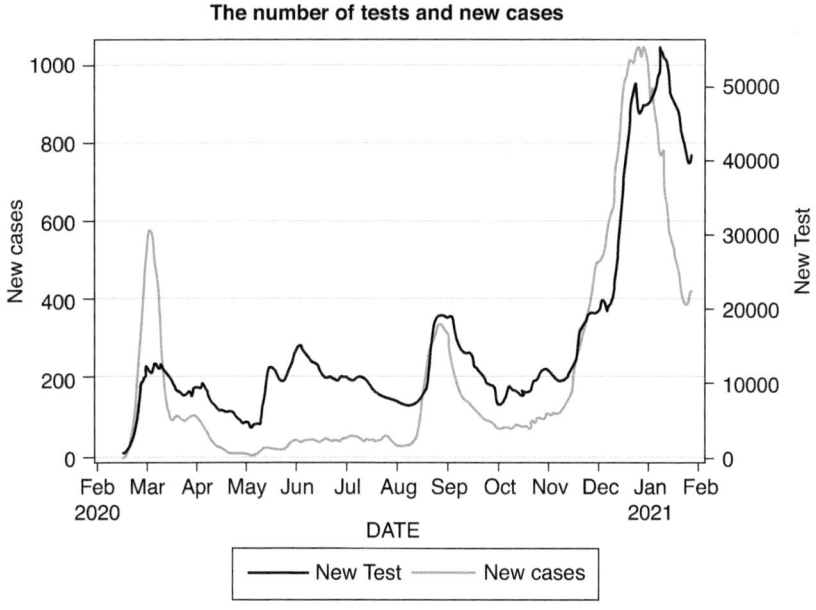

Figure 7.4 The number of tests and new cases.

Source: Adapted from Korea Center for Disease Control & Prevention. Analyzed by Ko Lab.

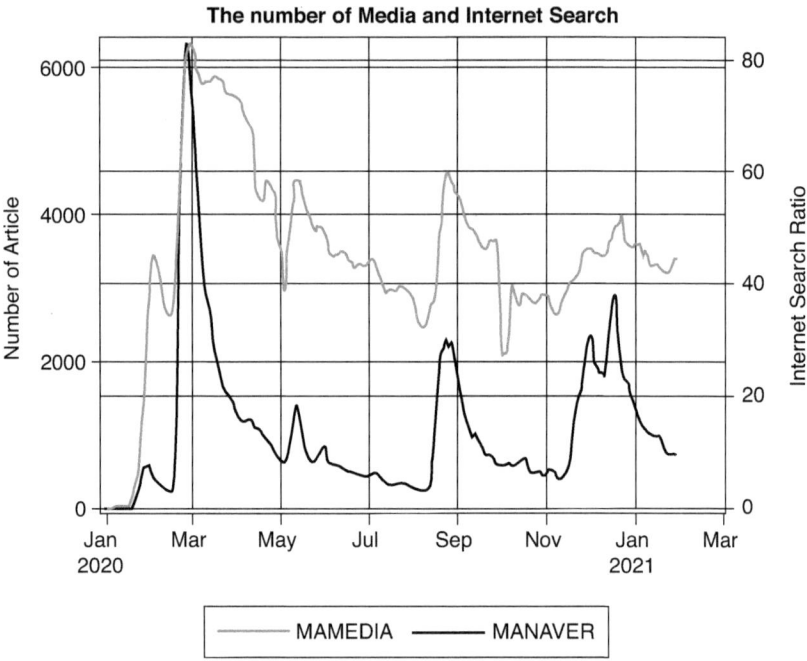

Figure 7.5 NAVER search trends and media articles about COVID-19.

Source: Adapted from Ko et al. (2022).

South Korean government increased the number of tests conducted by almost 60,000 per day while the new infection cases were slightly above 1,000. Some argued that the increased number of tests caused more infection cases to be caught, but Figure 7.4 shows the number of confirmed cases increased before the number of tests did. In conclusion, comprehensive testing was an effective tool for flattening the curve in the early stage of the pandemic, but not in 2022, as shown in Figure 7.1. Instead, medical service availability and vaccination were more effective at maintaining a low fatality rate.

The public's perception of COVID-19 risk is another factor explaining its strong compliance with the South Korean government's COVID-19 response policy. As Ko et al. (2022) argue, South Koreans started searching for the keywords "COVID-19" and "Wuhan virus" on the NAVER search engine, the most popular in South Korea, since it began its rampant spread in 2020. As shown in Figure 7.5, risk awareness was very high in early 2020 and the internet searches rose again when the new wave drew public attention. Notably, Google, the most globally popular search engine, showed somewhat different patterns than NAVER, but they both showed three co-occurring peaks. Overall, the public's attention to COVID-19 continually changed according to the unfolding of the pandemic.

Summing up, the infection and fatality rates, the supply of medical services, the frequency of COVID-19 testing, and people's risk awareness changed over time. Our knowledge of the seriousness of COVID-19 should be updated over time accordingly. The thousands of infection cases in 2022 were no longer enough to justify social distancing despite having been so in early 2020. Comprehensive testing was effective in flattening the infection curve in the early stage of the pandemic, but policy shifts to target reducing infection rates in the most vulnerable groups, such as the elderly, though vaccination and medical facility expansion were more effective in later stages. Moreover, the public's perception of COVID-19 risk was not static but changed over time. Hence, we can conclude that the South Korean government's successful response was not the result of the consistent application of a single standard. Instead, it was agile and flexible, which was important considering the rapidly evolving nature of the pandemic.

7.3   Policy Responses and Administrative Capacity

7.3.1   *Learning from Experiences and Communities*

The disaster response capacity has proven to be closely related to the degree of preparedness, which includes measures such as a clear legal chain of command, the mobilization of public resources, manuals for multiagency coordination, standard operation procedures, proper maintenance of and training in response organizations, and securing the requisite supplies and equipment. Although many scholars claim that the MERS crisis in 2015 was a primary factor in South Korea's successful response to the COVID-19 pandemic (), its preparation measures were developed through intentional effort over a longer period of time.

SARS started in 2003 in China. Then it spread to Hong Kong, Singapore, Vietnam, and North America, horrifying many countries due to its high contagiousness and fatality rate. Interestingly, the South Korean government even brought in military medical staff to control SARS transmission at airports and other entry points on March 16, 2003, right after noticing that China had a suspicious pneumonia case. People were unaccustomed to such intensive communicable disease control, and many complained that the government had overreacted. However, there were no infections and no fatalities from SARS in South Korea, which South Koreans the importance of quickly responding to emerging epidemics.

The South Korean government established an agency to manage epidemics based on its SARS response experience. During the SARS crisis, point-of-entry screening and quarantining were not well coordinated, and different agencies managed both measures. Information-sharing among agencies was also difficult due to bureaucratic red tape and organizational siloing. Responding to criticism, the South Korean government enhanced its institutional capacity by establishing the Korea Center for Disease Control and Prevention (KCDC) to integrate research, border screening, and quarantining in the face of disease and epidemics in 2004.

The South Korean government also changed legal structures and created a new organization. During the MERS response in 2015, the South Korean government did not publicly disclose the hospital where a patient was hospitalized and did not share this information with other organizations. Hospitals did not share patients' information promptly with the government, and there was no system for voluntary reporting of suspicious patients. Moreover, the tracking system of patients and their contacts was not well-established. Consequently, one super-spreader infected almost 90 people. Of course, there was a justification for not disclosing the hospital's name. As South Korea has a stringent privacy protection law and private information is only sharable under strict conditions, keeping the infected patients' hospital names private was considered necessary to protect patients' privacy and the hospitals that were treating them. To resolve this tension, the South Korean government revised the Infectious Disease Control and Prevention Act (IDCPA) to allow it to introduce standard operating procedures for tracking patients. Following the revision of the IDCPA, the South Korean government was able to legally track confirmed patients' contacts and places they visited during the COVID-19 crisis in 2020 without serious debate over privacy issues.

South Korea's SARS and MERS experiences still have not resolved the issue of communication and collaboration. During the MERS crisis, hospitals, medical experts, and local governments played significant roles in detecting and treating patients, but their authorities and channels for participating in policy-making were ambiguous. They were not sure where the response command center was. The Presidential office, the Prime Minister's office, the Minister of Public Health and Welfare, and the Commissioner of the KCDC chaired the different disaster response committees at different levels. The KCDC did not exert leadership in these situations because it was reluctant to take political responsibility. In response to this situation, the South Korean government revised the IDCAP again in 2018 to resolve the confusion about who was responsible. The 2018 revision of the IDCAP made clear that the KCDC is the command center during disaster response.

Response manuals were developed and revised during the COVID-19 crisis. Based on its SARS and MERS experience, the South Korean government prepared a COVID-19 response manual and revised it 15 times from January 2000 to December 2020. The early version of the manual was concise at 24 pages and mainly duplicated the MERS response manual. However, the last edition, version 9.4, published in December 2020, was 230 pages long and offered more accurate information and specific guidelines. The manual clarified each actor's responsibilities and reduced the coordination costs by clarifying uncertainty over responsibilities and setting standard operating procedures.

Table 7.1 Infection control system of South Korea

Entry Prevention	Response to Confirmed Cases	Early Patient Detection
• Entry ban on travelers from Hubei • Special entry procedures • Provision of travel history to healthcare providers	• Epidemiological investigations • Disclosure of each patient's whereabouts • Self-isolation of all contacts • On-site quarantining	• Expansion of diagnostic testing • Expansion of screening clinics • Specimen collection via drive-through and mobile facilities and door-to-door visits • Diagnostic testing for patients with pneumonia, etc.

Treatment of COVID-19 Patients	Treatment of Non-COVID-19 Patients	Resource-securing and Support
• Patient classification and bed allocation by severity • Therapeutic supply management • Clinical testing of and R&D for therapies	• Operation of government-designated COVID-19 protection hospitals • Permission for receiving prescriptions by phone and by proxy	• Living and treatment support centers and patient beds • Healthcare staff • Protective gear and supplies

⇧   ⇧   ⇧

- Seamless cooperation among the central disease control headquarters, central disaster and safety countermeasure headquarters, and local disaster and safety countermeasure headquarters
- Disclosure of information promptly and transparently and provision of counseling by the 1339 hotline and at public health centers
- Reinforcement of government measures such as face mask-wearing
- Compensation for infection prevention efforts by those put under isolation, their employers, and healthcare institutions

Source: The Republic of Korea (March 31, 2020), "Tackling COVID-19: Health, Quarantine and Economic Measures of South Korea," http://kostat.go.kr/file_total/COVID19_5_1.pdf)

The learning from MERS and response experiences during the early stage of the COVID-19 pandemic helped South Korea establish an infection control system consisting of entry prevention, case confirmation, early patient detection, treatment, and resource sharing. These activities are organized and coordinated under the leadership of the KCDC, which takes in innovative ideas from the outside (Table 7.1).

Policy responses to COVID-19 have been based on the utilization of information communication technologies. South Korea did not close its borders but rather adopted an intensive testing and quarantining policy for incoming international travelers. In airports, travelers had to take a COVID-19 test and were sent to special quarantine facilities if the test result was positive. Short-term travelers who had negative test results were also quarantined in these facilities. All incoming international travelers were asked to install the COVID-19 monitoring app on their cell phones and report on their health condition daily for 14 days. The South Korean government paid for the cost of testing. It also delivered necessities and food to those under quarantine. According to the Ministry of the Interior and Safety, among the 324,600 total people who were quarantined between February 19 and June 10, 2020, only 0.16% were known to have violated control rules.[1] Such strong compliance is very impressive, given that South Korea relied on voluntary compliance far more than China or other European countries that adopted lockdown policies.

South Korea's infection control system required the whole-community's participation and so was

a means by which residents, emergency management practitioners, organizational and community leaders, and government officials [could] collectively understand and assess the needs of their respective communities and determine the best ways to organize and strengthen their assets, capacities, and interests.

(FEMA, 2011: p.3)

For instance, many innovative ideas came from experts in the field. Given an exponential increase in infected patients, the city of Daegu did not have enough treatment facilities. The municipal government tried to use vacant beds in public and private hospitals, but this plan increased infection risk and resulted in the inefficient deployment of medical staff. Thus, medical experts proposed the idea of developing residential treatment centers, which significantly reduced hospitals' medical service demand. Universities, private companies, and public enterprises provided residential facilities to take care of patients with mild symptoms. Thanks to these centers, local governments were able to avoid the collapse of their medical service systems due to excessive demand.

Similarly, many people had to visit hospitals to take an infection test, increasing hospitals' burden. A group of doctors and local governments proposed and adopted the idea of drive-through testing. These ideas were ultimately adopted by the South Korean government as standard procedures.

7.3.2   Risk Communication and Institutional Governance

Risk communication and institutional governance are also critical to efficient disaster response (Comfort, 2019; Moynihan, 2009) as disaster response networks consist of many actors, relationships, and continuous interactions in which resources and information are produced, exchanged, and used. For example, when a doctor detects a suspicious patient, he or she has to report the case to the local government, the KCDC, the Ministry of Health and Welfare, and medical associations. The report is delivered by telephone, fax, email, and other networks. E-government systems allow for this information to be quickly collected in databases. Case reports are also used to track people who have come into contact with infected patients and design social distancing policies. Collaboration and whole-community responses are not possible if the central government does not share information with local governments, hospitals, and other network actors. Some argued that the government distorted the seriousness of COVID-19, but objective data analyzed by experts quickly refuted this claim.

The evolutionary nature of the pandemic required appropriate risk communication, which was challenging. The primary formal channel for risk communication was the government's official responses, as defined by the IDCPA. According to the law, Korea's National Infectious Disease Risk Alert System has four levels. The national responses were supposed to change according to the risk alert level issued and adjusted by the Minister of Health and Welfare. At level 4, the Central Disaster and Safety Countermeasure Headquarters becomes the national response command center. Meetings chaired by the Prime Minister must include all relevant ministries of the central government and the heads of local governments. Between late February and late April, meetings were held every day with few exceptions (ROK, 2020: p. 30). The Prime Minister received direct reports from the heads of local government and relevant ministries regarding the pandemic. The Prime Minister then ordered the director to resolve local governments' problems, coordinate central government ministries, and execute agile policy responses to identified problems. Moreover, meetings are opened to many communication channels between the leaders of governments, ministries, and agencies. Many heads of local governments stated that the Prime Minister's meetings helped resolve equipment and contact-tracing expert shortages (Figure 7.6).

One notable change that occurred during the COVID-19 pandemic was the empowerment of local governments. After SARS and MERS, the South Korean government repeatedly emphasized the importance of establishing a command center. However, this emphasis on centralized command and control failed to reflect how localities had differing infection rates. For instance, Jeonbuk Province had a small number of infection cases, but they still had to close schools as ordered by the national government during the early stages of COVID-19. Many of these policies were unnecessary for certain areas, so the central government gave more discretion to local governments to design and implement their own response policies in the later stages of the pandemic. Despite the flexibility of intergovernmental relationships, the autonomy of local government was still limited. One symbolic example was the city of Daegu's social distancing policy implemented on January 17, 2021. As Daegu had fewer infection cases than the Seoul metropolitan area, it allowed more than five people to meet together in restaurants and extended business hours to 11 PM. However, the central government was upset that it did so without consulting with the central

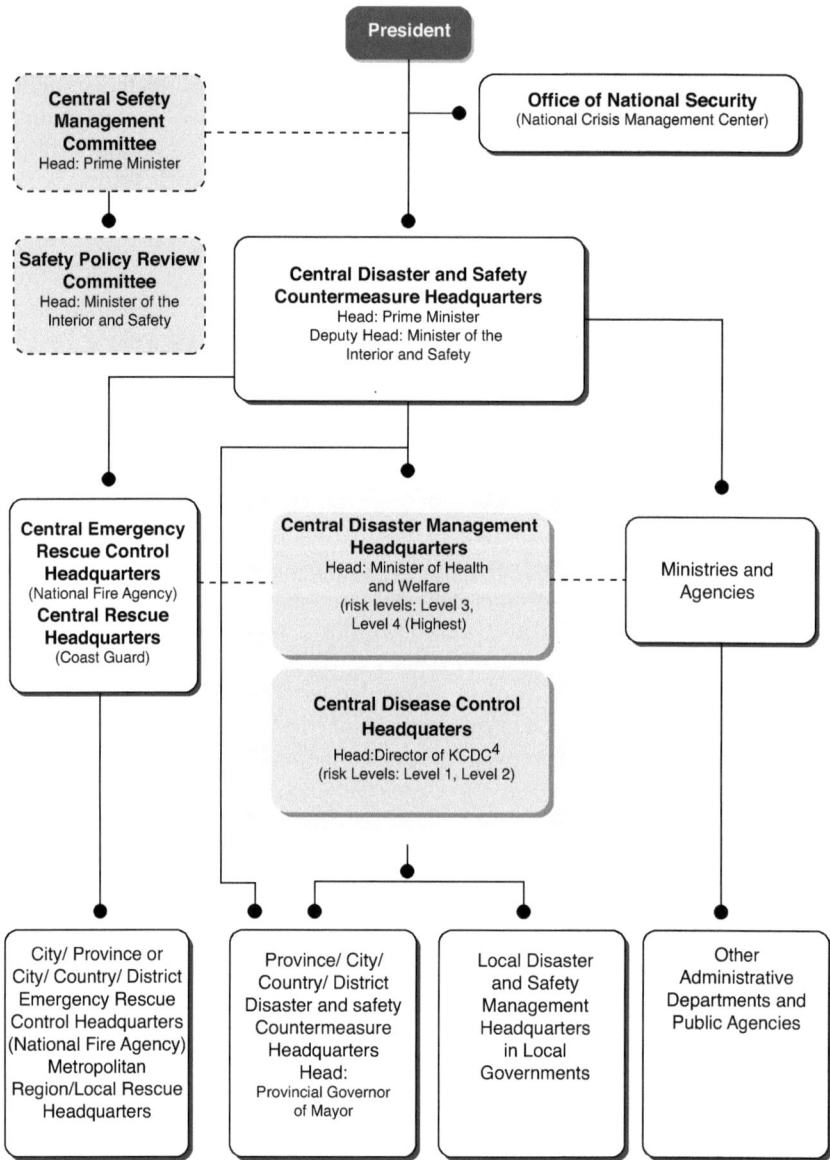

Figure 7.6 The governance structure at risk alert level 4.

Source: Adapted from ROK (2020: 33).

government first, so the Daegu government had to repeal its policy a day later. This example shows how the central government still wanted to control local governments and wanted them to follow national rules.

7.3.3   Social Distancing Policies

Because of the absence of vaccines and treatment drugs for COVID-19, social distancing policies were more critical during the COVID-19 pandemic than in the face of other transmittable diseases. After China admitted the spread of COVID-19, South Korean society debated the possibility of banning travelers from China. The KCDC was aware of the potential risk of COVID-19, so it installed thermal scanners at airports to detect suspicious patients from China on January 3, 2020. However, when the first confirmed patient, a Chinese person from Wuhan, was announced to have entered the country on January 20, 2020, many Koreans called for closing the borders to Chinese travelers. Initially, this seemed to be the best solution, but the South Korean government did not close the border and instead reinforced the entry-point quarantine requirement.

Moreover, the South Korean government did not adopt a lockdown policy even when severe infection cases were found in the city of Daegu in late February 2020. Even when more than 1,000 new cases were reported during the third wave, which occurred from December 2020 to January 2021, the South Korean government did not impose a lockdown on cities or ban travel. Public transportation, such as buses, taxis, and subways, were operated under official COVID-19 control measures. Doing so prevented massive layoffs and negative economic impacts that would have fallen especially heavily on low-income groups.

The South Korean government did not have specific social distancing policies before June 28, 2020. Initially, the government did not use the term "social distancing policy." Instead, it implemented response policies such as school closing, enforcing working from home, and preventing social gatherings. While there were only around 400 infection cases per day, the South Korean government implemented social distancing policies that suspended the operation of religious facilities; some types of indoor activity facilities, such as dance halls, health clubs, and martial arts training centers; and entertainment facilities, such as bars, clubs, and karaoke rooms on March 22, 2020. At the time, the government wanted to totally prevent COVID-19 transmission, so there was no concept of a tolerable transmission rate. As a result, social distancing policies were extended. Initially, social distancing policies were planned to last two weeks, but they were extended for an additional two weeks on April 7. The justification for the extension was that there were still around 100 new daily infection cases, which was minor compared to the rates of other countries. In May 2020, the Seoul Metropolitan government strongly prohibited the operation of entertainment facilities because of the community infection outbreaks that originated in the nightclubs of Itaewon. However, the number of infection cases per day was less than 50. While such social distancing policies perhaps reduced infection numbers and anger at politicians, they came at a hefty price for businesses.

The predictability of policies was very low because the government did not provide any scientific evidence about the cost-effectiveness of social distancing policies. As Ko and Hong (2020) found, South Korea did not have many infection cases, so it was not cost-effective to increase testing frequency. Instead, policies should have been designed to reduce fatalities, not new infections. However, this policy transition did not happen until COVID-19 vaccines were widely available in 2021.

Social distancing policies changed over time. A more systematic social distancing policy was introduced on June 28, 2020. As shown in Table 7.2,

Table 7.2 Three-level social distancing policy implemented on June 28, 2020

	Level 1	*Level 2*	*Level 3 (Lockdown)*
Average daily community infections for two weeks	Less than 50 people	50 to less than 100 people	100 people or more
Key message	Comply with quarantine rules, but daily economic activities are permitted	Avoid unnecessary outings and using multi-purpose facilities	All activities other than essential economic activities are prohibited
Gatherings	Allowed, but recommended to comply with quarantine rules	Up to 50 people indoors and 100 people outdoors	No more than 10 people
Sporting events	Limit the number of spectators	No spectators	Stop all sporting events
Public facilities	Operated with interventions if necessary	Shut down	Shut down
Schools	In-person attendance permitted and remote classes offered	Reduction of in-person attendance and increased remote classes	Remote classes only or school closure
Workplaces	Flextime and working from home encouraged	Flextime and working from home more strongly encouraged	Except for essential personnel, all public employees are to work from home

Source: The Ministry of Health and Welfare (MOHW).

it had three levels that were activated according to the number of infection cases. Level 3 was to be activated when the two-week average daily confirmed cases exceeded 100. However, the thresholds were critiqued because they were not based on any scientific explanation and were considered too restrictive. The effectiveness of the school closing policy has never been scientifically examined. The government asked people to reduce mobility and physical contact.

The three-tier social distancing policy was revised on November 7 as the number of infection cases rapidly increased. In the revised version, levels 1 and 2 were further divided into levels 1, 1.5, 2, and 2.5, and the threshold for activating level 3 was increased to 800 new cases. Furthermore, the new guidelines considered hospitals' capacities, the relative increase in new cases, and regional differences in infection rates. On December 16, the level 3 threshold was passed for the first time as the one-week average number of new cases exceeded 800. However, the South Korean government did not activate level 3 because of the predicted serious negative impact of the lockdown on the economy. The South Korean government's experience showed that increasing the social distancing level was not easy, and its effects varied according to regional, political, and economic situations.

Social distancing was not strongly correlated with the number of new confirmed cases. As shown in Figure 7.7 and Figure 7.8, social distancing policies, such as workplace closing and canceling public events, changed over time. The changes in the social distancing level were not correlated with the number of infection cases. For instance, the daily new cases were relatively small from April to June of 2020, but the South Korean government maintained a high social distancing level during this time. Also, the severity of public event regulations changed more frequently than that of workplace closing.

Despite the merits of incremental and flexible social distancing policy changes, it is difficult to decide when to activate a given level. For instance, although the government allowed restaurants to operate during level 2.5, health clubs had to close. The government failed to explain why health clubs were riskier than restaurants.

7.3.4   *Economic Subsidies*

The pandemic incurred economic hardships. Many governments introduced safety net programs such as job retention programs, extensions to unemployment insurance, extensions to means-tested programs, targeted transfers to specific groups, universal transfers, tax cuts, and housing subsidies. Like other OECD countries,[2] the South Korean government established two types of emergency relief funds. The first type compensated businesses and families

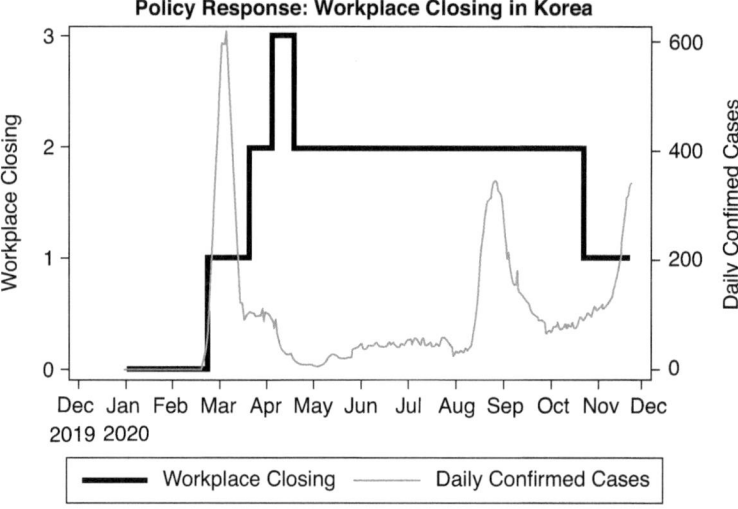

Figure 7.7 Workplace closing intensity.

Source: Adapted from Asia Regional Information Center, Seoul National University (2020).

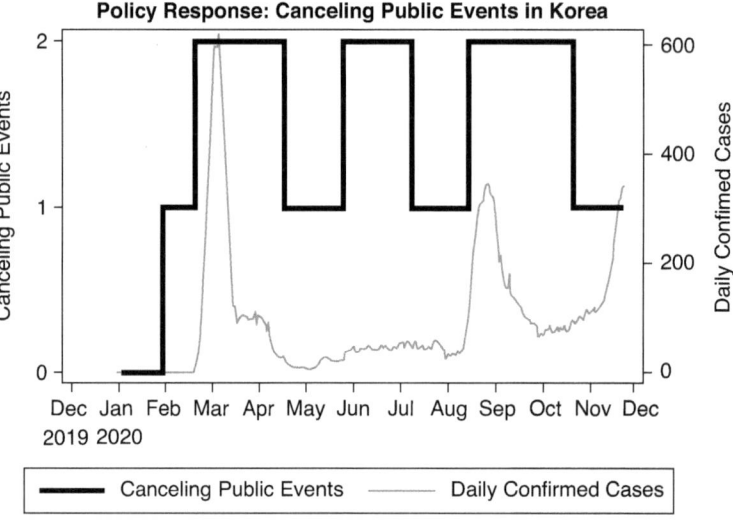

Figure 7.8 Public event canceling intensity.

Source: Adapted from Asia Regional Information Center, Seoul National University (2020).

that experienced costs due to distancing policies that limited people's rights. Many businesses, such as restaurants, health clubs, and movie theaters, could not be fully operational due to government regulations. Relief funds compensated these businesses for losses caused by complying with government policy. The second type offered subsidies to all residents.

The South Korean government used both universal and targeted transfers. Universal transfers were offered because it was difficult to identify beneficiaries and the amount that they should receive because losses were difficult to calculate. Also, the administrative costs of selecting beneficiary families were high. Most importantly, targeted transfers required a significant amount of time to implement and so failed to meet people's needs. Hence, the government provided universal transfers through the first wave of relief funds but shifted to targeted transfers through the second and third waves of relief funds.

Notably, the amount of the relief funds was largest in 2022 when the government started lowering the social distancing level. Around USD 62 billion was approved for the supplementary budget. Given the urgency of people's needs, it was unclear why the government spent more money in 2022 than in 2020. As the presidential and local government elections occurred in 2022, people suspect that the funds were released to increase voters' political favor (Figure 7.9).

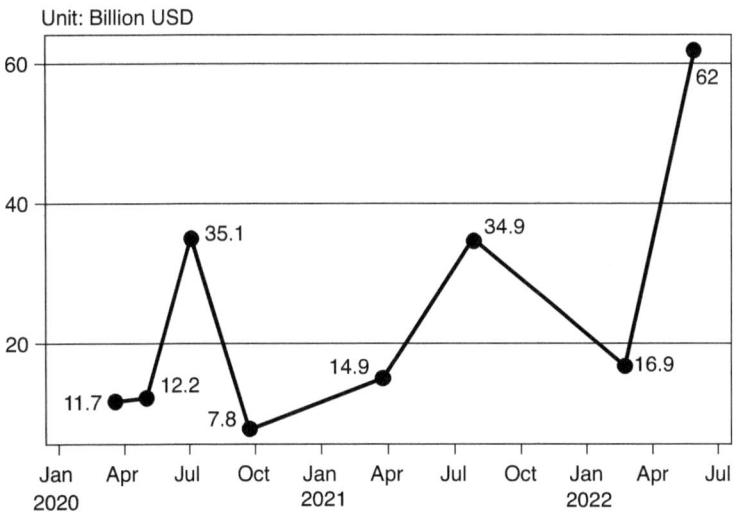

Figure 7.9 The size of the supplementary budget used for relief funds.

Source: Adapted from Ministry of Economy and Finance.

7.3.5 *People's Compliance*

The success of disaster response does not depend on a single actor if we assume that the disaster response network is complex (Perrow, 1984). The disaster management cycle, which consists of preparedness, response, recovery, and mitigation, involves multiple actors and different types of interactions at each stage of the cycle. Because the systems involved are connected and dynamic, civil society's role is critical.

One of the roles that civil society played during the COVID-19 pandemic was raising the issue of privacy and protecting minority groups. In February 2020, the South Korean government started to use texting and the internet to share information. During the MERS crisis, the government did not share details about patients and the hospitals that treated them, which led to the spread of fake news. To avoid this situation, the South Korean government established the Office of Risk Communication to create guidelines about how and when to share information. While this organization tried to minimize privacy violations, the government published patients' ages, genders, and workplaces. However, the government did not give any justification as to why such information was necessary to effectively respond to the COVID-19 pandemic at the expense of people's privacy. Facing the growing risk of privacy violations, civil rights groups protested against government policy. As a result, the National Human Rights Commission of Korea admitted that there was a problem and revised the government's information disclosure guidelines to not publish the age, gender, address, and workplace name of the infected on March 14, 2020.

Non-government experts play a significant role in developing platforms for sharing information about mask availability and infection and fatality rates. There was a significant mask shortage at the end of February 2020 and the government announced that it would fully control face mask distribution on March 5, 2020. Despite the announcement, people did not have information about the availability of masks in the pharmacies. As South Korea has public health insurance, most medical service information about hospitals and pharmacies was collected by the Health Insurance Review and Assessment (HIRA) and National Health Insurance Service (NHIS). Despite this information's availability, the government could not develop functional mobile apps. It was estimated that it took almost three months to contract out the development of apps because of bureaucratic processes. This period was cut to a week after non-government experts became involved. The Ministry of Science and ICT asked HIRA and NHIS to share information, which the National Information Agency cleaned and added geographical information. Then, the data was shared through Open API and non-government experts quickly developed mobile software apps that shared the locations of pharmacies and stores and their stocks of masks. This cooperative effort showed the potential of civil society to agilely respond to the pandemic.

According to a press release from the Prime Minister's Office on July 10, 2020, as of June 23, 2020, more than 660,000 people had volunteered by participating in a variety of response activities such as making face masks, controlling the spread of COVID-19, and helping the needy. Because of the social distancing policy, other volunteers provided online education. Volunteers' activities were strategically organized through a volunteer organization network through which nonprofit organizations worked closely with the Ministry of Interior and Safety. Another important set of groups was associations of doctors and nurses. According to the Korean Nurses Association, around 4,000 nurses, accounting for almost 2% of South Korea's practicing nurses, volunteered in Daegu in March 2020.[3] Doctors shared information about the pandemic through social network services. Their idea exchanges resulted in the adoption of drive-through testing and residential treatment centers.

Civil society's responses originated with individual people. Despite significant increases in cases in February, August, and December 2020, there was no panic-buying in South Korea. The shortage of face masks was serious in early March 2020, but people followed the government's distribution rule. The primary reason that the people were able to stay calm during the crisis was that they could access transparent information. For instance, in the first week of April 2020, interregional express traffic dropped to 60.2% of its level in the third week of January 2020 (KOTI, 2020). However, highway traffic only decreased by 3.3% in the same period. These figures indicate that people avoided public transportation to avoid contact with others and decided to use their cars to travel between regions. Within cities, people used their cars, bicycles, and other forms of transit. Such behavioral changes suggest that people found ways to resolve the inconveniences caused by COVID-19 in their daily lives. These choices were not enforced by the government but instead resulted from creative problem-solving efforts by individuals.

Figure 7.10 shows mobility changes in the Seoul metropolitan region and nationwide. The perpendicular line shows the social distancing level. There greatest number of infection cases in South Korea occurred on March 1 of 2020 and transit and retail use were at their lowest on this day. At the time, the government's social distancing policy remained at level 1. These figures suggest that the reduction in mobility was not because of government regulation. Instead, people voluntarily reduced their mobility regardless of the government's policy.

Finally, in October 2021, the South Korean government organized a recovery committee to discuss how to prepare for the post-COVID-19 era. The committee was chaired by the Prime Minister and consisted of many subcommittees with 31 non-government representatives from business, hospitals, academia, culture and sports organizations, and local governments. These representatives expressed their concerns and suggested ideas to the recovery committee. Involving these people in the recovery committee helped the government design COVID-19 response policies (Figure 7.11).

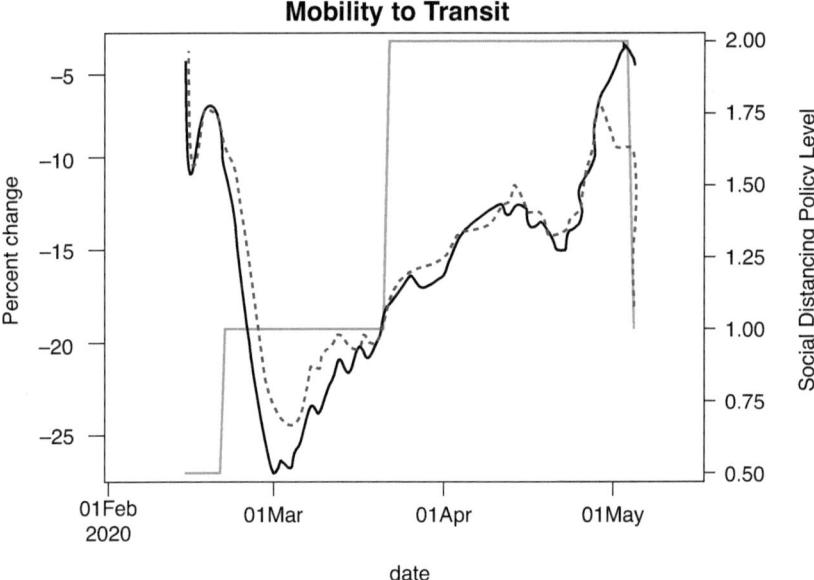

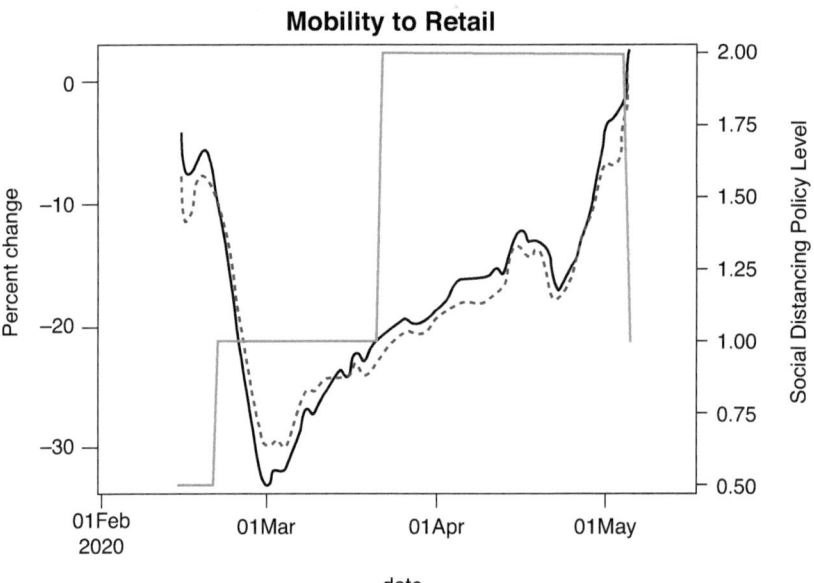

Figure 7.10 Mobility changes and social distancing policy.

Source: Adapted from Google, COVID-19 Community Mobility Reports. https://www. google.com/covid19/mobility/.

Note: The dashed line is for the Seoul metropolitan area and the solid line is for the national level. The perpendicular line shows the social distance policy level.

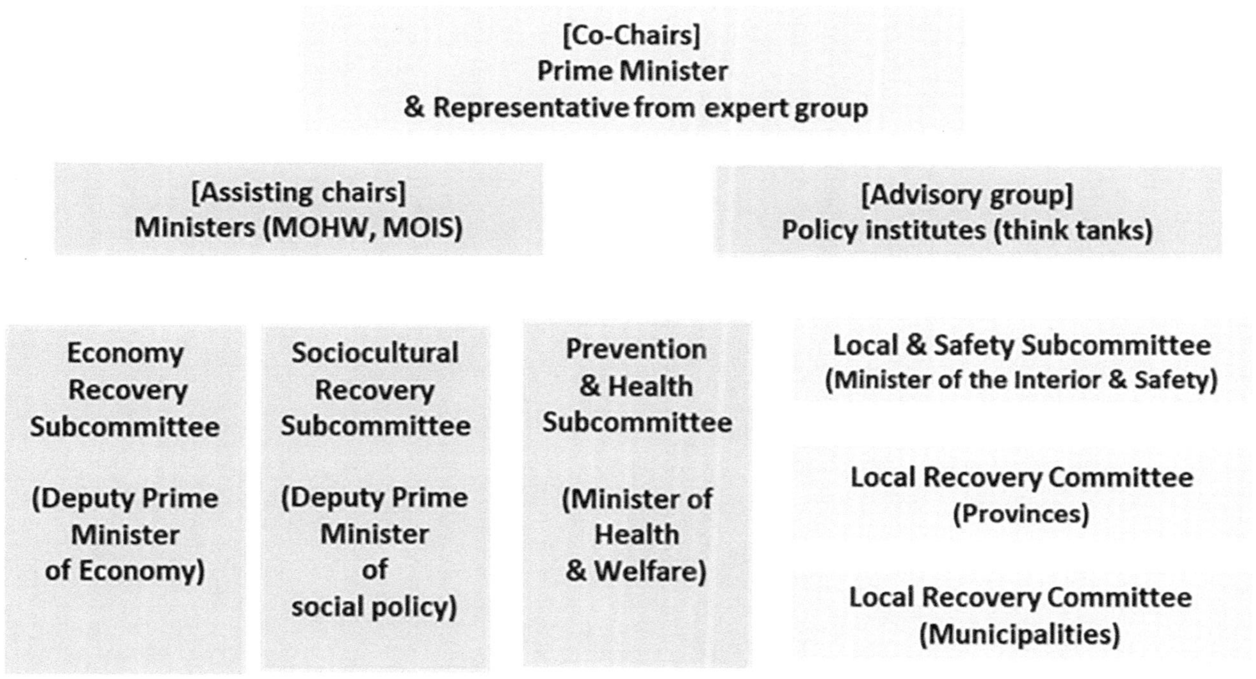

[Co-Chairs]
Prime Minister
& Representative from expert group

[Advisory group]
Policy institutes (think tanks)

[Assisting chairs]
Ministers (MOHW, MOIS)

Economy Recovery Subcommittee

(Deputy Prime Minister of Economy)

Sociocultural Recovery Subcommittee

(Deputy Prime Minister of social policy)

Prevention & Health Subcommittee

(Minister of Health & Welfare)

Local & Safety Subcommittee
(Minister of the Interior & Safety)

Local Recovery Committee (Provinces)

Local Recovery Committee (Municipalities)

Figure 7.11 The recovery committee structure.

Source: Adapted from Regulations on the Establishment and Operation of the Covid-19 Recovery Committee, 437 Presidential Instruction §3 and §8. https://www.law.go.kr/admRulSc.do?menuId=5&subMenuId=43&tabMenuId=193&query=%EC%9D%BC%EC%83%81%ED%9A%8C%EB%B3%B5#liBgcolor4.

7.4 Conclusions

The COVID-19 pandemic was an unprecedented event, yet it has underscored the need to enhance the response capacities of administrative systems in anticipation of future crises. A reflection on South Korea's handling of the pandemic highlights the critical role of flexibility in emergency management. Some observers might interpret South Korea's experience as support for strong government leadership, akin to the authoritarian measures implemented by China. This interpretation is based on the assumption that the government functions as the primary director of the response system, with the public expected to comply with governmental directives for the sake of protecting the collective interest. Citizens were called upon to relinquish certain freedoms, privacy, and other rights in the effort to control the spread of COVID-19. However, policies characterized by authoritarianism and a lack of transparency ultimately exacerbated the severity of the pandemic. For instance, because of the Chinese government's strict control of information, the people of Wuhan endured heavy casualties, the size of which remains unknown. Furthermore, while many countries adopted strong social distancing policies, only a few of them controlled the spread of COVID-19. There is no evidence that governments can process information better than non-government actors. Although governments possess greater authority than other actors, they are not necessarily the best at responding to disasters. Too much emphasis on strong government leadership can result in the retreat of democracy. Disaster response should not be used to justify excessively strong government.

Opposite to the interpretation of authoritarian approach, South Korea's experience shows the value of collaboration among the government, people, and private companies. The South Korean government's disaster response experiences have shown it the importance of sharing information, thinking about risk, and collaboration. The revisions of laws and guidelines can be seen as attempts to find more effective ways to communicate and coordinate actors in the disaster response network. People voluntarily wore face masks, reduced their travel, and developed apps and other information-sharing technologies. These efforts contributed to the success of government policies. The government alleviated the shortage of medical facilities, established residential treatment centers, and used the facilities of universities, private companies, and public enterprises with their voluntary cooperation. Thousands of volunteers also joined in COVID-19 control activities. Most importantly, millions of taxpayers implicitly endorsed the government's use of their money to take the future burden of taxes. Although populist politicians have argued that the COVID-19 relief funds were only possible because of their generosity, they would not have been possible without taxpayers' contributions.

The whole-community approach emphasizes the importance of communication and coordination over command and control. For instance, during disasters in the past, local government leaders could not directly access the Prime Minister or other key decision-makers in the central government. However, the Central Disaster and Safety Countermeasure Headquarters, led by the Prime Minister, allowed local governments to share innovative ideas and their difficulties with the central government. The Prime Minister can cut through bureaucratic red tape.

The rapid development of test kits, requiring the wearing of face masks, drive-through testing, advanced reporting and tracking systems, residential treatment centers, and risk communication led by doctors and experts were factors that contributed to South Korea's successful response to the pandemic. These factors would not have contributed as strongly or existed at all if the government was incompetent. Even if the President or other political leaders strongly desired to control the pandemic, the disaster response system would have failed if the administrative system was of poor quality and bureaucrats were incompetent. Certain strategies that were effective in the early stages of the pandemic, such as social distancing, were less effective in later stages. Therefore, the most important lesson that can be learned from South Korea's experience is that no single factor or actor is responsible for successful disaster response. The whole-community approach should be valued over strong command and control by the government.

Notes

1 *Yeonhap News*, June 14, 2020, https://www.yna.co.kr/view/AKR2020 0612042800530. Accessed March 6, 2021.
2 OECD (2020). "Supporting people and companies to deal with the COVID-19 virus: Options for an immediate employment and social-policy response," *ELS Policy Brief on the Policy Response to the COVID-19 Crisis*. Paris: OECD, http://oe.cd/covid19briefsocial. Accessed May 19, 2020.
3 https://www.medifonews.com/news/article.html?no=152712

References

Abbey, E. J., Khalifa, B. A. A., Oduwole, M. O., Ayeh, S. K., Nudotor, R. D., Salia, E. L., et al. (2020). The Global Health Security Index is not predictive of coronavirus pandemic responses among Organization for Economic Cooperation and Development countries. *PLoS One*, 15(10), e0239398. https://doi.org/10.1371/journal.pone.0239398.

Addison, H. J. (2009). Is administrative capacity a useful concept? Review of the application, meaning and observation of administrative capacity in political science literature. *LSE Research Paper*, 1–21.

Comfort, L. K. (2019). *The dynamics of risk: Changing technologies and collective action in seismic events* (Vol. 27). Princeton, NJ: Princeton University Press.

Fema, A. (2011). *Whole community approach to emergency management: Principles, themes, and pathways for action.* Washington, DC: Federal Emergency Management Agency, US Department of Homeland Security.

Hannan, M. T., & Freeman, J. (1977). The population ecology of organizations. *American Journal of Sociology*, 82(5), 929–964.

Ko, K., Chang, S., & Lee, S. (2022). The impact of inter-crisis learning on the risk cognition and the utilization of information technologies in Korea. In Comfort, Louise & Rhodes, Mary Lee eds. *Global risk management: The Role of Collective Cognition in Response to COVID-19* (pp. 65–83). New York: Routledge.

Ko, K., & Hong, M. (2020). Estimation of the impact of comprehensive covid-19 testing in South Korea: A cost-benefit analysis using the extended seir model. *Journal of Policy Studies*, 35(3), 141–168.

Ko, K., Park, H. H., Shim, D. C., & Kim, K. (2021). The change of administrative capacity in Korea: Contemporary trends and lessons. *International Review of Administrative Sciences*, 87(2), 238–255.

KOTI. (2020). COVID-19 and its impact on transportation and logistics. https://www.koti.re.kr/main/covid19/, accessed on February 23, 2021.

Lee, M., & You, M. (2020). Psychological and behavioral responses in South Korea during the early stages of coronavirus disease 2019 (COVID-19). *International Journal of Environmental Research and Public Health*, 17(9), 2977.

Moynihan, D. P. (2009). The network governance of crisis response: Case studies of incident command systems. *Journal of Public Administration Research and Theory*, 19(4), 895–915.

Perrow, Charles (1984). *Normal accidents: Living with high-risk technologies* (Revised edition, 1999). Princeton, NJ: Princeton University Press.

ROK. (2020). *All about Korea's response to COVID-19.* Seoul, The Republic of Korea: Ministry of Foreign Affairs.

8 Japan's Responses to COVID-19

Kohei Suzuki and Kentaro Sakuwa

8.1 Introduction

This chapter explores how Japan responded to and mitigated the spread of COVID-19, mainly focusing on the early period of the pandemic from 2020 to early 2021. The COVID-19 pandemic has posed unprecedented challenges to policy makers all over the world. The coronavirus pandemic can be understood as a wicked problem for policy makers (Ansell et al. 2020, Steen and Brandsen 2020, van den Oord et al. 2020), characterized by "unclear problem definitions, complex causalities, conflicting goals and lack of standard solutions" (Ansell et al. 2020, 2). As Moon (2020) argues, the COVID-19 outbreak has tested governments' abilities to solve wicked policy problems; in particular, governments have faced new challenges in preparing for, mitigating, and responding to the threats posed by contagious diseases. It is noteworthy to observe the significant variations in how governments have responded to and handled these unprecedented policy challenges. Some countries seem to have managed the COVID-19 crisis more effectively and swiftly than others in terms of several infection-related indicators (Van der Wal 2020). Although it is premature to draw any conclusions at this point, some countries—especially those in the Asia Pacific region, including South Korea, Taiwan, New Zealand, Australia, and possibly Singapore—seem to have controlled coronavirus more effectively than other countries (An and Tang 2020, Bromfield and McConnell 2020, Dunlop et al. 2020, Huang 2020, Jamieson 2020, Moon 2020, Van der Wal 2020).[1]

Despite the media attention that Japan received from around the world at the beginning of the pandemic due to the mishandling of the outbreak on the Diamond Princess cruise ship (Sturmer and Asada 2020, McCurry 2020), very little scholarly attention has been paid to the unique features of Japan's pandemic response or the specific challenges posed by the coronavirus in the Japanese context (Shimizu and Negita 2020). Given the volume of published studies on other Asia Pacific countries in the fields of public

DOI: 10.4324/9781003362760-8

administration and political science, the paucity of research on Japan's pandemic approach is especially glaring.[2] Despite several unfavorable conditions for controlling the COVID-19 pandemic—which include Japan's proximity to Wuhan, population density, and comparatively small number of ICU and PCR test laboratories for an industrialized nation (Inoue 2020)—Japan seems to have been relatively successful in responding to and mitigating the spread of COVID-19 compared to other industrialized democratic countries (Shimizu et al. 2021). Japan has recorded much lower numbers of confirmed cases and associated death numbers than other countries in Europe and North America. However, Japan's response, which we characterize as a "cautious and self-restraint-based approach"(Moon et al. 2021), seems different from the relatively proactive, agile, and collaborative governmental responses by the abovementioned countries (An and Tang 2020, Bromfield and McConnell 2020, Dunlop et al. 2020, Huang 2020, Jamieson 2020, Moon 2020, Van der Wal 2020).

We argue that the Japanese government's policy is characterized by a cautious and restraint-based approach that relies on citizens' self-restraint behavior and personal hygiene practices rather than on enforcing strict, legally binding measures and proactively testing and tracing potentially infected individuals (Moon et al. 2021). Unlike many Western countries (including the United States, Australia, and New Zealand), Japan never implemented strict lockdown measures or imposed financial penalties on violators. Instead, the Japanese government took a "mild lockdown" approach that was non-punitive (Sugaya et al. 2020). Starting with the declaration of a state of emergency in April 2020, the Japanese government has largely relied on citizens' voluntary self-restraint behavior (jishuku in Japanese), requesting that citizens refrain from going out or attending mass gatherings (Muto et al. 2020) and that retail, dining, and entertainment industries shorten business hours or cancel large events. Unlike Hong Kong, Taiwan, and Singapore, Japan did not conduct extensive and proactive contact tracing (An and Tang 2020). Furthermore, unlike South Korea, Japan has not employed a proactive and aggressive testing policy (Moon et al. 2021). Instead, Japan has "focused on controlling clusters of more than five COVID-19 cases and preventing environmental transmission in the three Cs: closed spaces, crowded spaces, and close contact settings" (Shimizu et al. 2020, 1).

Most Japanese citizens seem dissatisfied with how the Japanese government has handled the pandemic (Gallup International Association 2020b, Jiji Tsushin 2020, Nihon Keizai Shimbun 2020a). But in spite of relatively loose corona measures, reliance on citizens' self-restraint, and low citizen satisfaction, Japan still seems to have managed the pandemic effectively compared with other industrialized democratic countries. In fact, Japan's success in managing the coronavirus appears inexplicable in Western media; Japan was initially considered the "most likely case" for disastrous results due to its high population density, lack of virus testing, soft approach without financial penalties, and the widespread media perception that Japan mishandled the Diamond Princess cruise ship situation in February 2020 (Sturmer and Asada 2020, McCurry 2020).

The purpose of this chapter is not to analyze how Japan's pandemic approach has led to a small number of infections and fatalities. Our purpose, rather, is to delineate the distinctive features of Japan's reaction to the COVID-19 pandemic and the associated institutional contexts for Japan's response. The first section looks at several objective performance indicators of governments' responses to the pandemic and examines to what extent Japan has controlled the coronavirus in comparison to other countries. The second section explains the institutional contexts for Japan's pandemic approach. The third section considers how Japan handled the COVID-19 pandemic and the characteristics of Japan's approach, followed by a concluding section.

8.2   Assessment of Japan's National Response to the COVID-19 Pandemic

Researchers should be careful when comparing the effectiveness of different government's COVID-19 measures due to several potential measurement issues in cross-national research: large variations in definitions of confirmed COVID-19 cases and related deaths; different testing policies and types of tests used and other potential biases that may render cross-national comparisons less reliable. However, as far as we can see from the data used in existing comparative studies, Japan seems to have controlled the COVID-19 pandemic relatively well compared to other industrialized democratic countries in Europe and North America, but not as well as many other countries in the Asia Pacific region.

Figure 8.1 shows a graph of cumulative confirmed COVID-19 cases/million people and COVID-19-related deaths/million people in the nine countries examined in this book. We also add United Kingdom, the Netherlands, and Canada as examples of OECD member countries in Europe and North America and add Taiwan and Australia as Asia Pacific region countries. As seen from the left graph of Figure 8.1, Japan records a much lower number of infected cases per million people (3,473.82) than other developed countries including the United States (87,609.07), Sweden (67,822.82), the Netherlands (66,254.24), the United Kingdom (62,327.52), Germany (29,941.95), Canada (23,639.32), and Finland (11,201.26). However, Japan's number is not as low as those of other Asia Pacific countries such as South Korea (1,810.39), Australia (1,139.06), New Zealand (498.73), Thailand (378.81), Taiwan (40.69), and Vietnam

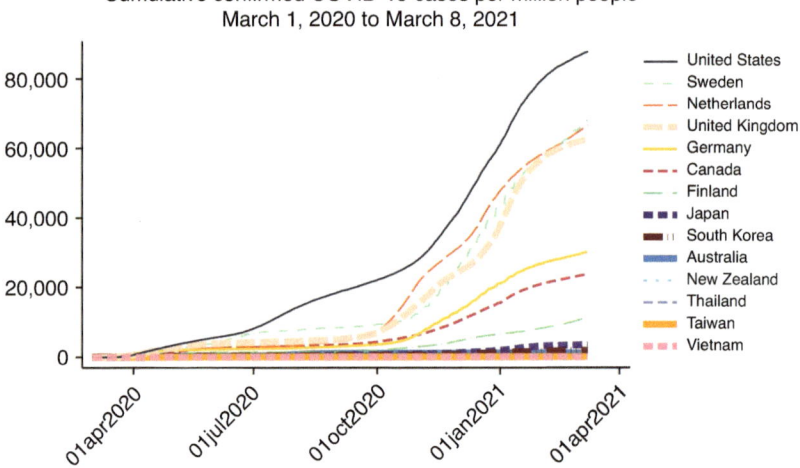

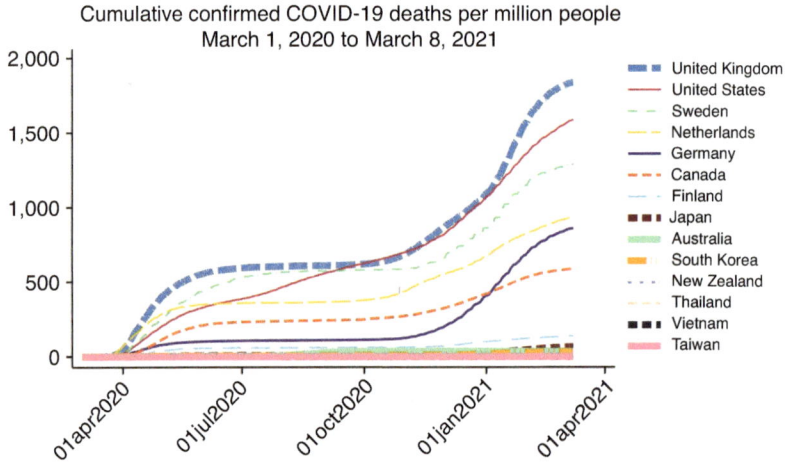

Figure 8.1 Cumulative confirmed COVID-19 cases and deaths per million people.
Source: Adapted from Our World in Data – CSSE at Johns Hopkins University 2021a, 2021b).

(25.81) (as of March 7, 2021). Cumulative confirmed COVID-19 deaths/ million people in Japan are 65.27, which is much lower than the United Kingdom (1,837.43), the United States (1,586.18), Sweden (1,287.52), the Netherlands (931.55), Germany (859.16), and Finland (138.43). However, Japan has not been able to mitigate COVID-related deaths as successfully as Australia (35.65), South Korea (32.03), New Zealand (5.39), Thailand (1.22), Taiwan (0.42), and Vietnam (0.36) (See Figure 8.1). These figures suggest that Japan has not been able to control COVID-19 infections and related deaths as effectively as some countries in the Asia-Pacific region. However, Japan still controlled the coronavirus better than several developed countries in Europe and North America.

One of the distinctive features of Japan's pandemic approach is to not actively conduct widespread COVID-19 testing for asymptomatic people; this approach is opposed to the widespread testing of asymptomatic people in countries such as South Korea, the United States, and China. This approach results from Japan's limited administrative and testing capacity (Moon et al. 2021, Shimizu et al. 2020). In Japan, 61.15 people are tested per 1,000 people as of Feb 28, 2021 while this number is 128.27 in South Korea, 395.33 in the Netherlands, and 7.34 in Taiwan (CSSE at Johns Hopkins University 2021c).[3] In fact, it has been reported that doctors' and citizens' requests for Polymerase chain reaction (PCR) tests are often rejected by public health centers due to the lack of testing capacity in Japan (Shimizu et al. 2020). In early 2020, only people who with a fever of 37.5C or higher for four days or longer were eligible for PCR testing in order to allow elderly people and those with severe symptoms such as difficulty breathing to receive a consultation based on the guidance of the Ministry of Health, Labor and Welfare (Nikkei Asia 2020, The Japan Times 2020). The Japanese government downplayed the need for PCR testing, and the government's scientific advisors rejected the need for extensive testing without scientific evidence (Shimizu et al. 2021). These strict testing guidelines were somewhat relaxed later on. However, the availability of PCR tests in Japan has remained lower than in many other countries.

As Figure 8.2 shows, the ratio of confirmed cases in Japan ranges roughly between 0.03 and 0.10 though the figure was initially higher, sometimes going beyond 0.10. This means that there are about 3 to 10 confirmed cases found per one hundred tests for COVID-19. Japan's fatality rate in 2020 was 0.023, which is a little higher than that of the United States (0.048); however, this rate is still much lower than that of many other Western European countries, such as France (0.18), Belgium (0.159), Italy (0.144), United Kingdom (0.139), the Netherlands (0.12), and Spain (0.095), among others (Worldometers 2020).

When we look at the cumulative number of the share of positive cases in the number of total tests as of February 14, 2021, Japan's number seems to be high (5.9%) when compared to Germany (5.9%), the United Kingdom (5.1%), Canada (3.6%), Finland (1.6%), South Korea (1.4%), Thailand (1.0%), Taiwan (0.6%), Australia (0.2%), and New Zealand (0.1%). The Netherlands's share is 16.3%, and the U.S.'s share is 8.6% (OurWorldInData.org 2021c). However, due to differences in the performances and types of COVID-19 tests across countries and even within countries, it is not possible to draw any definitive conclusions at this time.

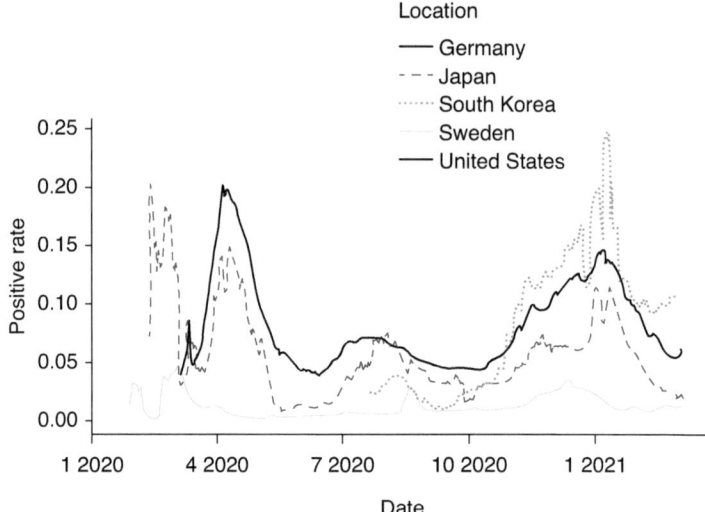

Figure 8.2 Positive confirmed case rates.

Source: Adapted from Hasell, J., Mathieu, E., Beltekian, D. et al. A cross-country database of COVID-19 testing. *Sci Data* 7, 345 (2020)).

Furthermore, one of the features of Japan's pandemic approach is that it does not actively conduct widespread COVID-19 testing for asymptomatic people. This testing policy may partly explain Japan's relatively high rate of positive tests.

Japan never imposed a strict lockdown, a process that requires enforced mobility and activity restrictions and mandatory quarantines with financial penalties for violations (as seen in countries such as New Zealand, Australia, the United Kingdom, the Netherlands, and Germany). Instead, Japan implemented "mild lockdowns" using non-binding request-based approaches to reduce mobility and certain types of public activities and relying on citizens' self-restraint behaviors to control the pandemic (Moon et al. 2021, Parady et al. 2020, Sugaya et al. 2020). The Government Stringency Index (GSI) created by Hale et al. (2020), which is a composite index measure to score the strictness of government policies, illustrates the relative looseness of Japan's measures. The index is a composite measure of nine indicators: school closures; workplace closures; cancellation of public events; restrictions on public gatherings; closures of public transport; stay-at-home requirements; public information campaigns; restrictions on internal movements; and international travel controls (OurWorldIn-Data.org 2021b). The index ranges from 0 to 100. Higher values show stricter responses. For instance, lower values indicate no measures or more recommendations to proceed with the above measures while higher values indicate stricter measures such as compulsory closures or restrictions. Figure 8.3a shows the trend of GSI since January 2020 and compares Japan with some European and North American countries while the right graph compares Japan with Asia Pacific region countries. Most countries tightened COVID-19 measures in March 2020. Japan's score is much lower than the scores of European and North American countries, demonstrating Japan's relatively relaxed measures to prevent infections. Finland seems to have followed the same path as Japan in terms of the strictness of corona measures after August 2020; however, the Finnish government took stricter measures than Japan before July 2020. Figure 8.3b suggests that Japan's measure have been less strict than those of other Asia-Pacific region countries (including Vietnam, South Korea, Australia, and Thailand) in most periods of the pandemic so far. Taiwan also seems to impose less strict COVID-19 measures. New Zealand has employed both stricter and more relaxed measures depending on conditions.

As for the economic impacts of COVID-19, Japan recorded a slight increase in its unemployment rate of 0.43 percentage points from 2.35% in 2019 to 2.78% in 2020. South Korea records only a 0.16 percentage point increase from 3.78 % to 3.94%. However, Japan's increase in the unemployment rate is much lower than in the United States (4.42), Canada (3.83), and Sweden (1.53), and it is lower than the OECD member countries' average (1.72) (OECD 2021). Japan, however, seems to have experienced a larger decline in GDP/capita when looking at the percentage decline of GDP relative to GDP in the second quarter of 2020 to the same quarter in 2019 with adjustment for inflation. Japan records a 10% decrease in GDP/capita compared to the United Kingdom (–21.7%), Canada (–13.5%), Germany (–11.7%), OECD (–10.9%), United States (–9.5%), the Netherlands (–9%), Sweden (–8.3%), Finland (–5.2%), South Korea (–3%), and Taiwan (–0.6%) (OurWorldInData.org 2021a).

Despite these surprisingly low rates of infection and fatality, responses to the Japanese government's initiatives have been mixed. According to the Gallup International polling conducted at the end of March 2020, only 23% of respondents were satisfied with the Japanese government's responses to the pandemic, placing Japan second from the bottom of 17 countries. Citizens in other countries reported significantly higher rates of satisfaction with the government: Austria (88%), India (83%), Malaysia (77%), the Netherlands (79%), South Korea (74%), United Kingdom (49%), Germany (47%), and the United States (42%). Only Thailand scored lower than Japan (20%) (Gallup International Association 2020b).[4] In the third wave of the Gallup International Survey conducted in the beginning of June 2020, Japanese citizens' satisfaction with the government approach increased from 23% to 34%. However, this result was

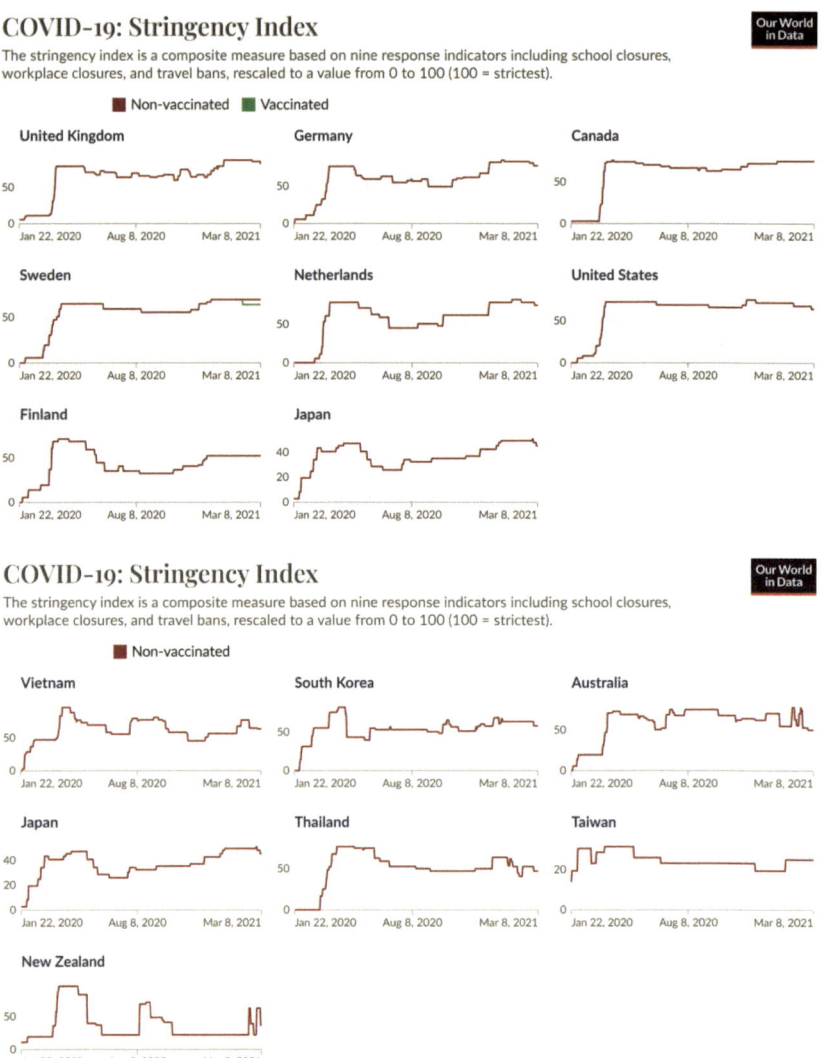

Figure 8.3 Trend of Government Stringency Index (a and b).

Source: Adapted from Hale et al. (2020). Data collected from OurWorldInData.org (2021b).

still much lower than in other countries such as Malaysia (94%), South Korea (85%), Austria (75%), India (76%), and the Philippines (59%), and it was even lower than in the United States (40%) and United Kingdom (38%) (Gallup International Association 2020a). Public opinion polls conducted by Japanese media also show low rates of citizen satisfaction with the Japanese government's handling of the virus (38% in Nihon Keizai Shimbun (2020a) and 37.4% in Jiji Tsushin (2020)).[5] Citizen confidence in the national government in general has been low in Japan compared to in other democratic countries (OECD 2019).[6] Therefore, it is not clear to what extent such a high rate of dissatisfaction accurately reflects Japanese citizens' assessment of government initiatives and strategies for the pandemic. However, Japan's relative success in virus containment does not seem to match citizens' evaluations of the government.

In sum, Japan seems to have managed the pandemic more effectively than several European and North American countries in terms of its numbers of coronavirus infection cases and fatalities. However, Japan does not seem to have been as successful in containing the disease as other Asia Pacific countries. Japan's pandemic measures appear relatively loose, based on citizens' self-restraint behaviors and lack of a clear legal basis, when compared to other industrialized democracies and several Asia-Pacific countries.

8.3   Institutional Contexts of Japan's Pandemic Approach

Social science scholars have often pointed out that institutional settings and arrangements influence the choice of policy tools and strategies for problem-solving; furthermore, these contexts determine the "logic of appropriateness," or the social norms and expectations that influence social and individual responses to a crisis (March and Olsen 2013, Pierre 2020, Kuhlmann et al. 2021). This section identifies the institutional contextual factors that may have influenced the way the Japanese government managed the COVID-19 pandemic. These factors include (1) institutional constraints on the prime minister's leadership, (2) limited administrative capacity and pandemic unpreparedness, and (3) bureaucratic professionalism and closedness.

8.3.1   *Institutional Constraints on the Prime Minister's Leadership*

The first institutional factor we examine is institutional constraints on the prime minister's leadership. Japan is an advanced democratic country, similar to many other countries studied in this book. Japan has a parliamentary system, not a presidential system. Scholars of Japanese politics have often pointed out the weak leadership of Japanese prime ministers and the institutional constraints on the prime minister's leadership (Krauss and Pekkanen 2015, Takenaka 2019). These institutional constraints on the prime minister's leadership include the strong veto power of the parliamentary Upper House; the powerful influence of the ruling party on the selection of prime minister; short leadership selection cycles; and the fragmented and decentralized vote gathering, party leadership, and policy-making processes of the ruling party (Liberal Democratic Party of Japan) (Estévez-Abe and Kim 2014, Krauss and Pekkanen 2015). Since Japanese prime ministers are not re-elected directly by citizens but instead by the ruling political party, this leadership selection process creates "a strong incentive to appeal to the majority of the fellow Diet members from the same party" (Estévez-Abe and Kim 2014, 672). The weak leadership of the prime minister was especially remarkable from 1955 to 1993, a period marked by the formation of the perennially ruling LDP until it finally lost power to a coalition of smaller, reform-oriented opposition parties (Krauss and Pekkanen 2015). A serious of institutional reforms beginning in 1994 (including electoral and administrative reforms) expanded the prime minister's power (Takenaka 2019). However, compared to leaders in other countries that seem to have successfully managed the pandemic such as New Zealand, South Korea, and Taiwan, Japanese prime ministers (Abe and Suga) seem to lack strong leadership.[7]

The institutional and political settings in Japan with respect to the COVID-19 response are characterized by stronger restrictions upon the administration and prime minister's leadership. First, Japan does not have an independent government agency that controls responses to infectious diseases; the ad hoc Novel Coronavirus Response Headquarters (NCRH) is the highest authority for COVID-19 responses. Japan has only the National Institute of Infectious Disease (NIID), which is responsible for research and administrative support. Without having experienced the MERS virus, the Japanese government was not well prepared for COVID-19. The prime minister headed the central COVID-19 response headquarters (i.e., Novel Coronavirus Response Headquarters), under which two major ministers played critical roles as vice heads. Second, the Japanese legal tradition does not allow for the exercise of emergency powers by the government. The ruling LDP's proposals to expand the government's emergency powers faced strong opposition by bar associations, law professors, and news organizations despite the Abe administration's electoral popularity (Repeta 2020). Third, economic policy has been central to the LDP, especially under Abenomics. During the 2011–2016 period, donations grew for five straight years, with nearly 90% going to the LDP. This steep rise in LDP donations reflects annual calls since 2014 by the Japan Business Federation, also known as Keidanren, for member companies to make contributions (Nikkei 2017). The centrality of economic policy and these connections with the business community underlies the political circumstances surrounding the Abe administration.

The Abe administration was further concerned about the potential impact of COVID-19 on the Tokyo 2020 Olympics, which was eventually postponed to the following year based on negotiations between the Japanese government and the International Olympic Committee (IOC) concluded on March 25, 2020. Until the postponement decision was made, the Abe administration had appealed strongly for hosting the Summer Olympic Games as scheduled. In his statement to the parliament on February 6, 2020, Prime Minister Abe made clear that his administration would not cancel or delay the Tokyo 2020 Olympics despite international concerns about COVID-19 (Reynolds and Hirokawa 2020). The political environment surrounding the Tokyo 2020 Olympic Games appeared to influence the somewhat passive initial responses of the Abe administration to COVID-19. In fact, the number of confirmed cases began to rise sharply after the postponement decision was made (Moon et al. 2021).

8.3.2 Limited Administrative Capacity and Pandemic Unpreparedness

Existing studies frequently emphasize the importance of government capacity in preventing the spread of COVID-19 (Dunlop et al. 2020, Mazzucato and Kattel 2020, Woo 2020). Government capacity has been considered one of the key factors for a high quality of government and good governance (Fukuyama 2013, Im and Choi 2018, Im and Hartley 2017, D'Arcy and Nistotskaya 2018, 2020) along with the concept of government impartiality (Nistotskaya 2020, Rothstein and Teorell 2008, Suzuki and Demircioglu 2020). Although definitions of capacity and levels of government organization studied vary (e.g., state, administration, and organization), "capacity" essentially refers to the government's "ability to perform work" (Yu-Lee 2002, 1 as cited in Christensen and Gazley (2008)). Organizational capacity in the public sector has been defined as the "government's ability to marshal, develop, direct and control its financial, human, physical and information resources" (Ingraham et al. 2003, p. 15 as cited in Christensen and Gazley (2008)). In the context of governmental responses to COVID-19, scholars focus on several aspects of government capacity (such as the operational, fiscal, and analytical) to prevent the spread of COVID-19 (Woo 2020). Scholars have also examined governments' competences and capabilities to "galvanize its administration and society into action and execute its decisions effectively" (Capano et al. 2020, 298) and government capacities to communicate and collaborate with key stakeholders and citizens (Dunlop et al. 2020, Van der Wal 2020).

Several scholars have pointed out the insufficient operational capacity of Japan's health care resources in relation to its measures against COVID-19, including the shortage of labor in the Ministry of Health, Labor and Welfare; inadequate laboratory capacity for coronavirus testing; and low ICU capacity (Inoue 2020, Kitamura 2020, Sensho 2020, Shimizu et al. 2020). Furthermore, the excessive work hours of career bureaucrats (including those who are in charge of pandemic control) has been also pointed out (Kitamura

2020, Populi 2021). Furthermore, media has reported on the increasing number of young bureaucrats who leave or wish to quit because of excessive working hours and difficulty in maintaining a work-life balance (Nagata 2020, The Japan Times Editorial Board 2020). In fact, despite the widespread image of a strong Japanese bureaucracy (Aoki 2018, Johnson 1982, Matsunami 2018), scholars have revealed the declining and smaller size of the Japanese bureaucracy compared to other industrialized democratic countries (Kitamura 2020, Maeda 2014, Nakamura and Kikuchi 2011). The OECD (2020) average for employment in the general government as a percentage of total employment was 18.06% in 2015, while Japan's rate was only 5.94%, the smallest among the 27 countries in the data set and behind Korea (7.61%). Norway records 29.97%, followed by Denmark (29.13%), Sweden (28.59%), and Finland (24.85%). The overall number of personnel in the Japanese central government has significantly declined after several government reforms (Nakamura 2012), from 6.09% in 2007 to 5.94% in 2015.

Furthermore, recent experiences of fighting similar diseases such as SARS (Severe Acute Respiratory Syndrome) and MERS (Middle East Respiratory Syndrome) may have influenced the operational capacities of governments to prevent pandemics (Capano et al. 2020). Unlike South Korea, Hong Kong, Taiwan, Singapore, and China (which all recently experienced SARS or MERS), Japan did not suffer from these viruses, perhaps leading to the Japanese government's lack of preparedness in the face of the COVID-19 pandemic (An and Tang 2020, Capano et al. 2020, Moon 2020).

8.3.3 Bureaucratic Professionalism and Closedness

Another institutional context that may have influenced Japan's reaction to the pandemic is the structural characteristics of the national bureaucracy. It is well known that the administrative characteristics of bureaucracy vary significantly across countries (Dahlström and Lapuente 2017, Hammerschmid et al. 2016, Kuhlmann and Wollmann 2019, Painter and Peters 2010, Suzuki and Demircioglu 2019). Types of national bureaucracy may partly explain different government responses to the pandemic. Although there are several dimensions of bureaucracy, we focus on the degree of political influence in bureaucratic decision-making and the degree of openness/closedness in the personnel system, following previous studies (Bekke and Meer 2000, Dahlström et al. 2012a, b, Dahlström and Lapuente 2017, Lapuente and Suzuki 2020, Lœgreid and Wise 2007, Suzuki and Hur 2020, 2021).

While government responses to the coronavirus pandemic seem to be highly influenced by political decisions in some countries, such as the United States and Brazil, this has not been the case in other countries.

In fact, the degree of political influence in bureaucratic decision-making differs significantly across countries (see, for example, Dahlström and Lapuente (2017) and Suzuki and Demircioglu (2019)). Results of previous empirical studies suggest that a meritocratically recruited bureaucracy (as opposed to a bureaucracy that is vulnerable to political intervention in personnel matters) and an impartial bureaucracy are strong predictors of favorable macro-level outcomes such as low levels of corruption, higher economic growth, improved health outcomes, government effectiveness, and innovation (Evans and Rauch 1999, Cingolani et al. 2015, Dahlström and Lapuente 2017, Nistotskaya and Cingolani 2016, Suzuki and Demircioglu 2019, Povitkina and Bolkvadze 2019).

The modern Japanese bureaucracy has been characterized by a large degree of bureaucratic autonomy and relative independence from politics in terms of personnel matters (Ginsburg 2001, Johnson 1982, Nakamura 2012, Rothacher 1993). However, this high autonomy and independence from politics seem to have been declining recently (Maeda 2018, Nakamura 2012). Overall, though, Japan's national bureaucracy remains at the top of bureaucratic professionalism from a comparative perspective. Figure 8.4 shows countries sorted by degree of bureaucratic professionalism using the QoG Expert survey (Dahlström et al. 2015a).[8] Higher levels of professionalism indicate more politically neutral public administrations (Suzuki and Demircioglu 2019). Japan's bureaucracy, ranked 6th out of the 119 sample countries, demonstrates high insulation and autonomy from political interference, at least in terms of the recruitment and promotion of bureaucrats. New Zealand, Ireland, Norway, Hong Kong, Denmark, and Sweden are also at the top of bureaucratic professionalism.[9]

Although there have been problems with relationships between politicians and bureaucrats, including medical experts (such as loose policy coordination between expert meetings and decision-makers and politicians that prioritize the interests of the tourism industry ahead of public health), there seems to have been little excessive political intervention or arbitrary political decision-making that ignored scientific evidence by the Japanese government as seen in Brazil and the United States.

Some countries which appear to have been relatively successful in containing the infection seem to have taken agile, flexible, and collaborative approaches, as seen in New Zealand, Australia, South Korea, and Taiwan (An and Tang 2020, Bromfield and McConnell 2020, Huang 2020, Jamieson 2020, Moon 2020, Van der Wal 2020). In contrast, Japan's pandemic response seems to be characterized by cautious, somewhat rigid, sluggish responses, with little policy coordination and harmonization (Moon et al. 2021, Shimizu and Negita 2020). We argue that this reaction may be partly due to Japan's rigid bureaucratic structure. Another dimension for classifying bureaucratic structures is to look at the "closed" or "open" nature of the civil service system (Bekke and Meer 2000, Dahlström et al. 2012b, Lægreid and Wise 2015). "Open" systems are flexible in recruiting and promoting public officials, with a focus on selecting the best candidate for each position (i.e. position-based systems). "Closed" systems, in contrast, feature formalized entries into the public service, seniority systems, and lifetime employment (i.e. career-based systems) (Dahlström et al. 2012b, Lægreid and Wise 2015). In closed systems, promotions tend to follow rules of seniority rather than reflecting merit or performance (Bekke and Meer 2000, Gualmini 2008). Job mobility between the public and private sectors is limited in closed systems. Closed bureaucracies tend to be highly legalistic and formalistic in internal decision-making processes (Lapuente and Suzuki 2020).

Like France, Japan's civil service is a closed career-based system with limited lateral entry, with an emphasis on internal and seniority-based promotion. Rather than to the civil service as a whole, Japanese civil servants are strongly attached to the ministry that hired them (Maeda 2018). Partly due to such strong "ministerial loyalism," Japanese bureaucrats often demonstrate poor cross-ministerial coordination. This problem of "vertical administration" (tatewari gyosei) is regarded as a major source of administrative inefficiency (Mishima 2017). Figure 8.5 shows countries sorted by degree of bureaucratic closedness using the QoG Expert survey (Dahlström et al. 2015a).[10] Japan records the highest level of bureaucratic closedness among 113 sample countries. On the other hand, New Zealand, Sweden, and the Netherlands have relatively open structures. Australia appears around the middle.[11] Taiwan and South Korea, which have been depicted as countries with agile and collaborative pandemic responses, also have high closedness structure scores (Moon 2020, Huang 2020). However, the remarkably high closedness of Japan's bureaucratic structure may be one of the institutional factors that shaped Japan's distinctive pandemic response.

8.4 Japan's COVID-19 Containment Policy

The first phase of Japan's response, from the onset to June 2020, was led by the Expert Meeting of Scientists and the Response Headquarters. The Cabinet decided to set up the Novel Coronavirus Response Headquarters (NCRH) led by Prime Minister Abe on January 30, 2020, when Japan had 11 cumulative confirmed cases. The Ministry of Health, Labour and Welfare (MHLW) was the main bureaucratic actor involved in decision-making. On February 16, 2020, the Japanese government established the Novel Coronavirus Response Expert Meeting, which is chaired by the head of the National Institute of Infectious Disease (NIID). The Expert Meeting, consisting of related scientists, provided scientific findings and

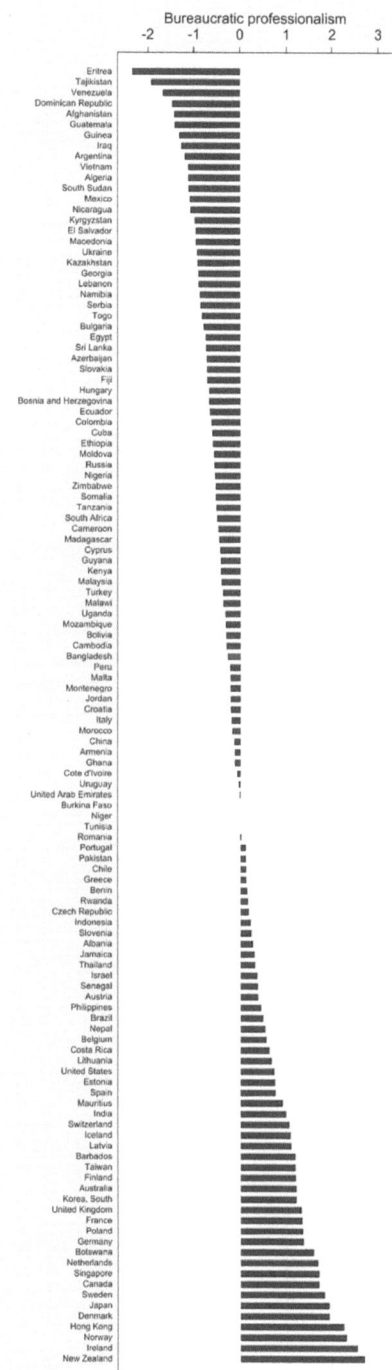

Figure 8.4 Bureaucratic professionalism.

Source: Adapted from Dahlström, C., Teorell, J., Dahlberg, S., Hartmann, F., Lindberg, A., & Nistotskaya, M. (2015). *The QoG expert survey dataset II.* Retrieved from: https://www.qogdata.pol.gu.se/dataarchive/qog_exp_15_codebook.pdf.

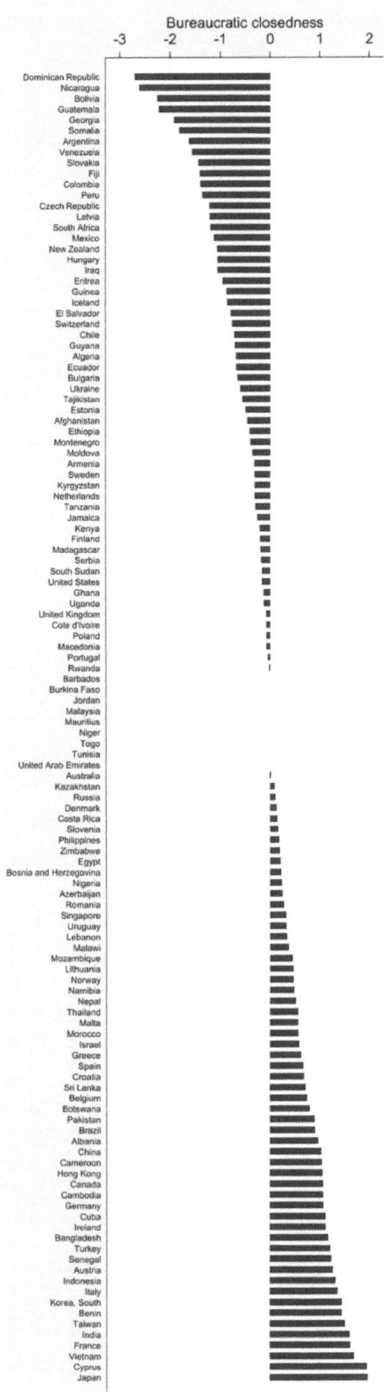

Figure 8.5 Bureaucratic closedness.

Source: Adapted from Dahlström, C., Teorell, J., Dahlberg, S., Hartmann, F., Lindberg, A., & Nistotskaya, M. (2015). *The QoG expert survey dataset II.* Retrieved from: https://www.qogdata.pol.gu.se/dataarchive/qog_exp_15_codebook.pdf.

offered policy advice to the Prime Minister and the Cabinet on matters related to COVID-19. Later, the Novel Coronavirus Response Headquarters was officially established as the related law was passed on March 26, 2020. The NCRH, led by the Prime Minister, is supported by two major ministers, the Chief Cabinet Secretary and the Minister of the MHLW. During this period, the first state of emergency was enacted between April 7 and May 25.

In the second phase starting in July 2020, the COVID response policy was driven by the newly-formed Subcommittee on Novel Coronavirus Disease Control. Along with continued requests for citizens to stay at home, the government launched stimulus packages named "Go To Travel" in late July and "Go To Eat" in September in the midst of the second wave of increased cases of new infections. The third phase of Japan's reaction centers on stopping the Go To Travel campaign (on December 28, 2020) and requests that restaurants and bars shorten business hours under the second state of emergency declared on January 7, 2021.

Japan was relatively passive and cautious in the initial phase in identifying those who were subject to COVID-19 testing and tracing potentially infected individuals, partially due to its concern about the potential impact of the coronavirus on the 2020 Tokyo Olympics, as well as the nonexistence of an independent administrative agency for disease control and prevention. As noted earlier, there is not much evidence to suggest that the Japanese government's response to infectious diseases is necessarily quicker or more effective than that of other countries. Policy decisions lack clear leadership. Japan's homogeneous and closed career-based bureaucratic system (Aoki 2018, Dahlström and Lapuente 2017, Mishima 2017) appears to be ill-equipped to deal with this unprecedented crisis, and government attempts to control the disease were request-based rather than punitive. On February 3, 2021, the parliamentary Upper House finally passed bills related to COVID-19 which allows the government to impose financial penalties when restaurants fail to comply with orders to shorten business hours, or when coronavirus patients refuse to be hospitalized (Johnston 2021, Nihon Keizai Shimbun 2021).

Like Korea, the Japanese government established an advisory committee led by their prime minister. However, the Japanese government has been less successful than Korea in terms of formulating a proactive response and communicating the management of COVID-19. Japan's mismanagement of an outbreak on the British-flagged Diamond Princess cruise ship in February 2020 drew criticism from national and international press. The sudden announcement on February 27 that all of the country's schools should close starting March 2 also confused teachers and parents (Rich et al. 2020) since it was presented as a request rather than a mandate. While in the Korean government school-related decisions were made by the Ministry of Education based on consultations with KCDC and expert groups, in Japan the decision to close schools was left to local authorities and schools. Parents were not informed of school closures until the following week on Friday afternoon. Around 60% of households with children under the age of 18 in Japan are dual-income households (Kuga 2020) and schools were not prepared to shift to digital teaching, resulting in further uncertainty among teachers and families (O'Donoghue 2020).

This lack of transparency, strong political leadership, or effective communication among stakeholders in the decision-making process drew criticism from the public (NHK 2020). Failure to take the minutes of the Novel Coronavirus Expert Meeting, which advises the government from a medical point of view, led to further criticism (Takahashi 2020). Consequently, many polls show that Prime Minister Abe's approval rate has continued to fall since the outbreak of COVID-19 in January 2020. Other incidents of administrative mismanagement and prosecutor scandals may also have affected Abe's declining rate of support (Sugiyama 2020). However, the high rate of popular dissatisfaction with government measures against COVID-19 should be one of the major reasons for this drop.

The government lifted the state of emergency in all prefectures on May 25, 2020. However, local governments, such as Tokyo's, implemented a gradual reopening of economic activities. All requests (with a few exceptions) for suspending businesses have been lifted as of June 19 although stores and businesses are still asked to implement measures to prevent coronavirus infections and to conduct health checkups of employees (Jiji Press 2020b).

Japan's public health capacities when the coronavirus outbreak started were apparently not ideal in many regards. There were relatively fewer intensive care unit beds in comparison to other OECD countries. According to a report by the Health Policy Bureau, Ministry of Health, Labor and Welfare, there were only 5.6 intensive care unit (ICU) beds per population as of 2017, which is fewer than the United States (34.7), Germany (29.2), Italy (12.5), and the United Kingdom (6.6). In addition to the lack of public health capacities, research budgets on infectious diseases have been constantly cut at national level over the last decade. The research budget of the National Institute of Infectious Diseases (NIID), the leading national research institute, dropped from about 6 trillion yen in 2009 to about 4 trillion in 2018. The number of researchers decreased from 325 in 2010 to 306 in 2018, an approximately 5.8% cut (Kawata 2020). Consequently, public health capacities were quite limited at the beginning of the crisis.

As explained in Moon et al. (2021), the role of experts in crisis management is relatively limited in that they "advise" the policy making of the administration and bureaucracy; however, the experts neither make decisions nor implement policies. The closed employment system of civil servants and limited use of external experts may be one reason for passive use of experts in the policy-making process. Japan also lacks an independent decision-making body led by experts similar to the Center for Disease Control and Prevention (CDC) in the United States or KCDC in Korea. The NIID is an outpost agency of the MHLW and was not granted decision-making autonomy. Professor Kentaro Iwata of Kobe University, an infection control specialist, pointed out that Japan's lack of "scientific decision-making by an independent team of professionals" caused problems during the quarantine on the Diamond Princess cruise ship in February (Osaki 2020a). The Novel Coronavirus Expert Meeting led by NIID Director Takaji Wakita is a collective of academics and infectious disease experts; however, its role was limited to offering advice. In fact, the nationwide closures of schools "requested" by Prime Minister Abe was not even advised by the Expert Meeting (Nihon Keizai Shimbun 2020b). Administrative experts in Japan also criticized the unclear division of roles in infection disease control between the parties involved, including the prime minister, minister in charge, chief cabinet secretary, and expert meetings. It is also reported that the government relies on experts' opinions and that experts informally "control" policy decisions despite their lack of status as an independent decision-making body, as explained below (Makihara 2020).

New tools of control and policing were implemented; many of these measures, however, were not compulsory. Since the government declared a state of emergency in seven prefectures (including Tokyo and Osaka) on April 7, the Abe administration called on citizens to perform "self-restraint" (jishuku in Japanese) activities without direct inter-human contact, with the goal of decreasing contacts by 80%. Following this declaration, local governments "requested" targeted industries, ranging from museums and schools to bars and nightclubs, to suspend business. These rules were requests and there were no penalties for non-compliance; the administration has consistently been reluctant to enforce measures that restrict private rights. On June 15, PM Abe insisted that introducing penalties should be considered with great caution (Yomiuri Shimbun 2020). However, such requests have been effectively enforced even without legal penalties. Although the reasons for this effectiveness have not been systematically explained, it is sometimes attributed to Japan's unique culture of social norm compliance. In extreme cases, stores that legally continued business were insulted and pressured to stop operations by local citizens called jishuku keisatsu, or "self-restraint police" (Fujii and Hata 2020). Rule breakers of the new social norms (including mask-wearing, staying at home, and suspending business) were often harassed by these local citizens (Katafuchi et al. 2020, Moon et al. 2021, Osaki 2020b).

This reliance on self-restraint can also be attributed to Japan's unique constitutional regime. The contemporary Japanese constitution lacks explicit emergency provisions, and there has been strong resistance to legislation that would give the government emergency power. The pre-war Imperial Constitution had emergency provisions that led to abuses of power during "national crises" such as the Great Kato Earthquake of 1923 and the wars of the 1930s–1940s. Therefore, the legal basis for compulsory measures during a crisis is severely limited (Oya 2020).

Financial packages were also offered in Japan. These packages included 100 thousand yen (about 935 USD) of individual financial aid and up to 1 million yen (about 9,350 USD) of the Subsidy Program for Sustaining Businesses (METI 2020). The government also offered two reusable cloth face masks per household, which were sent by mail. However, it took almost two months for the government to complete this delivery of face masks to most households in Japan (Jiji Press 2020a).

8.5   Conclusion

We argue that the Japanese government policy is characterized by reliance on self-restraint behavior and individual hygiene practices rather than enforcing strict, legally binding measures and proactively testing and tracing individuals. First, Japan did not implement strict lockdown measures involving penalties. Instead, the Japanese government took a "mild lockdown" approach. Instead of imposing strict COVID-19 measures, the Japanese government has largely relied on citizens' voluntary self-restraint behavior (jishuku in Japanese), requesting that citizens refrain from going out or attending mass gatherings and requesting that retail, dining, and entertainment industries shorten business hours or cancel large events.

Moreover, the ruling party's economic interests, including the Olympic games, are often strongly reflected in policies, seemingly due to the specific institutional contexts characterized by the lack of emergency power and centralized leadership at both the expert- and executive-levels. Thus, Japan's response to the spread of COVID throughout the two rounds of the state of emergency is cautious and restrained, although the actual performance—how the enacted policy influenced the spreading of COVID-19— needs further examination.

This chapter explains Japan's pandemic approach and the institutional contexts that may partly explain the distinctiveness of Japan's policy. Cross-national comparative studies are needed to understand in detail the relationship between national institutional factors, the nature of the government's corona control, and corona-related outcome measures. A further challenge is that it is difficult to compare COVID-19 related outcome measures across countries due to differences in testing policies, testing abilities, and the reliability of COVID-19 related statistics. Future studies should undertake such tasks as the data become available.

Notes

1 For example, the European Union Council's set epidemiologically safe countries outside the Schengen Area amid the COVID-19 pandemic. The EU Council advises the member states to lift travel restrictions at the country boarders for residents of the countries in the list. The safe countries list includes Australia, New Zealand, Rwanda, Singapore, South Korea, Thailand, and China (if China lifts entry restrictions for European travelers) as of January 28, 2021. Canada and Japan along with other several countries were originally in the safe countries list in June 2020, but were excluded later (Schengen VisaInfo.com 2021).

2 See, for example, Hur and Kim (2020), Kim (2020), Lee et al. (2020), Moon (2020), Park and Maher (2020) for South Korea, Huang (2020), Liao et al. (2020), Lin et al. (2020), Yen (2020) for Taiwan, Cai et al. (2021), Hu et al. (2020), Santos (2021) for China, Jamieson (2020) for New Zealand, and Bromfield and McConnell (2020), Wallace and Dollery (2021) for Australia. See, for example, Fraser and Aldrich (2021) and Moon et al. (2021) as examples of already published works examining Japan by public administration and political science scholars. See Inoue (2020), Shimizu and Negita (2020), Shimizu et al. (2020), Shimizu et al. (2021) for summaries of Japan's approach by health policy scientists.

3 Test numbers in the United Kingdom, the United States, Canada, Finland, Australia, Germany, New Zealand, Thailand, and Vietnam show only number of tests performed per 1000 people, not number of people tested.

4 Participants were asked to select responses from "strongly agree" to "strongly disagree" as well as "do not know" for the question, "How strongly do you agree or disagree with the following statements?—I think the Government is handling the Coronavirus well." Respondents who selected "strongly agree" or "agree" were considered satisfied citizens.

5 Those respondents who selected "rate it highly (*hyouka suru*)" were considered satisfied.

6 Confidence in national government in Japan was 38% in 2018 (24% in 2007) while in South Korea it was 39% (24%), Switzerland 85% (63%), India 75% (82%), Netherlands 66% (66%), the United States 31% (39%), and the United Kingdom 42% (36%), where the percentage is representative of the number of respondents who selected "yes" to the question, "Do you have confidence in national government?" (OECD 2019).

7 Prime Minister Abe, followed by Prime Minister Suga, announced his resignation on August 28, 2020.

8 Professional bureaucracy is an index variable created based on a principal component analysis of the following statements: (1) When recruiting public sector employees, the skills and merits of the applicants decide who gets the job, (2) When recruiting public sector employees, the political connections of the applicants decide who gets the job, (3) The top political leadership hires and fires senior public officials. Cronbach's alpha is 0.88. We reversed the scale of the index to show that higher values mean less political influence in personnel policies. Please see Dahlström et al. (2015b) for details of the QoG Expert Survey.

9 Japan also records high level of meritocracy in the 3rd wave of the QoG Expert Survey that was recently released (Nistotskaya et al. 2021).

10 Closed bureaucracy is also an index variable created based on the following statements: (1) Public sector employees are hired via a formal examination system, (2) Senior public officials are recruited from within the ranks of the

public sector, (3) Once one is recruited as a public sector employee, one remains a public sector employee for the rest of one's career. Cronbach's alpha is 0.70, which is relatively low. However, it is still at an acceptable level of reliability.

11 Japan also records a high level of closedness in the 3rd wave of the QoG Expert Survey (Nistotskaya et al. 2021).

References

An, Brian Y., and Shui-Yan Tang. 2020. "Lessons from COVID-19 responses in East Asia: Institutional infrastructure and enduring policy instruments." *The American Review of Public Administration* 50 (6–7):790–800.

Ansell, Christopher, Eva Sørensen, and Jacob Torfing. 2020. "The COVID-19 pandemic as a game changer for public administration and leadership? The need for robust governance responses to turbulent problems." *Public Management Review* 23 (7):949–960.

Aoki, Naomi. 2018. "Japan's bureaucracy in international perspective." In *Global encyclopedia of public administration, public policy, and governance*, edited by Ali Farazmand, 1–5. Cham: Springer International Publishing.

Bekke, Albertus Johannes Gerhardus Maria, and Frits M. Meer. 2000. *Civil service systems in Western Europe*. Cheltenham: Edward Elgar Publishing.

Bromfield, Nicholas, and Allan McConnell. 2020. "Two routes to precarious success: Australia, New Zealand, COVID-19 and the politics of crisis governance." *International Review of Administrative Sciences* 87 (3):518–535.

Cai, Changkun, Weiqi Jiang, and Na Tang. 2021. "Campaign-style crisis regime: how China responded to the shock of COVID-19." *Policy Studies* 43 (3):599–619. doi: 10.1080/01442872.2021.1883576.

Capano, Giliberto, et al. 2020. "Mobilizing policy (in) capacity to fight COVID-19: Understanding variations in state responses." *Policy and Society* 39 (3):285–308.

Christensen, Robert K., and Beth Gazley. 2008. "Capacity for public administration: Analysis of meaning and measurement." *Public Administration and Development: The International Journal of Management Research and Practice* 28 (4):265–279.

Cingolani, Luciana, Kaj Thomsson, and Denis de Crombrugghe. 2015. "Minding Weber more than ever? The impacts of state capacity and bureaucratic autonomy on development goals." *World Development* 72:191–207.

CSSE at Johns Hopkins University. 2021a. "COVID-19 data repository: Cumulative confirmed COVID-19 cases per million people." Accessed March 8, 2021. https://ourworldindata.org/coronavirus-data-explorer?zoomToSelection=true&time=2020-03-01..latest&country=USA~DEU~JPN~KOR~VNM~SWE~THA~NZL~FIN&region=World&casesMetric=true&interval=total&perCapita=true&smoothing=0&pickerMetric=location&pickerSort=asc.

CSSE at Johns Hopkins University. 2021b. "COVID-19 data repository: Cumulative confirmed COVID-19 deaths per million people." Accessed March 8, 2021. https://ourworldindata.org/coronavirus-data-explorer?zoomToSelection=true&time=2020-03-01..latest&country=USA~DEU~JPN~KOR~VNM~SWE~THA~NZL~FIN&region=World&deathsMetric=true&interval=total&perCapita=true&smoothing=0&pickerMetric=location&pickerSort=asc.

CSSE at Johns Hopkins University. 2021c. "COVID-19 data repository: Cumulative COVID-19 tests per 1,000 people." Accessed March 9, 2021. https://ourworldindata.org/coronavirus-data-explorer?zoomToSelection=true&time=2020-03-01..latest&country=USA~SWE~DEU~FIN~JPN~KOR~NZL~THA~VNM~TWN~GBR~NLD~CAN~AUS&region=World&testsMetric=true&interval=total&perCapita=true&smoothing=0&pickerMetric=location&pickerSort=asc.

D'Arcy, Michelle, and Marina Nistotskaya. 2018. "The early modern origins of contemporary European tax outcomes." *European Journal of Political Research* 57 (1):47–67. doi: 10.1111/1475-6765.12214.

D'Arcy, Michelle, and Marina Nistotskaya. 2020. "State capacity, quality of government, sequencing and development outcomes." In *Oxford handbook of the quality of government*, edited by A Bågenholm, M Bauhr, M Grimes and B Rothstein. Oxford: Oxford University Press.

Dahlström, Carl, and Victor Lapuente. 2017. *Organizing the Leviathan: How the relationship between politicians and bureaucrats shapes good government*. Cambridge: Cambridge University Press.

Dahlström, Carl, Victor Lapuente, and Jan Teorell. 2012a. "The merit of meritocratization: Politics, bureaucracy, and the institutional deterrents of corruption." *Political Research Quarterly* 65 (3):656–668.

Dahlström, Carl, Victor Lapuente, and Jan Teorell. 2012b. "Public administration around the world." In *Good government: The relevance of political science*, edited by Sören Holmberg and Bo Rothstein, 40–67. Cheltenham: Edward Elgar Publishing.

Dahlström, Carl, Jan Teorell, Stefan Dahlberg, Felix Hartmann, Annika Lindberg, and Marina Nistotskaya. 2015a. The QoG expert survey dataset II. In *Gothenburg, Sweden: Quality of Government Institute*. Gothenburg, Sweden. Retrieved from https://www.qogdata.pol.gu.se/dataarchive/qog_exp_15_codebook.pdf.

Dahlström, Carl, Jan Teorell, Stefan Dahlberg, Felix Hartmann, Annika Lindberg, and Marina Nistotskaya. 2015b. "The QoG expert survey II report." The QoG Working Paper Series.

Dunlop, Claire A., Edoardo Ongaro, and Keith Baker. 2020. "Researching COVID-19: A research agenda for public policy and administration scholars." *Public Policy and Administration* 35 (4):365–383.

Estévez-Abe, Margarita, and Yeong-Soon Kim. 2014. "Presidents, prime ministers and politics of care-why Korea expanded childcare much more than Japan." *Social Policy & Administration* 48 (6):666–685.

Evans, Peter, and James E Rauch. 1999. "Bureaucracy and growth: A cross-national analysis of the effects of 'Weberian' state structures on economic growth." *American Sociological Review* 64 (5):748–765.

Fraser, Timothy, and Daniel P. Aldrich. 2021. "The dual effect of social ties on COVID-19 spread in Japan." *Scientific Reports* 11 (1):1596. doi: 10.1038/s41598-021-81001-4.

Fujii, Ryo, and Takeru Hata. 2020. "Kyugyo semaru 'jishuku keisatsu' dema kakusan de kyaku gekigen—sutoresu de kishimu shakai [The 'restraint police' are pressing for closure. The number of customers plummeted due to the spread of the hoax.].” *Yomiuri Shimbun*, May 13, 2020. Accessed June 17, 2020. https://www.yomiuri.co.jp/national/20200513-OYT1T50231/.

Fukuyama, Francis. 2013. “What is governance?” *Governance* 26 (3):347–368.

Gallup International Association. 2020a. “3rd wave of the gallup international survey on the corona crisis.” Accessed March 11, 2021. https://www.gallup-international.com/fileadmin/user_upload/surveys/2020/Covid-19Wave-3-1.pdf.

Gallup International Association. 2020b. “The coronavirus: A vast scared majority around the world.” Accessed June 11, 2020. https://www.gallup-international.com/wp-content/uploads/2020/03/GIA_SnapPoll_2020_COVID_Tables_final.pdf.

Ginsburg, Tom. 2001. “Dismantling the developmental state”? Administrative procedure reform in Japan and Korea.” *The American Journal of Comparative Law* 49 (4):585–625.

Gualmini, Elisabetta. 2008. “Restructuring Weberian bureaucracy: Comparing managerial reforms in Europe and the United States.” *Public Administration* 86 (1):75–94.

Hale, Thomas, Samuel Webster, Anna Petherick, Toby Phillips, and Beatriz Kira. 2020. *Oxford COVID-19 government response tracker*. Blavatnik School of Government. Retrieved from: https://www.bsg.ox.ac.uk/research/research-projects/oxford-covid-19-government-response-tracker.

Hammerschmid, Gerhard, et al. 2016. *Public administration reforms in Europe: The view from the top*. Cheltenham: Edward Elgar Publishing.

Hu, Qian, Haibo Zhang, Naim Kapucu, and Wu Chen. 2020. “Hybrid coordination for coping with the medical surge from the COVID-19 pandemic: Paired assistance programs in China.” *Public Administration Review* 80 (5):895–901.

Huang, Irving Yi-Feng. 2020. “Fighting against COVID-19 through government initiatives and collaborative governance: Taiwan experience.” *Public Administration Review* 80 (4):665–670.

Hur, Joon-Young, and KyungWoo Kim. 2020. “Crisis learning and flattening the curve: South Korea’s rapid and massive diagnosis of the COVID-19 infection.” *The American Review of Public Administration* 50 (6–7):606–613.

Im, Tobin, and Youngmi Choi. 2018. “Rethinking national competitiveness: A critical assessment of governmental capacity measures.” *Social Indicators Research* 135 (2):515–532.

Im, Tobin, and Kris Hartley. 2017. “Aligning needs and capacities to boost government competitiveness.” *Public Organization Review* 19:119–137.

Ingraham, Patricia W., Philip G. Joyce, and Amy K. Donahue. 2003. *Government performance: Why management matters*. Baltimore: Johns Hopkins University Press.

Inoue, Hajime. 2020. “Japanese strategy to COVID-19: How does it work?” *Global Health & Medicine* 2 (2):131–132.

Jamieson, Thomas. 2020. ““Go Hard, Go Early”: Preliminary lessons from New Zealand’s response to COVID-19.” *The American Review of Public Administration* 50 (6–7):598–605.

Jiji Press. 2020a. “Abeno masuku haihu, hobo kanryou shingatakorona [Abeno mask distribution almost complete: Novel coronavirus].” *Jiji Press*, June 15, 2020. Accessed March 28, 2021. https://www.jiji.com/jc/article?k=2020061500902&g=pol.

Jiji Press. 2020b. "To no kyugyo yosei ga zenmen kaijo shinjukuku 'yorunomachi' sekkyoku kensa-shingata korona [The Tokyo Metropolitan Government's request to close the office was fully lifted. Shinjuku City actively inspects the "nightlife district" - the new corona." *Jiji Press*, June 9, 2020. Accessed June 27, 2020. https://www.jiji.com/jc/article?k=2020061801221&g=eco.

Jiji Tsushin. 2020. "Naikakushiji 38%, fushiji 61% Shingatakorona taiou 6 wari hyoukasezu jiji yoronchousa [Cabinet approval rate 38%, disapproval rate 61%. 60% of the respondents did not evaluate the government responses to new coronavirus." Accessed June 11, 2020. https://www.jiji.com/jc/article?k=2020060600324&g=pol.

Johnson, Chalmers. 1982. *MITI and the Japanese miracle: The growth of industrial policy, 1925–1975*. Stanford, CA: Stanford University Press.

Johnston, Eric. 2021. "Japan's new virus law: Fines for noncompliance and support for hard-hit firms." *The Japan Times*, February 4, 2021. Accessed April 4, 2021. https://www.japantimes.co.jp/news/2021/02/04/national/new-virus-law-explainer/.

Katafuchi, Yuya, Kenichi Kurita, and Shunsuke Managi. 2020. "COVID-19 with stigma: Theory and evidence from mobility data." *Economics of Disasters and Climate Change* 5:71–95.

Kawata, Atsushi. 2020. "Kokuritsu kansenken gemba wa himei: rekidai seikenka de jinin yosan den [The National Institute of infectious diseases struggles after budget and personnel cuts]." *Tokyo Newspaper*, March 7, 2020. Accessed June 16, 2020. https://www.tokyo-np.co.jp/article/14466.

Kim, Pan Suk. 2020. "South Korea's fast response to coronavirus disease: Implications on public policy and public management theory." *Public Management Review* 23 (12):1736–1747.

Kitamura, Wataru. 2020. "Nihon no gyousei wa surimu sugiru [Japanese administration is too small]." *Chuo Kouron*, 134:42–51.

Krauss, Ellis S., and Robert J. Pekkanen. 2015. "Possible futures of political leadership: Waiting for a transformational Prime Minister." In *Possible futures of political leadership: Waiting for a transformational PrimeMinister*, edited by Baldwin Frank and Allison Anne, 282–303. New York: New York University Press.

Kuga, Naoko. 2020. *Shingata korona, kyukoude kosodatekatei daikonranno mittsuno haikei* [Three reasons why the novel corona virus and school closures are wreaking havoc on families raising children]. https://www.nli-research.co.jp/files/topics/64068_ext_18_0.pdf?site=nli.

Kuhlmann, Sabine, Hellström, M., Ramberg, U., & Reiter, R. 2021. "Tracing divergence in crisis governance: Responses to the COVID-19 pandemic in France, Germany and Sweden compared." *International Review of Administrative Sciences* 87 (3):556–575.

Kuhlmann, Sabine, and Hellmut Wollmann. 2019. *Introduction to comparative public administration: Administrative systems and reforms in Europe*. Cheltenham: Edward Elgar Publishing.

Lægreid, Per, and Lois Recascino Wise. 2015. "Transitions in civil service systems: Robustness and flexibility in human resource management." In *Comparative civil service systems in the 21st century*, edited by Theo Toonen, Frits van der Meer and Jos Raadschelders, 203–222. New York: Palgrave.

Lapuente, Victor, and Kohei Suzuki. 2020. "Politicization, bureaucratic legalism, and innovative attitudes in the public sector." *Public Administration Review* 80 (3):454–467.

Lee, Sabinne, Changho Hwang, and M. Jae Moon. 2020. "Policy learning and crisis policy-making: Quadruple-loop learning and COVID-19 responses in South Korea." *Policy and Society* 39 (3):363–381.

Liao, Wei-Jie, Nai-Ling Kuo, and Shih-Hsien Chuang. 2020. "Taiwan's budgetary responses to COVID-19: The use of special budgets." *Journal of Public Budgeting, Accounting & Financial Management* 33 (1):24–32. doi: 10.1108/JPBAFM-07-2020-0128.

Lin, Ching-Fu, Chien-Huei Wu, and Chuan-Feng Wu. 2020. "Reimagining the administrative state in times of global health crisis: An anatomy of Taiwan's regulatory actions in response to the COVID-19 pandemic." *European Journal of Risk Regulation* 11 (2):256–272. doi: 10.1017/err.2020.25.

Lœgreid, Per, and Lois Recascino Wise. 2007. "Reforming human resource management in civil service systems: Recruitment, mobility, and representativeness." In *The civil service in the 21st century*, edited by Jos C. N. Raadschelders, Theo A. J. Toonen and Frits M. Van der Meer, 169–182. London: Palgrave Macmillan.

Maeda, Kentaro. 2014. *Shimin wo yatowanai kokka [A state not actively employing its citizens]*. Tokyo: Tokyo University Press.

Maeda, Kentaro. 2018. "The Japanese civil service." In *Global encyclopedia of public administration, public policy, and governance*, edited by Ali Farazmand, 1–9. Cham: Springer International Publishing.

Makihara, Izuru. 2020. *Maenomerino "senmonka chiimu" gaaburidasu shingatakorona heno abeseikenno mijukuna taiou [The Abe administration's inexperienced response to the new corona uncovered by its lean-forwarding 'expert team']*. Ronza.

March, James G., and Johan P. Olsen. 2013. The logic of appropriateness. In *The Oxford handbook of political science*, edited by Robert E. Goodin. New York: Oxford University Press Inc.

Matsunami, Jun. 2018. "Politico-administrative relationships in Japanese context." In *Global encyclopedia of public administration, public policy, and governance*, edited by Ali Farazmand, 1–5. Cham: Springer International Publishing.

Mazzucato, Mariana, and Rainer Kattel. 2020. "COVID-19 and public-sector capacity." *Oxford Review of Economic Policy* 36 (Suppl. 1):S256–S269.

McCurry, Justin. 2020. "From near disaster to success story: How Japan has tackled coronavirus." *The Guardian*. Accessed June 11, 2020. https://www.theguardian.com/world/2020/may/22/from-near-disaster-to-success-story-how-japan-has-tackled-coronavirus.

METI. 2020. "Keizai sangyoshou no shiensaku [METI's support measures]." Accessed June 20, 2020. https://www.meti.go.jp/covid-19/index.html.

Mishima, Ko. 2017. "A big bang for Japanese Mandarins? The civil service reform of 2014." *International Journal of Public Administration* 40 (13):1101–1113.

Moon, Jae M., et al. 2021. "A comparative study of COVID-19 responses in South Korea and Japan: Political nexus triad and policy responses." *International Review of Administrative Sciences* 87 (3):651–671.

Moon, Jae M. 2020. "Fighting Against COVID-19 with agility, transparency, and participation: Wicked policy problems and new governance challenges." *Public Administration Review* 80 (4):651–656.

Muto, Kaori, et al. 2020. "Japanese citizens' behavioral changes and preparedness against COVID-19: An online survey during the early phase of the pandemic." *PLoS One* 15 (6):e0234292.

Nagata, Kazuaki. 2020. "Taro Kono looks to pinpoint what is demotivating young Japanese bureaucrats." *The Japan Times*, October 3, 2020. Accessed March 17, 2021. https://www.japantimes.co.jp/news/2020/10/03/national/taro-kono-motivation-bureaucrats/.

Nakamura, Akira. 2012. "Asian model of government re-examined in the aftermath of the global economic crunch: A Japanese perspective from the experience of the triple disasters in March 2011." *International Review of Administrative Sciences* 78 (2):239–259.

Nakamura, Akira, and Masao Kikuchi. 2011. "Japanese public administration at the crossroads: Declining trust in government and civil service reform in the age of fiscal retrenchment." In *International handbook on civil service systems*, edited by Andrew Massey, 282–304. Northampton, MA: Edward Elgar Publishing.

NHK. 2020. "Naikaku Shijiritsu [Cabinet approval ratings]." Accessed June 13, 2020. https://www.nhk.or.jp/senkyo/shijiritsu/.

Nihon Keizai Shimbun. 2020a. "Korona taiou hyoukasezu 55% yoronchousa naikakushijiritsu yokobai 49% [Disapproval rate for government's response to corona 55%, cabinet approval rate unchanged at 49%]." Accessed June 11, 2020. https://www.nikkei.com/article/DGKKZO58921710Q0A510C2MM8000/.

Nihon Keizai Shimbun. 2020b. "Nihon wa senmonka no shireito-soshiki nashi kengen to sekinin no meikakuka fukaketsu [Absence of expert leadership in Japan: Clear delineation of authorities and responsibilities needed]." *Nihon Keizai Shimbun*, April 21, 2020. Accessed June 18, 2020. https://www.nikkei.com/article/DGXMZO58271700Q0A420C2EA2000/.

Nihon Keizai Shimbun. 2021. "Financial penalty for refusal of shortened working hours and hospitalization. Revised Special Measures Law, etc. enacted [Jitan nyuuin no kyohi ni karyou. Kaisei tokusohou nado seiritsu]." *Nihon Keizai Shimbun*, February 3, 2021. Accessed April 4, 2021. https://www.nikkei.com/article/DGXZQODE030ZQ0T00C21A2000000/.

Nikkei Asia. 2020. "Japan to scrap 37.5 C fever rule for PCR testing." *Nikkei Asia*, May 6, 2020. https://asia.nikkei.com/Spotlight/Coronavirus/Japan-to-scrap-37.5-C-fever-rule-for-PCR-testing.

Nikkei. December 1, 2017. "Japan's ruling party gets lion's share of business donations: Automakers association was the single largest donor to Shinzo Abe's LDP in 2016."

Nistotskaya, Marina. 2020. "Quality of Government (QoG) as impartiality: Review of the literature on the causes and consequences of QoG." *KIPA Public Policy Review* 1:25–49.

Nistotskaya, Marina, and Luciana Cingolani. 2016. "Bureaucratic structure, regulatory quality, and entrepreneurship in a comparative perspective: Cross-sectional and panel data evidence." *Journal of Public Administration Research and Theory* 26 (3):519–534.

Nistotskaya, Marina, et al. 2021. "The quality of government expert survey 2020 (Wave III): Report." *QoG Working Paper Series* 2:1–59. doi: 10.18157/qoges2020.

O'Donoghue, J. J. 2020. "In era of COVID-19, a shift to digital forms of teaching in Japan." *The Japan Times.* https://www.japantimes.co.jp/news/2020/04/21/national/traditional-to-digital-teaching-coronavirus/.

OECD. 2019. *Government at a glance 2019.* Paris: OECD Publishing.

OECD. 2020. Government at a Glance – 2017 Edition: Public employment and pay. Accessed October 9, 2020. https://stats.oecd.org/Index.aspx?QueryId=78408; https://stats.oecd.org/Index.aspx?QueryId=78408#.

OECD. 2021. "Unemployment rate (indicator)." https://data.oecd.org/unemp/unemployment-rate.htm.

Osaki, Tomohiro. 2020a. "Coronavirus outbreak highlights need for independent CDC-style body in Japan." *The Japan Times*, February 24, 2020. Accessed June 27, 2020. https://www.japantimes.co.jp/news/2020/02/24/national/niid-cdc-japan/#.Xu1pH2j7Suk.

Osaki, Tomohiro. 2020b. "Japan's 'virus vigilantes' take on rule-breakers and invaders." *The Japan Times*, May 13, 2020. Accessed June 27, 2020. https://www.japantimes.co.jp/news/2020/05/13/national/coronavirus-vigilantes-japan/.

OurWorldInData.org. 2021a. "Economic decline in the second quarter of 2020." Accessed March 9, 2021. https://ourworldindata.org/covid-health-economy.

OurWorldInData.org. 2021b. "Government stringency index." Accessed March 11, 2021. https://ourworldindata.org/policy-responses-covid#government-stringency-index.

OurWorldInData.org. 2021c. "The share of COVID-19 tests that are positive." Accessed March 12, 2021. https://ourworldindata.org/coronavirus-data-explorer?zoomToSelection=true&time=2020-03-01..latest&country=USA~SWE~DEU~FIN~JPN~KOR~NZL~THA~VNM~TWN~GBR~NLD~CAN~AUS&region=World&positiveTestRate=true&interval=total&perCapita=true&smoothing=0&pickerMetric=location&pickerSort=asc.

Oya, Takehiro. 2020. "Naze Nihon wa Jishuku no Onegai Shika Dekinai noka: Oya Takehiro san (hotetsugakusha) no Baai." Online article. https://nhkbook-hiraku.com/n/n0e6820c4d2a5.

Painter, M., and B. Peters, eds. 2010. *Tradition and public administration.* London: Palgrave Macmillan.

Parady, Giancarlos, Ayako Taniguchi, and Kiyoshi Takami. 2020. "Travel behavior changes during the COVID-19 pandemic in Japan: Analyzing the effects of risk perception and social influence on going-out self-restriction." *Transportation Research Interdisciplinary Perspectives* 7:100181.

Park, Sungho, and Craig S. Maher. 2020. "Government financial management and the coronavirus pandemic: A comparative look at South Korea and the United States." *The American Review of Public Administration* 50 (6–7):590–597. doi: 10.1177/0275074020941720.

Pierre, Jon. 2020. "Nudges against pandemics: Sweden's COVID-19 containment strategy in perspective." *Policy and Society* 39 (3):478–493.

Populi, Vox. 2021. "VOX POPULI: Extreme work hours crushing staff in seat of Japanese power." *The Asahi Shimbun*, March 9, 2021. Accessed March 17, 2021. http://www.asahi.com/ajw/articles/14252874.

Povitkina, Marina, and Ketevan Bolkvadze. 2019. "Fresh pipes with dirty water: How quality of government shapes the provision of public goods in democracies." *European Journal of Political Research* 58 (4):1191–1212

Repeta, Lawrence. April 14, 2020. "The coronavirus and Japan's Constitution." *The Japan Times.* Accessed February 3, 2021. https://www.japantimes.co.jp/opinion/2020/04/14/commentary/japan-commentary/coronavirus-japans-constitution/

Reynolds, I. and T. Hirokawa. 2020. "Japan's Abe says Olympics won't be postponed amid virus fears. *Bloomberg.* https://www.bloomberg.com/news/articles/2020-02-06/japan-s-abe-says-olympics-won-t-be-postponed-amid-virus-fears?embedded-checkout=true

Rich, Motoko, Ben Dooley, and Makiko Inoue. February 27, 2020. "Japan shocks parents by moving to close all schools over coronavirus." *The New York Times.* https://www.nytimes.com/2020/02/27/world/asia/japan-schools-coronavirus.html.

Rothacher, Albrecht. 1993. *The Japanese power elite.* New York: St. Martin's Press.

Rothstein, Bo, and Jan Teorell. 2008. "What is quality of government? A theory of impartial government institutions." *Governance* 21 (2):165–190.

Santos, Niedja de Andrade e Silva Forte dos. 2021. "Multi-level governance tackling the COVID-19 pandemic in China." *Brazilian Journal of Public Administration* 55 (1):95–110.

SchengenVisaInfo.com. 2021. "EU's list of epidemiologically safe countries amid COVID-19." Accessed March 9, 2021. https://www.schengenvisainfo.com/eu-list-of-epidemiologically-safe-countries-amid-covid-19/.

Sensho, Yasuhiro. 2020. "Hitodebusoku to gyoumu kata de kasumigaseki houkai no pinchi [Shortage of labor and overwork will cause the collapse of Kasumigaseki]." *Chuou Kouron* 134:52–57.

Shimizu, Kazuki, and Masashi Negita. 2020. "Lessons learned from Japan's response to the first wave of COVID-19: A content analysis." *Healthcare* 8 (4):426.

Shimizu, Kazuki, Yasuharu Tokuda, and Kenji Shibuya. 2021. "Japan should aim to eliminate Covid-19." *BMJ* 372:n294. doi: 10.1136/bmj.n294.

Shimizu, Kazuki, et al. 2020. "Resurgence of Covid-19 in Japan." *BMJ* 370:m3221. doi: 10.1136/bmj.m3221.

Steen, Trui, and Taco Brandsen. 2020. "Coproduction during and after the COVID-19 pandemic: Will it last?" *Public Administration Review* 80 (5):851–855.

Sturmer, Jake, and Yumi Asada. 2020. "Japan was feared to be the next US or Italy. Instead their coronavirus success is a puzzling 'mystery'." *ABC News.* Accessed June 11, 2020. https://www.abc.net.au/news/2020-05-23/japan-was-meant-to-be-the-next-italy-on-coronavirus/12266912.

Sugaya, Nagisa, et al. 2020. "A real-time survey on the psychological impact of mild lockdown for COVID-19 in the Japanese population." *Scientific Data* 7 (1):1–6.

Sugiyama, Satoshi. 2020. "Abe's influence takes a hit with prosecutor scandal and bill reversal." *The Japan Times.* Accessed June 13, 2020. https://www.japantimes.co.jp/news/2020/05/24/national/politics-diplomacy/japan-shinzo-abe-gambling-prosecutor/.

Suzuki, Kohei, and Mehmet Akif Demircioglu. 2019. "The association between administrative characteristics and national level innovative activity: Findings from a cross-national study." *Public Performance & Management Review* 42 (4):755–782.

Suzuki, Kohei, and Mehmet Akif Demircioglu. 2020. "Is impartiality enough? Government impartiality and citizens' perceptions of public service quality." *Governance* 34 (3): 727–764. doi: 10.1111/gove.12527.

Suzuki, Kohei, and Hyunkang Hur. 2020. "Bureaucratic structures and organizational commitment: Findings from a comparative study of 20 European countries." *Public Management Review* 22 (6):877–907.

Suzuki, Kohei, and Hyunkang Hur. 2021. "Revisiting the old debate: Citizens' perceptions of meritocracy in public and private organizations." *Public Management Review* 24 (8):1226–1250. doi: 10.1080/14719037.2021.1895545.

Takahashi, Fumiya. 2020. "Korona senmonka kaigi, gijiroku sakuseisezu, rokuonmo nashi. naikakukanbou 'jiyuuna giron dekinai'[Corona expert meeting, no minutes taken, no recording. Cabinet Secretariat, 'Free discussion impossible']." *HuffPost Japan*. Accessed June 15, 2020. https://www.huffingtonpost.jp/entry/story_jp_5ed0544ec5b6aeca900edccb.

Takenaka, Harukata. 2019. "Expansion of the Prime Minister's power in the Japanese Parliamentary system: Transformation of Japanese politics and institutional reforms." *Asian Survey* 59 (5):844–869.

The Japan Times. 2020. "Japanese government, criticized for low testing rates, eases guidelines for seeking virus tests." *The Japan Times*, May 9, 2020. https://www.japantimes.co.jp/news/2020/05/09/national/japan-criticism-relaxes-coronavirus-testing-guidelines/.

The Japan Times Editorial Board. 2020. "Work-style reform needed at the government's center." *The Japan Times*, August 20, 2020. Accessed March 17, 2021. https://www.japantimes.co.jp/opinion/2020/08/20/editorials/work-style-reform-japan-government/.

van den Oord, Steven, et al. 2020. "Network of networks: Preliminary lessons from the Antwerp Port Authority on crisis management and network governance to deal with the COVID-19 pandemic." *Public Administration Review* 80 (5):880–894.

Van der Wal, Zeger. 2020. "Being a public manager in times of crisis: The art of managing stakeholders, political masters, and collaborative networks." *Public Administration Review* 80 (5):759–764. doi: 10.1111/puar.13245.

Wallace, Andrea, and Brian Dollery. 2021. "Municipal responses to COVID-19: The case of library closures in New South Wales local government." *Brazilian Journal of Public Administration* 55 (1):84–94.

Woo, JJ. 2020. "Policy capacity and Singapore's response to the COVID-19 pandemic." *Policy and Society* 39 (3):345–362.

Worldometers. (2020). Retrieved from https://www.worldometers.info/

Yen, Wei-Ting. 2020. "Taiwan's COVID-19 management: Developmental state, digital governance, and state-society synergy." *Asian Politics & Policy* 12 (3): 455–468. doi: https://doi.org/10.1111/aspp.12541.

Yomiuri Shimbun. 2020. "Kyugyoyosei ni bassoku hiteiteki shusho "shiken ni okina seiyaku" [Prime Minister talks against penalties on violation of business suspensions, "Severe Restrictions on Private Rights"]. *Yomiuri Shimbun*, June 16, 2020. Accessed June 16, 2020. https://www.yomiuri.co.jp/politics/20200615-OYT1T50134/.

9 Thailand's Responses to COVID-19 and the Acceleration of Public Sector Reform

Ora-orn Poocharoen and Phanuphat Chattragul

9.1 Introduction

Thailand's response to the pandemic has been relatively successful in controlling the spread of the virus. The World Health Organization (WHO) praised its community health system as a best practice (Pornbanggird & Angskul, 2020). Despite the relative success, along the way, pockets of the population were critical of policy choices and implementation. The country's control of the virus came hand in hand with continuous oppression and centralization of power by the government. Before focusing on the policies and performance of Thailand that have led to such overall praise and tensions in the country, it is essential to understand Thailand's context at the time of the outbreak.

Firstly, Thailand is the first country outside China to report a confirmed case of COVID-19. Due to its proximity, Thailand is one of the most popular destinations for visitors from China. Before COVID-19, inbound Chinese visitors to Bangkok accounted for around 40% of international overnight arrivals in 2018 (Mastercard, 2019). Second, Thailand's economy relies heavily on global tourism, from which 20% of the country's total GDP originated in 2019 (Theparat, 2019). The country was already struggling to shift itself out of the middle-income trap, rapidly aging society, and deteriorating environment. Thus, Thailand was one of the first countries that felt the direct impact of the spread of the virus and the choice of lockdown.

Third, the political backdrop at the time of the pandemic in Thailand was very much a self-censored and government-obeying atmosphere. Since the latest coup d'état in 2014, Thailand's democracy has faltered into closed autocracy, especially after the 2017 Constitution was adopted. During the pandemic, Thailand faced numerous large-scale political protests against the military-backed government and the monarch. The government used social-distancing measures and emergency decrees to cleverly contain protests throughout the pandemic.

DOI: 10.4324/9781003362760-9

Lastly, Community Health Workers (CHWs) in Thailand play an essential role in implementing government policies at the local level. The country has been relying on these CHWs since the 1970s to help mitigate the impact of deadly diseases (e.g., HIV/AIDS, Ebola, and avian influenza) in local communities (Geissler & Prince, 2020; Tejativaddhana et al., 2020). Most of CHWs are well-trained to operate under a state-agent mentality that underlines a centralized chain of command (Sudhipongpracha & Poocharoen, 2021). The system of community health workers is an essential component of good practice in times of emergencies that Thailand can offer the international community.

During the initial phases of the pandemic during the year 2020, Thailand was praised by some rankings and indicators. On July 25, 2020, Thailand ranked first, best recovery from the COVID-19 outbreak by the Global COVID-19 Index (GCI). The country scored the Recovery Index of 81.55 out of 100 (The Government Public Relations Department (Thailand), 2020). On the same ranking on May 9, 2021, Thailand's Recovery Index dropped to 56.95, marking the country's rank to be 64th out of 180 countries in the world (PEMANDU Associates, 2021). Based on the same dashboard, Thailand's COVID-19 Severity Rating is number 2, and the score of the Severity Index is 11.36. This means that Thailand was considered to be in the group of countries that were coping with the crisis with a low percentage of infections and resulting deaths per population (PEMANDU Associates, 2021).

In sum, Thailand belongs to the group of countries that controlled the spread of the virus relatively well. The outcomes are related to the relatively decisive and stringent non-pharmaceutical interventions (NPIs) by the autocratic military-backed government. In addition, the government utilized the network of community health workers and launched digital applications for Test, Trace, Isolate, and Support (TTIS) processes. Prior to the pandemic, Thailand already had universal healthcare coverage for its people. This factor helped to leave no one behind, especially during the vaccination process. Thai people in general trust health experts, and many value public health over short-term economic growth. It also helped that Thais do not greet each other by shaking hands or hugging in public. The above lists of factors will be elaborated on in this chapter. Following this introductory section, the second part of this chapter covers a description of the phases of COVID-19 and key government responses. The third section offers distinct factors that explain the performance of the Thai case. The last section provides lessons for other countries and suggests future research topics.

9.2   Government Response to COVID-19 Key Phases

This section provides a description and analysis of policy responses according to the phases of the pandemic in Thailand. The Thai experience can be divided into five phases. The first three phases, which were between January 2020 and March 2021, mark the first year of the pandemic, which was full of unknowns and unavailability of vaccines (see Figure 9.1). The fourth and fifth phases of the pandemic in Thailand, which were between May 2021 and September 2022, saw a substantially large increase in the number of cases that were a mix of old and new, less deadly variants. At the same time, vaccines were being rolled out. Until finally the government ended the Emergency decree and fully opened the country in September 2022.

Thailand is the first country outside China to detect a COVID-19 index case on January 12, 2020, which is the start of the first phase of the outbreak in Thailand. Before the pandemic, Thailand and Chinese business ties were growing exponentially. As the demand for connections increased, many airlines launched direct flights connecting Chinese cities to Thailand. Wuhan alone was directly connected to four Thai airports, Suvarnabhumi, Don Mueang, Chiang Mai, and Phuket. Moreover, other regional airports such as Pattaya's U-Tapao airport also received charter flights from the Chinese city (Reuters, 2020). However, after the index case was confirmed, most flights from Wuhan and then cities in China were subjected to heavy screening by the Immigration Bureau personnel under the supervision of the Department of Disease Control, yet they were not halted from entering Thailand unless the Chinese government suspended travel from China themselves. As a result, the cases in Thailand gradually rose.

At first, the transmission was traceable since it was limited among those in close contact with travelers from China (Bangkok Post & Reuters, 2020). This escalated into clusters of outbreaks since no lockdown measures took place and public spaces were still accessible by all. However,

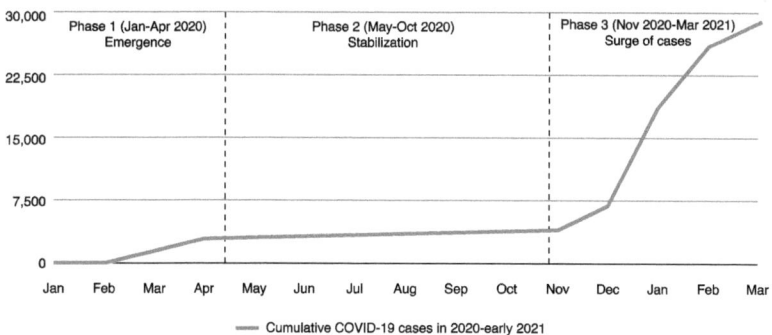

Figure 9.1 The first three phases of the pandemic in Thailand in the year 2020 to early 2021.

Source: Adapted from WHO COVID-19 Dashboard – processed by Our World in Data, 2022.

in the locations where the infection took place, provincial governments including Bangkok Metropolitan Administration would order the closure of public venues and businesses, while the others such as educational institutions and private sectors chose to close their own on-site spaces and migrated to online settings. This abrupt closure caused tens of thousands of workers and students to return home, to other provinces, which dispersed the risk of infection across the country. As the outbreak became more serious, from the end of March 2020 through early April 2020, the national government declared a state of emergency, a curfew, and a nationwide lockdown which included suspension of all future flights into the country on March 26 and April 3, and 4, 2020, respectively. Community Health Workers (CHWs) also followed and helped to enforce the national government's order. Their action included monitoring the returnees from the infected and high-risk areas. This practice continued throughout the major outbreaks in 2020 and 2021.

After the strict lockdown was enforced by the national government in April 2020, the outbreak was suppressed and contained inside quarantine facilities that were set up by medical experts. By mid-May 2020, local transmitted infection rates had dropped to near-zero which led to the decision to ease restrictions (Kuhakan, 2020). Though public venues, businesses, and educational institutions were allowed to open again under COVID-19 preventive measures, the emergency decree was renewed numerous times. The emergency decree was finally dismissed on September 30, 2022. By the end of May 2020, the domestic transmission was non-existent, and 14-day-stay in state quarantine or self-paid Alternative State Quarantine (ASQ) was mandatory for all travelers and this measure continued throughout 2020.

As the country enjoyed a period of reported zero cases of COVID-19, the country lost substantial income from the tourism industry. The government used economic stimulus packages to boost the domestic economy. Interestingly, this was the first time in history that subsidies were delivered directly to the people via digital applications. Considering the mobile phone internet user penetration rate of over 73% in 2020 (Statista Research Department, 2021), the national government took this opportunity to finally transform Thailand into a digital society. The national government offered universal stimulus packages for Thais on a first come, first served basis via the application called Paotang, an electronic wallet containing a co-payment subsidy that users could top-up with their own money as well as receive payment from the government. This application by the Ministry of Finance is more successful than the vaccine tracking application launched by the Ministry of Health.

These applications help to create governmental databases which benefit future policy in terms of target and coverage. The packages included Rao

Tiew Duay Gun ("We travel together") and Kon La Krueng ("Half-Half") scheme that encouraged domestic travel and spending. However, despite living in a COVID-19-free bubble, Thailand, as a country that is heavily dependent on international travel, gradually had to open. Consequently, on the first of October 2020, Thailand Special Tourist Visa (STV) was introduced targeting long-stay tourists that had to undergo 14-day in quarantine before ultimately entering Thailand. As tourists had to pay for the ASQ by themselves and had to go through complicated visa processes, a trip to Thailand was costly and not convenient.

The period from November 2020 onwards is succinctly a game changer of the COVID-19 pandemic in Thailand. Since before the pandemic broke out, Thailand's low-skilled jobs had been held by migrant workers from neighboring countries, especially from Myanmar. Since Thailand and Myanmar share over 2,400 kilometers of border, there are many ways to enter Thailand, both legally and illegally. As each national government shut down its border due to COVID-19, people can still cross borders through natural passages. At the end of November 2020, a group of migrant workers was detained, and some tested positive for COVID-19. Thai government thus promptly ordered quarantine for those in close contact. Nonetheless, this effort was too late, especially after the outbreak in mid-December in Samut Sakhon, the center of the country's fishing industry. Later, clusters of outbreaks sprouted in Rayong's gambling den which later spread to Bangkok. On December 30, 2020, Thailand banned new year gatherings countrywide which was followed by the closure of all schools in January 2021. This situation was continuously exacerbated especially after the third wave of outbreak surge hit Thailand in April 2021. This incident, coming from migrant workers, highlights Thailand's weak human security system for non-Thais, especially vulnerable groups such as migrants.

Figure 9.2 depicts the change in the number of confirmed cases in Thailand from its first case found on January 11, 2020, to May 7, 2021. As of May 7, 2021, the confirmed cases were 78,855 in total, and the number of deaths was recorded as 363 (Emergency Operations Center, Department of Disease Control (Thailand), 2021a). The figure shows that in the first phase there were some confirmed cases. Then, in the second phase, most of the year 2020, the COVID-19 cases in Thailand were relatively low. However, toward the end of the year, in the third phase, there was a rise in confirmed cases. In the following first quarter of the year 2021, there is a spike of rising cases which marks the fourth phase. The fourth and fifth phases had an exponential number of cases (see Figure 9.2). In the end, Thailand had about 4.6 million people of reported cases (see Figure 9.3). However, the number of severe cases was not high. The number of deaths stood at 32,771 deaths (see Figure 9.2). Also, by that time vaccines were rolling in and most governments around the world, including WHO had much

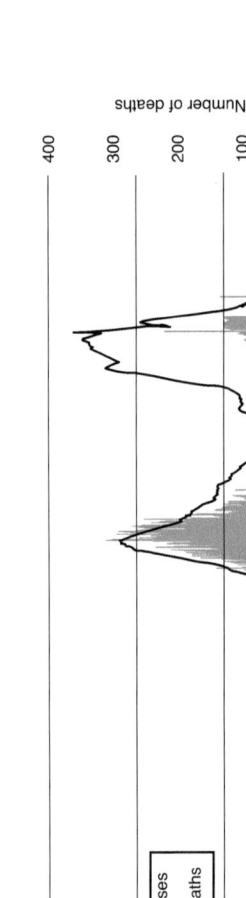

Figure 9.2 Number of confirmed cases and deaths in Thailand 2020–2022.

Source: Adapted from WHO COVID-19 Dashboard – processed by Our World in Data, 2022.

better knowledge about the virus and how to contain the spread and treat patients. The world was moving into the phase of how we live with the virus. In the next section, the policy interventions are described and analyzed. It is divided into non-pharmaceutical interventions; test, trace, isolate, support (TTIS); hospital and health care; and vaccination programs.

9.2.1 NPIs (Non-Pharmaceutical Interventions)

Thailand detected the first case of COVID-19 after China in January 2020. As the government took nationwide lockdown measures and screening, as shown in Figure 9.3, the situation was under control mostly throughout the year 2020. Non-pharmaceutical interventions (NPIs) have paid a significant role in this COVID-19 suppression. These interventions include screening, social distancing, mandatory mask-wearing, and lockdowns that were fiercely implemented throughout the entire country. As Thailand is a unitary state with a highly centralized governance system, policy decisions thus were made by the central government and all 77 provinces would comply, especially in health emergencies. The government set up the Center for COVID-19 Situation Administration (CCSA) to advise, make decisions, and communicate to the public throughout the pandemic.

The nature of Thailand is such that ministries usually comply with the decision that is backed up by recommendations from experts and advisors in each field, who are often members of the government's advisory board. Advisory advice is often not challenged by other ministries or local governments. Since the advice is believed to be scientific and evidence-based, civil societies also usually do not reject expert advice. Moreover, for COVID-19, in the beginning, most agreed that strict measures would help to protect everyone indiscriminately.

Moreover, Community Health Workers (CHWs) also operated under the government chain of command and organization silo, which also did not contradict the national government plan even at the operational level (Sudhipongpracha & Poocharoen, 2021, p. 246). These CHWs are thus "private street-level bureaucrats (private SLBs)" as they follow directions given by public health authorities to fill the void of clinically trained healthcare personnel shortages (Jaskiewicz & Tulenko, 2012; Geissler & Prince, 2020; Sager et al., 2014, p. 483). During the first wave of COVID-19 in Thailand (January–April 2020), CHWs acted as implementing agents in conducting contract tracing and in the dissemination of public information about preventive measures against COVID-19 (Smith, 2020). As CHWs work in their own areas of residence, they thus could employ a "walking through communities" strategy, which helps promote information about preventive measures and mitigate the rumors and misinformation, among the general population and harder-to-reach community members

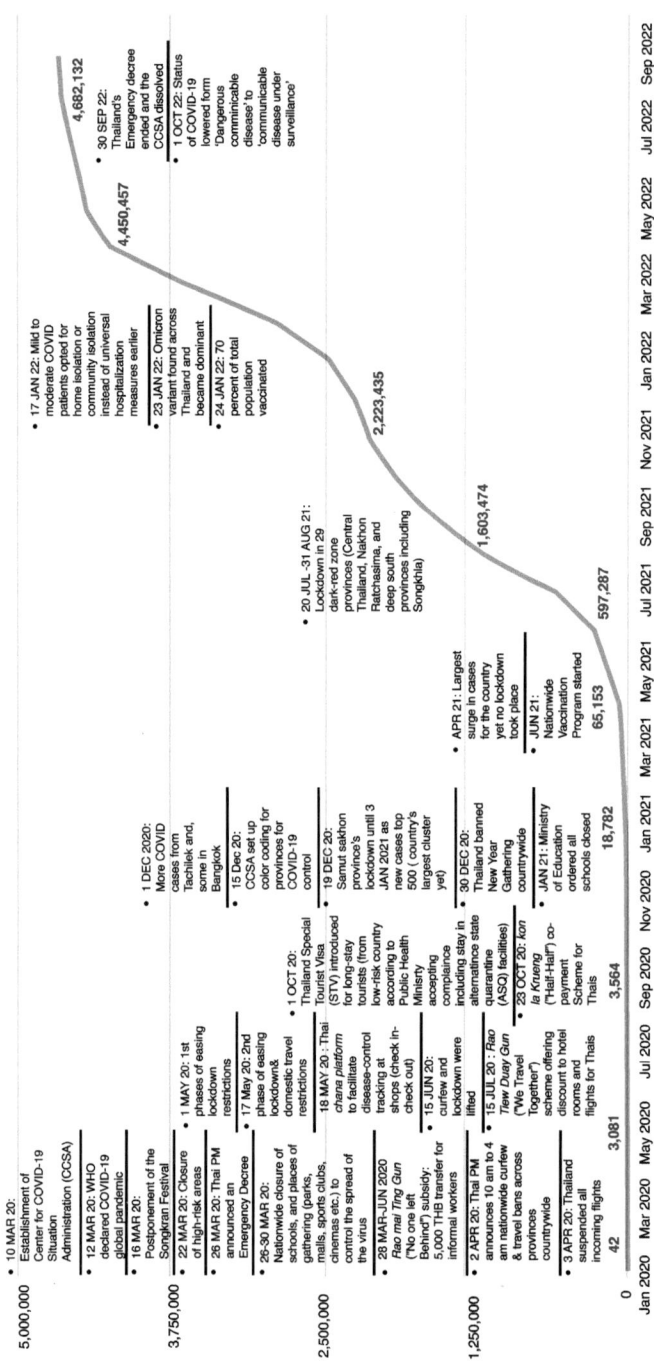

Figure 9.3 Cumulative COVID-19 cases timeline in Thailand and policy measures.

Source: Adapted from WHO COVID-19 Dashboard – processed by Our World in Data (2022), TERRABKK (2020), Bangkok Post (2020a, 2020b), Reuters (2020), Social Protection Toolbox (n.d.), TAT Newsroom (2020, 2021a, 2021b), Nation Thailand (2020), ThaiEmbassy.com (n.d.), National News Bureau of Thailand (2021), United Nations Thailand (n.d.), Thai PBS World (2022), Thailand Convention and Exhibition Bureau (2022), and Chulalongkorn University (2022).

(Sudhipongpracha & Poocharoen, 2021, p. 244). These factors hence contribute to Thailand's success in 2020.

Figure 9.4 below depicts the level of stringency practiced by the Thai government over time. We can see that the Thai government agencies together with the private sector started to use very stringent policies and measures (so-called whole-of-society approach) at the very beginning of the pandemic (World Health Organization & Ministry of Public Health (Thailand), 2020, pp. 14–19). Gradually, the level of stringency was adjusted and became relatively lower than at the beginning of the pandemic over time. This success stems from the early and widespread adoption of masking, hand hygiene, and social distancing helped prevent further community widespread (World Health Organization & Ministry of Public Health (Thailand), 2020, pp. 14–19).

It can be observed that the stringency index generally grew when there was an increase in new cases. The level of stringency was distinguishably high when lockdown measures were enforced, with April–May 2020, December 2020–January 2021, and July–August 2021 being three distinct periods. These periods of elevated stringency during 2020 and 2021 usually followed and coincided with the spike in new cases. However, as Thailand reached 2022, the level of stringency continued to drop despite the peak in new cases taking place in the first half of the year when the fatality rate was significantly lower, and more population was vaccinated against COVID-19 compared to the previous years. The next section elaborates on the policy responses of the Thai government in each phase.

9.2.1.1   First Phase (January–April 2020)

During the first phase of the pandemic, the first strands of the virus were found in Thailand and the government tried to make sense of the problem. It opted for rather severe lockdown policies from the start of the pandemic by enforcing a nationwide lockdown from April 3, 2020, under the authority of CCSA, around three weeks after WHO declared COVID-19 a global pandemic. The Thai government executed the following measures.

January 2020: Travelers from Wuhan brought COVID-19

a Temperature scanning at international airports on incoming passengers after the novel coronavirus (then COVID-19) outbreak is confirmed by the WHO on January 12, 2020.

February 2020: Travel ban on travel to and from Wuhan and COVID-19 risk areas

a Refusal of entry for visitors who may have had exposure to COVID-19.
b Passengers were screened at all ports. High-risk passengers were restricted from entering the country.

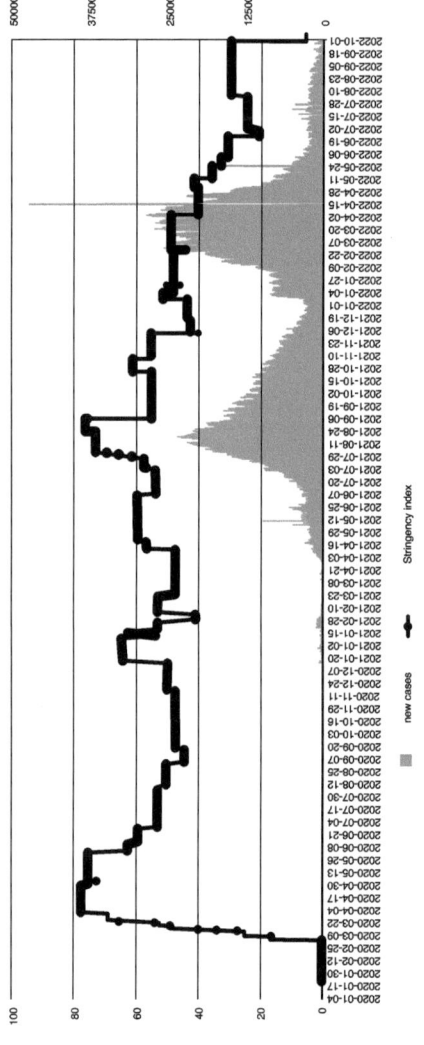

Figure 9.4 Thailand's new cases and stringency index over time.

Source: Adapted from The Oxford COVID-19 Government Response Tracker (OxCGRT), n.d.

c Department of Disease Control, Ministry of Public Health was the main body of decision-making and control measures for COVID-19. Immigration Bureau was asked to cooperate and disseminate information about COVID-19 spread through "health beware care" leaflets for incoming travelers (Royal Thai Government, 2020).

March 2020: A plateau of cumulative cases of untraceable origin

a March 1, 2020: Ministry of Public Health declared the first confirmed death from COVID-19 in Thailand.
b March 6, 2020 (+14 days): COVID-19 outbreak started in Thailand as a domestic transmission. The number of infections exceeded a hundred since March 15, 2020. Places with possible COVID-19 infections began to close, which include the Lumphini Boxing Stadium. The contacted population must take quarantine measures and isolate themselves from the general population.
c March 10, 2020: Center for COVID-19 Situation Administration (CCSA) was established as a principal body of all policy decisions and measures related to COVID-19. It is headed by the prime minister.
d March 12, 2020: World Health Organization declared COVID-19 as a global pandemic.
e March 16–22, 2020: Public venues, schools, and businesses across the country were ordered to close by the government. "Work From Home" was adopted by sectors where remote working is possible.
f March 26, 2020: Emergency Decree was issued by the prime minister.
g March 26–30, 2020: Nationwide closure of places of gatherings and businesses causing a mass exodus of people back to their homes in provinces around the country. Affected businesses registered for relief money under the scheme called *Rao Mai Ting Gun* (first come, first served basis).

April 2020: COVID-19 in control as Thailand went to a month-long nationwide lockdown

a April 3, 2020: Curfew from 10 pm to 4 am went into effect. Travel across provinces was banned. All incoming flights were suspended.
b April 13–15, 2020: Songkran festival holidays were canceled.

During this first phase, on March 10, 2020, the government set up the Center for COVID-19 Situation Administration (CCSA), which became the main body for decision-making and communication on COVID-19 throughout the pandemic. CCSA made daily announcements (in Thai and English) on television at noon time to keep the population updated on the situation and policies. Other communication channels include social media such as Facebook, Twitter, and LINE (Krusarnpisit, 2022, p.15).

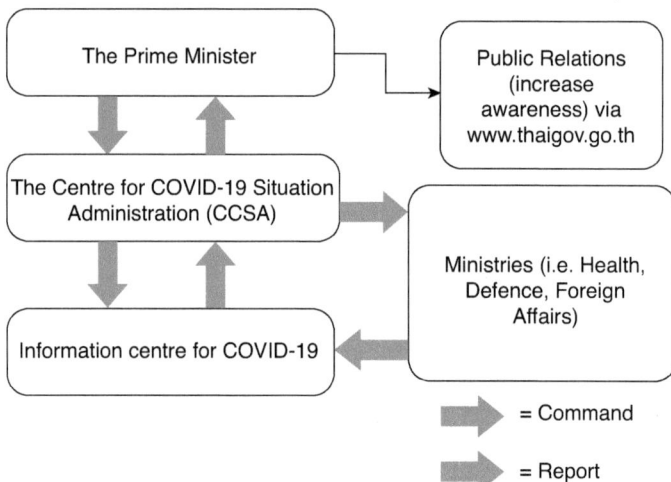

Figure 9.5 Center for COVID-19 Situation Administration (CCSA) chain of command.

Source: Adapted from Khaosod (2020).

The agency reported directly to the Prime Minister and coordinated with the relevant line ministries (Figure 9.5).

In this phase, the government, due to lack of experience, made several mistakes. The government failed to prevent shortages of surgical masks and issued inconsistent policies regarding international travel and quarantine measures resulting in contradicting measures implemented by government units (BBC Thai, 2020; Thansettakij, 2020). Later, this was rectified, and state quarantine measures were clearly designed. Due to surgical mask shortages, many sought substitutions by cutting their own mask from fabric pieces, which did not provide proper protection against COVID-19. Moreover, due to a brief period of inflated prices of masks, many also resorted to re-using the masks by washing or wearing them again. This period of turmoil could have been better if the government took measures like price-controlling, setting quotas as well as providing free masks which they failed to do.

The inequities of Thai society began to unveil themselves from this initial phase. It started with who got the masks and who did not. Later it included who got vaccines and who did not. And obviously, society is witnessing who will and will not survive the economic crisis of the pandemic.

9.2.1.2   *Second Phase (May to October 2020)*

During the second phase, the cases were under control thus, the government eased travel and lockdown restrictions. This followed the harsh travel restriction and lockdown in the first phase. All in all, this period reaped the rewards of the strict and heavy application of the NPIs measures earlier in the first phase. Moreover, the citizens also cooperated well with the government since there was visibly no protest regarding the NPIs measures including lockdown and social distancing.

May 2020: New cases dropped to near zero

a May11–17, 2020: Phases of easing of domestic travel restriction.
b May 1–31, 2020: 1st Extension of the Emergency Decree.
c May 18, 2020: Launching of Thai Chana, a contact tracing platform (in addition to paper registration) at shops for check-in and check-out.

June 2020: Recovery and stabilization

a June 1–30, 2020: 2nd Extension of the Emergency Decree.
b June 15, 2020: Curfew and lockdown were lifted.

July 2020: Cases dropped to zero and the rising need for more domestic spending.

a July 1–31, 2020: 3rd Extension of the Emergency Decree.
b July 8, 2020: The emergency decree was extended until September 30, 2020, despite zero domestic transmission.
c July 15, 2020: *Rao Tiew Duay Kan* travel stimulus package for Thai citizens (first come, first served basis).

August 2020: Medical coup "against political" protests.

a August 1–31, 2020: 4th Extension of the Emergency Decree.
b August 21, 2020: Despite no new domestic cases since mid-May, the CCSA decided to extend the Emergency decree to prevent incoming cases from abroad. There were restrictions on the movement of people, public gatherings, public buildings, and spaces. This extension had been criticized by international human rights groups as a tool for protest control (Macan-Markar, 2020).

September 2020: New Normal

a September 1–30, 2020: 5th Extension of the Emergency Decree.
b 'Relaxed' New normal: social distancing and mask-wearing became the new normalcy although there was no outbreak outside the contained clusters.

October 2020: Boosting the economy

a October 1–31, 2020: 6th Extension of the Emergency Decree.
b October 1, 2020: Special Tourist Visa (STV) introduced for long-stay tourists with a validity of 90 days (can be renewed twice).
c October 23, 2020: *Kon La Krueng* ("Half-Half") co-payment scheme for Thai citizens (first come, first served) was launched. The relief money was distributed digitally into each registered persona's *Pao Tang*, a digital wallet application.

During this phase, there was better coordination from the national level down to the provincial and local levels of governance. At the national level, as advised by CCSA, the Prime Minister issued nationwide policies and measures which were delivered through a single spokesperson (World Health Organization & Ministry of Public Health (Thailand), 2020, p. 17). At the provincial level, governors, who are appointed by the Ministry of Interior, would take lead to coordinate with related agencies and local governments in each province. Governors usually followed guidelines from the central government with some minor adaptations to fit the local context. At the very community and village level, Community Health Workers (CHWs), semi-volunteers financed by the government, played vital roles in fighting the pandemic by implementing government policies, raising awareness, encouraging compliance from citizens, and addressing community needs (Sudhipongpracha & Poocharoen, 2021, p. 235). Since the 1970s, CHWs have been a key player in delivering primary healthcare services to the population, particularly in rural areas where there are shortages of primary healthcare personnel (Geissler & Prince, 2020; Tejativaddhana et al., 2020). These pre-existing CHWs also reinforced the health care system in Thailand. Notwithstanding, challenges such as reversion to traditional organization reporting lines were not absent since the national plans and protocols were not clearly defined (World Health Organization & Ministry of Public Health (Thailand), 2020, pp. 14–15).

9.2.1.3 *Third Phase (November 2020–April 2021)*

During the third phase, Thailand faced the second wave of COVID-19. This second wave is characterized by the increase in COVID-19 cases within the border of Thailand, which had been absent since mid-May 2020. Based on the lessons learned that COVID-19 can be overcome by a prompt lockdown and strict control of movement, the government used more targeted lockdown measures, customized responses in each location, and softer tones of communication. The country faced mutated variants of COVID-19 which include the Delta variant, which brought a sharp rise in new cases from April

2021 onwards. This time the government did not apply lockdown measures. Instead, the government encouraged people and organizations to take self-care and self-regulatory measures such as shutting down and disinfecting their own facilities where COVID-19 was detected.

November 2020: COVID-19 cases were detected among migrants who entered Thailand through natural passages.

a November 1–30, 2020: 6th Extension of the Emergency Decree.
b Quarantine for those in contact with infected persons.

December 2020: The largest COVID-19 cluster since the start of the pandemic was founded in Samut Sakhon province in the areas where most migrant workers were concentrated.

a December 1–31, 2020: 7th Extension of the Emergency Decree.
b December 15, 2020: CCSA set up a color-coding map of provinces based on COVID-19 risks. Samut Sakhon and peripheral areas were marked as red which signified maximum control over COVID-19 and movements.
c December 19, 2020, to January 3, 2021: National government imposed a lockdown on Samut Sakhon province.
d December 30, 2020: New Year Gathering countrywide was banned.

January 2021 to April 2021: Cases rapidly increased as the lockdown was not implemented in every province and people infected were not strictly quarantined.

a January 1–31, 2021: 8th Extension of the Emergency Decree (February 9, March 10, April 11, and May 12, 2021, respectively).
b Targeted lockdowns in specific provinces.
c Fine and arrest for not wearing masks.
d Ministry of Education ordered all schools closed. Yet, other sectors' closures depended on each authority's discretion.
e Contact tracing for COVID-19: people with high risk were to test for COVID-19 as the pandemic began to break out domestically again. This started around late December 2020. Testing was not an obligation in the first phase. Whoever conceals or mutilates their timeline or information may be punished in this phase.

June 2021: The vaccination campaign started

a Continue school closures
b Work From Home

c Self-regulatory measures (no lockdown)
d Beginning of mass vaccination

During this phase, the government began to code provinces by colors on December 25, 2020, to illustrate the stringent levels of lockdown measures (Bangkok Post, 2020a). The general population had learned enough about the dos and don'ts regarding COVID-19. Thus, it became feasible to customize responses based on location and target population as it does not have to rely on a one-size-fits-all measure for the whole country. Nevertheless, these self-regulatory measures, later, ended up being a catastrophe in the middle of the year when lockdown and NPI measures were brought back stringently.

9.2.1.4   *Fourth Phase (May to December 2021): Third Wave of COVID-19 (Delta) and Vaccination Race against Time*

The Emergency Decree was renewed monthly throughout this phase (8 times). Thai population started receiving their first doses of COVID-19 vaccines; however, in terms of vaccination, there was a delay in ordering and distribution which caused millions to seek self-paid vaccines and they also had to wait for the government's authorization. The vaccination campaign continued throughout the year. Thailand's first shipments of vaccines were from China. In addition, Thailand did not join the COVAX program. This delayed the shipment of western or more trustworthy vaccines in the views of many Thais.

As the outbreak situation worsened in July 2021, Thailand issued a lockdown in 29 dark-red zone provinces from July 20 to August 31, 2021, which are Bangkok and 28 other provinces. Other remaining provinces were ordered to take the highest caution on those traveling from these high-risk provinces. By this time, the structure of the CCSA was expanded to incorporate many new authorities and decision-making bodies. Figure 9.6 below shows the elaborate diagram.

9.2.1.5   *Fifth Phase (January to September 2022): Omicron Variant, Home Isolation, and Personal Self-care*

In this last phase, the Emergency Decree was extended until September 30, 2022. Though more population than ever was infected by COVID-19, the government did not force lockdowns or movement control measures. This was because most COVID-19 patients who were infected with the Omicron variant experienced milder symptoms and lower fatality rates compared to the previous phase. By this time, the vaccination rate covered 70% of the total population.

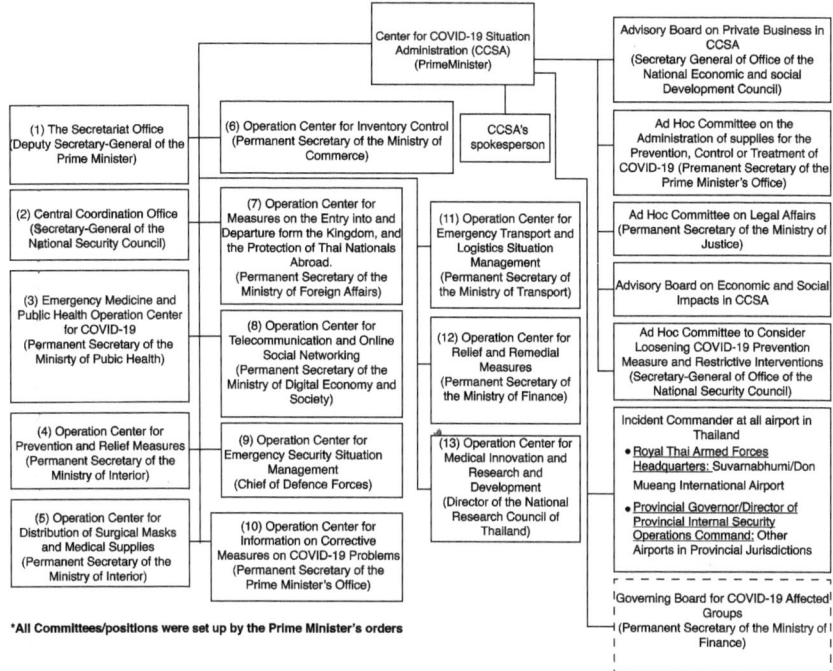

Figure 9.6 Elaborate diagram of the Center for COVID-19 Situation Administration (CCSA).

Source: Adapted from The Secretariat of the Prime Minister, n.d.

The government substantially shifted its policy from hospitalizing all COVID-19 patients in all previous phases to home and community isolation following the global trend. Patients with mild to moderate symptoms were asked to remain home until their conditions subsided. They would be given medications from medical centers in the areas and return to their home. The guidelines for self-care were directed and given by the National Health Security Office after the patient reported their own case to the district or local government of their residence.

9.2.2   *TTIS (Test, Trace, Isolate, Support)*

TTIS is deemed important for preventing uncontrollable outbreaks (Rajan et al., 2020). In the beginning, when test kits were not yet available to the public in Thailand, only hospitals provided testing services. Testing by hospitals was restricted only to those who had close contact with confirmed cases. All tests performed by the medical system are recorded properly. Doubts remain on how many positive cases Thailand actually had or has because not everyone came forward to get tested in medical facilities. This is due to several reasons. They include accessibility to medical facilities, costs of testing, not knowing the information, and some who did not have severe symptoms, did not think it was necessary.

ATK test kits were made available in hospitals and pharmacies in July 2021 (Hfocus, 2021). Then, in September 2021, it was recategorized as a non-medical good, which allowed it to be sold in general stores and online (Hfocus, 2021). This gave full access for citizens to test for the virus themselves. When test kits were fully available to the public, was when the government realized they could not maintain an accurate number of positive cases. Eventually, the effort to keep track stopped. As of September 2022, testing by medical staff is conducted only for people who need it for overseas travel purposes, enter restricted events.

Figure 9.7 demonstrates the number of tests per 1,000 people in Thailand. The graph shows that the number of tests performed continuously went up from April 2021 and continued high until May 2022. This aligns with the increased number of confirmed cases from April 2021 onwards. Therefore persons-under-investigation (PUIs) numbers went up from the contact tracing mechanism.

Figure 9.8 illustrates the share of the number of tests that are positive. It shows that, in the beginning, the government was very selective in doing the tests and the share of positive returns was very high. At one point in January 2020, the share was as high as 28.6%. Nevertheless, as the

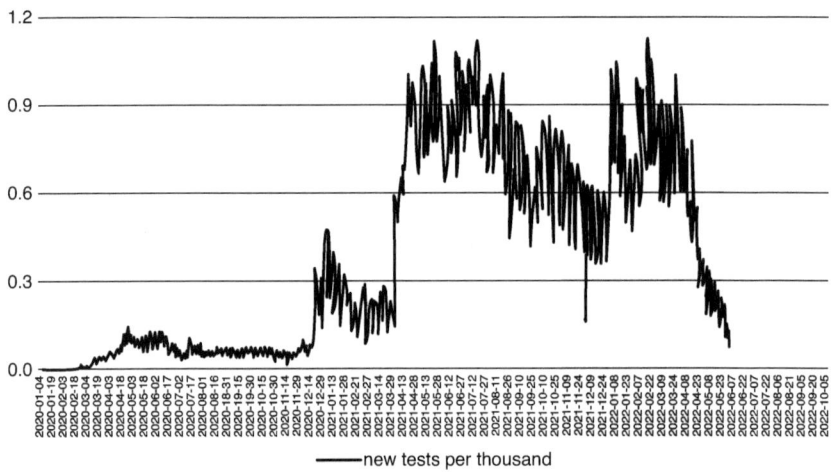

Figure 9.7 Daily new COVID-19 tests per 1,000 people.

Source: Adapted from WHO COVID-19 Dashboard – processed by Our World in Data, 2022.

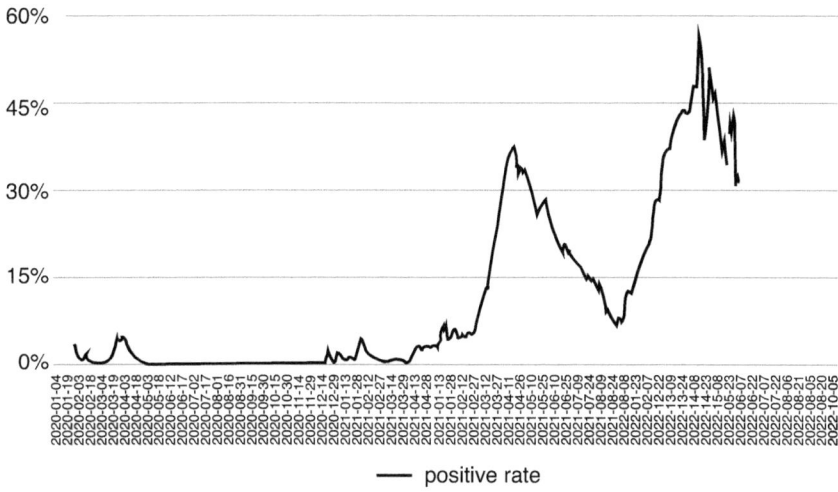

Figure 9.8 The share of daily COVID-19 tests that are positive.

Source: Adapted from WHO COVID-19 Dashboard – processed by Our World in Data, 2022.

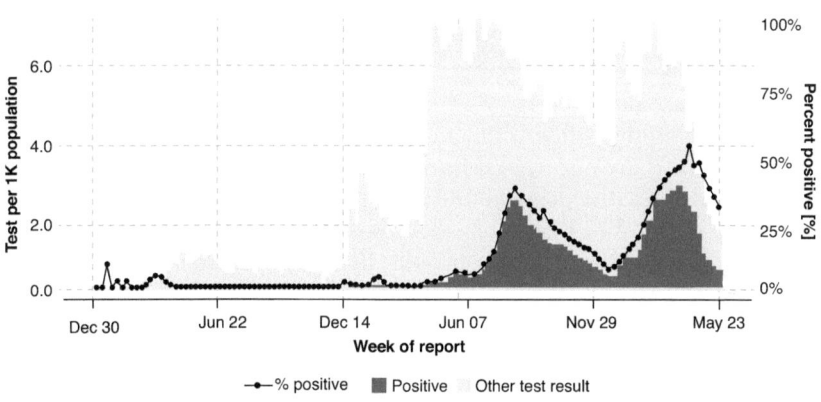

Figure 9.9 Shifts in testing strategy throughout the phases test measurement: samples tested.

Source: Adapted from WHO COVID-19 Dashboard – processed by Our World in Data, 2022.

number of available testing kits and testing centers expanded there were wider opportunities for testing for the population. As of April 24, 2021, the rate came down to 3.5%.

Figure 9.9 above depicts how the Thai government shifted its testing strategies from strategy 0 (no testing strategy) to 1 (only testing those with symptoms and fitting certain criteria) and then to 2 (anyone showing symptoms). However, despite the earlier investments in laboratory capacity, the accurate total number of tests performed nationwide is still an undetermined figure since there is no centralized diagnostic data system (World Health Organization & Ministry of Public Health (Thailand), 2020, pp. 25–26).

The Thai government quickly came up with two simple strategies for tracing covid cases. One was for everyone to sign in on paper when they enter shops and buildings. The information included full name and phone number. The second strategy was for people to check in and check out via an application called Thai Chana (Thais Win) when they entered and when they left buildings or public spaces. This was to trace citizens in general. This app was launched in May 2020. It was developed by Krungthai Bank, which used to be a state-owned enterprise. This same bank also owns other apps that are used to disburse subsidies to targeted groups in Thailand.

Another app introduced was called Moh Chana (Doctors Win). This app was developed by the Ministry of Health, Ministry of Digital Economy, and Society, in collaboration with Digital Government Development Agency, and a private entity called Code for Public (BBC Thai, 2021). It was launched in April 2020. This app was to help identify levels of risk of an individual based on their previous locations and symptoms. This app was not widely used by the public. It was officially closed on June 1, 2022 (BBC Thai, 2021).

In the beginning, when someone is confirmed of having COVID-19 it would be mandatory to reveal his/her past activities to medical authorities. This includes disclosing all the places they visited, restaurants they ate in, flights, trains, and buses that they took, including seat numbers. Such information would be shared officially by the government on television, and websites and the media would also echo the information. As experienced by other countries, such information soon became unhelpful because there was no way of preventing the spread of the virus. More importantly, the public soon realized that the tracing data collected by the government was not used systematically for decisions nor for improving services. Thus, as time went by, the public did not religiously follow this guideline. Finally, Thai Chana lose and was closed on October 1, 2022 (Thairath, 2022). The government announced that all data would be deleted according to the Privacy Data Protection Act.

At the very local and less urban locations, local governments and community health workers played important roles in keeping track of cases of those who needed to be in quarantine facilities and those who were self-isolating. Local governments and primary health care centers played vital roles in TTIS. They used simple methods of walking in communities, village meetings, and online apps such as LINE to provide information.

Thais are also accustomed to using Facebook to find information from their respective local governments. These are all in addition to the daily televised special news announcement that the government's team provides. These clear communication strategies helped to maintain coherency in policy implementation throughout the pandemic.

9.2.3 Healthcare

Based on the Ministry of Interior's open data source as of 2018, there were over 6,500 hospitals and community hospitals in Thailand. In total, there were approximately 740,000 beds (Ministry of Interior (Thailand), 2021). During the pandemic, the Thai government's policy was to have everyone who tested positive for the virus be hospitalized regardless of the symptoms (World Health Organization & Ministry of Public Health (Thailand), 2020, pp. 30–31). This is in stark contrast to some countries, where the confirmed cases could be quarantined and do self-care at home. In the first three phases (March to June 2020, July to September 2020, and October to December 2020), when there were adequate beds, patients stayed in normal hospitals.

Nonetheless, new cases emerged again in the fourth phase (January to March 2021) following the second wave of infection in December 2020, which later skyrocketed in April 2021 and reached a 7-day average of around 20,000 new cases in August 2021 (Department of Disease Control of Thailand, 2022), when there was a spike in the number of positive cases. Consequently, different provincial health authorities and the Bangkok Metropolitan set up over 1,000 field hospitals, which include semi-hospitals (Hospitel), a modified hotel for COVID-19 patients, to accommodate asymptomatic or very minor symptom cases (Emergency Operations Center, Department of Disease Control (Thailand), 2021b).

Thailand has universal healthcare coverage; thus, all Thais are eligible for treatment by public hospitals for COVID-19. Similar to other countries, the largest proportion of deaths is the group of those above 60 years old. In addition, the majority of people who die suffer from pre-existing health problems such as obesity, heart conditions, and high blood pressure. As of November 3, 2022, Thailand recorded 4,692,488 COVID-19 cases and a total of 32,955 deaths.

9.2.4 Vaccination and Vaccine Issues

Throughout 2020, Thailand's infection rate and the death toll were among the world's lowest. Between mid-May and late November 2020, no domestic transmission had been found in Thailand. This followed the nationwide lockdown and strict control of movement in April 2020, as well as the ban on free-flow entry into the country. The Emergency Decree was announced on March 26, 2020, which helped the national government and the CCSA to centralize the power. Nevertheless, the Emergency Decree was heavily criticized as being undemocratic especially when it comes to the COVID-19 vaccination and vaccine issues. As the number of cases remained low in the middle of 2020, the government was slow to order the vaccines as well as decided not to join the UN-backed COVID-19 Vaccines Global Access (COVAX), a global platform to ensure fair and equitable access to COVID-19 vaccines, which most countries of the world took part in.

The first target group that received the first lot of vaccines were frontline medical personnel, those above 60 years old, and those with specific illnesses (Chronic Respiratory Disease, Cardiovascular Disease, Chronic Kidney Disease, cerebrovascular disease, Cancers, Diabetes, Obesity, Human Immunodeficiency Virus, Psychiatric patient, Autistic patient, Patients who cannot take care of themselves and their caregivers) (Department of Disease Control of Thailand, 2021). When more vaccines arrived, the government rolled out the second target group, which were non-frontline medical personnel, the general population, those in the tourism industry, those who need to travel overseas, diplomats, international organization officers, international businessmen, long-term residents, and workers in factories and services (Department of Disease Control of Thailand, 2021).

Thailand's confidence in controlling COVID-19 had impacted their policy direction toward being a large-scale manufacturing hub of AstraZeneca (British Embassy Bangkok, 2020) since the need to acquire vaccines was not seen as urgent as other countries with higher transmission rates. The country signed an advance agreement with AstraZeneca to purchase 26 million doses of vaccine, which only covered 13 million people and was expected to arrive in the first quarter of 2021, as well as support local mass production of the doses by Siam Bioscience, owned by King Maha Vajiralongkorn (Kishimoto, 2021). Yet, as the situation started deteriorating in December 2020, Thailand failed to secure enough vaccines due to its over-reliance on AstraZeneca and a long queue of delivery in 2021. To address this shortage, the government thus turned to ordering vaccines from China as reinforcement. From February 24, 2021, Thailand started receiving many million doses from China which include Sinovac vaccines which will be the first batch of 2 million vaccines that will be administered throughout the country (Huaxia, 2021). Nevertheless, although there was a steady rise in new cases, Thailand did not join COVAX despite acknowledging the low vaccine supply (Sriring & Thepgumpanat, 2021; Ekvittayavechnukul, 2021). As AstraZeneca and other kinds of vaccines arrived later in an amount that was unable to cover the entire population of Thailand, two strategies were employed. The first strategy is "mixing series of

COVID-19 vaccines" started in July 2021, shortly after the acknowledgment of vaccine shortages, by mixing-and-matching doses of Sinovac and AstraZeneca vaccines since the latter dose would increase protection and build a high level of immunity against COVID-19 according to a preliminary Thai study (Thepgumpanat & Wongcha-um, 2021). Nevertheless, the practice of mixing the vaccine provided by the government has brought controversies among the general public due to its scientific proof inadequacy and concerns over safety after death following the jabs (Online Reporters, 2021a). Due to the uncertainties of vaccination procedures, over ten million Thais opted for self-paid vaccines which included Sinopharm and Moderna (Reuters, 2021; Online Reporters, 2021b). Nevertheless, the procurement and delivery of these alternative vaccines were delayed by state agencies which sparked complaints among the Thai public anticipating their first dose (Online Reporters, 2021c).

The national government's initial decision to rely on AstraZeneca and its most obvious support for Siam Bioscience, wholly owned by a subsidiary of the Crown Property Bureau for technology transfer to produce AstraZeneca, caused hot political debates among groups of people. This issue erupted after the surge in infections and months of youth-led protests between July and December 2020, whose agenda included the reform of the monarchy due to the expansion of lèse-majesté. As criticizing the royal family is illegal, speaking negatively about a company owned by King Maha Vajiralongkorn could be punishable by the law. Criticisms of the company include the lack of transparency over local production since the firm had no prior experience in vaccine production (Strangio, 2021). For instance, the leader of the dissolved progressive political party, Thanathorn Juangroongraungkit of Future Forward Party, was charged with lèse-majesté charges by the accusations he had made about the AstraZeneca vaccine production by Siam Bioscience (Post Reporters, 2021). The monarchy-owned firm reported a profit of nearly a 50-fold increase in profit in 2021 (Reuters, 2022).

In February 2021, Thailand successfully rolled out "Mohpromth" (Doctor Ready), which is an app for registering for vaccines, monitoring post-vaccination symptoms, and receiving digital vaccine certificates owned by the Ministry of Health. Initially, it was used only for medical personnel vaccination. In May 2021, it was open to the public. This application was developed from the LINE Official account called Ministry of Public Health Connect: MOPH Connect (Mohpromth, 2021). It was a channel of communication that began in 2018 for citizens to find out information on hospitals (public and private), clinics, and pharmacies, and to check medical insurance and rights. Citizens can also book hospital appointments, call for emergency 1,669 services, send GPS locations, donate to hospitals and get a tax refund, donate organs to the Red Cross,

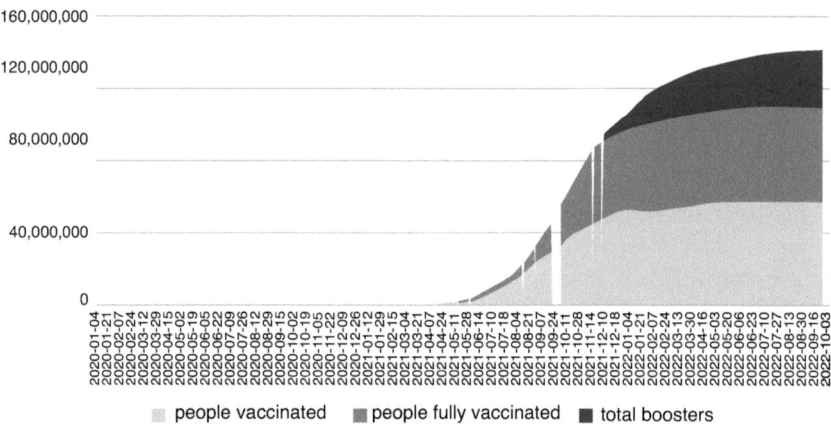

Figure 9.10 COVID-19 Vaccinations in Thailand by population.

Source: Adapted from WHO COVID-19 Dashboard – processed by Our World in Data, 2022

and general information on medicine and health. Pre-pandemic there were about 400,000 users of the online service (Mohpromth, 2021). This system tremendously helped to reduce congestion in vaccination sites, give priority to vulnerable groups, and prevent the wastage of vaccines.

By December 2021, Thailand had overcome the problem of vaccine shortages, and people can now choose vaccine types and vaccination procedures. This caused many Thais to sell the COVID-19 vaccination slots they purchased at private hospitals that had yet to arrive (Setboonsarng, 2021). By mid-2022, Thais were able to walk in for free COVID-19 vaccinations, indicating the surplus of vaccines available (Thai PBS, 2022a). In addition, Thailand also developed COVID-19 vaccines, with two home-grown vaccines, Chula-Baiya and Chula-Cov19, were still in Phase 2 trials as of February 26, 2022, and would be ready for use in the last quarter of 2022 (Tham, 2022). Figure 9.10 depicts the vaccination rate in Thailand. By November 3, 2022, 53,486,086 people, or 80.4% of the population, were fully vaccinated (Our World in Data, 2022).

9.3   Distinct Features of Thailand's Response of the COVID-19 Pandemic

The main features of Thailand during 2020s COVID-19 pandemic that explain its policy responses and results are investigated by dividing into four features. By way of presentation, it can be summarized as the four Cs: (1) cultural aspects related to social distancing and values of health; (2) centralized government and the political climate; (3) community health workers and the universal health system; and (4) consensus on the science of health issues.

9.3.1 Cultural Aspects

The first feature comprises several aspects of Thai culture. The first aspect is that most Thais value health over other important things in society. This is true, especially during the initial lockdown phases. There were pockets of people who questioned the trade-offs between economic and health benefits at the mid and later phases of the pandemic (see Boosabong & Chamchong, 2020 for discussion on this topic). Furthermore, Thais in general have great respect for medical doctors and tend to believe in doctors' advice. Thus, when told to wear masks, wash hands, and keep physical distance from doctors who are part of the government team, many Thais followed the public advice from the start (Bello, 2020). These are key interventions to prevent community spread (World Health Organization & Ministry of Public Health (Thailand), 2020, p. 27). Needless to say, in every society, there would be pockets of non-compliance people. Reasons for not complying include not knowing information, not taking the advice seriously, not believing the information, and not knowing which information to believe. These are the target groups that require specific policy communication tactics and messaging in order to be successful at getting accurate information across and accepted. For the general public, in Thailand, there did not seem to be many misunderstandings about the virus, how it spreads, and the symptoms. This is unlike some countries where high volumes of fake news and conspiracy theories proliferated. It is speculated that this is due to respect toward the medical field in general.

The way Thais greet, by putting two hands together at the chest or chin level, is the second cultural factor that might be an explanation for the relatively low levels of the virus spread. This is as opposed to other cultures where people shake hands, give hugs, and kiss hands, forehead, cheeks, and lips. This aspect covers not just the way Thais greet but also how Thais normally do not hug, kiss, hold hands, give pecks on the cheeks, or other physical gestures in public. Nevertheless, compared to other East Asian nations like Japan, the act of wearing a surgical mask is new for Thais. The exception would be in the Northern part of the country where prior to the pandemic people suffered from seasonal air pollution (PM2.5) for at least 5–10 years. Thus some were already accustomed to wearing face masks.

9.3.2 Centralized Government and the Political Climate

Thailand follows the constitutional monarchy system and is a unitary state. The current Thai government is highly centralized. After the most recent coup on May 22, 2014, the military took over and the 2017 constitution was promulgated. The current constitution strengthens the military's power in politics through appointed Senate members and oversight of administrative bodies, such as the constitutional court and the anti-corruption commission. Many critics observe the unfairness of the constitution and election laws, including the law to follow a national 20-year plan that is drafted by the military-backed regime. In 2016, Thailand went through its transition from the reign of Rama 9 to Rama 10. The transition of the monarch was a time of anxiety and uncertainty. It is perceived that the military and related elite class have an interest to maintain stability and power during and after this transition; hence, unlawful interventions were observed. In sum, Thailand has "relapsed into dictatorial administrative structures, political attitudes, and the military-led alliances" that resembled the past before the 1990s (Sopranzetti, 2016).

Conversely, on the political front, the country's liberal democracy index is falling rapidly. Based on the Varieties of Democracy (V-Dem) 2021 report, Thailand is one of the top 10 countries in the world that is "autocratizing." In 2010, Thailand was already categorized as an "electoral autocracy"; however, in 2020, it fell further into the "closed autocracy" category (V-Dem Institute, 2021). In the year 2020, the country witnessed numerous political protests offline and online covering grievances related mostly to the Thai Constitution, the power and role of the Senate, the harsh application of Lèse-majesté charges, and unfair play in electoral politics. Major anti-government Facebook groups proliferated. One of them being as large as 2 million members. Twitter and Clubhouse (audio only) are social media platforms used widely by both anti and pro-government supporters. Issues related to COVID-19 were prominent on online platforms (i.e., access to medical care, medical equipment, and vaccine) but were not the main issue for political protests on the streets.

Against this backdrop, during the pandemic, the Thai government has used traditional public policy and administrative tools to curb and control the pandemic. They are such as top-down orders from the central government to restrict movements, control of prices, shut down facilities, and other lockdown measures. Directly reporting to the Prime Minister, Thailand's Center for COVID-19 Situation Administration (CCSA) was set up to tackle the pandemic. To manage the lockdowns, the military extensively used the Emergency Decree on Public Administration in Emergency Situations 2005, rather than the more appropriate Contagious Disease Control Act 2015 (Boosabong & Chamchong, 2020). This gave extra power to security and military personnel which curbed people's rights to assemble. There was little room for local governments, civil society, and the private sector to play formal roles in the policies to curb the virus. There were strict media and social media control for anti-monarch sentiments. This in turn helped to curb political protests that were on the rise and curbed fake news related to COVID-19.

Considering the first factor of cultural aspects, people complied with those severe lockdown measures under the Contagious Disease Control Act anyway, but the government decided to use the emergency decree to control anti-government activities. Moreover, during an outbreak in Samut Sakhon, disease prevention authorities were reported to have excessively used their power in containing COVID-19 by sanitizing seemingly "unhygienic" places at their discretion (Princess Maha Chakri Sirindhorn Anthropology Center, 2021). Following the 100-day serious measures, the outbreak in Samut Sakhon stopped.

On the contrary, countries such as New Zealand, which is also a unitary state, practiced top-down centralized policies but it was with care and empathy. The state used the right laws, levels of strictness, and empathetic communication to gain acceptance from citizens. Thai military leaders often used threats, blame, and shame tactics to control the public's behavior, in addition to fines and arrest warrants. In a nutshell, Thailand's political and administrative features were highly centralized with high vertical coordination but lacked empathy. This feature worked for both controlling the virus and political opponents. However, in the long-term, this is not healthy for democratic development nor is it healthy for economic recovery for a more equitable society (Gleason & Baizakova, 2020).

9.3.3 Community Health Workers (CHWs)

The role of community health workers (CHWs) is crucial to Thailand's public health system. They are volunteers that are close to "private street-level bureaucrats" or "quasi-bureaucrats" (Sudhipongpracha & Poocharoen, 2021). They receive a small stipend of 1,000 baht from the government per month (about US$36) and are trained and governed centrally by the Ministry of Public Health. The current number is approximately 1.04 million volunteers. They were set up since the 1970s thus have long history in the administrative structure of local-level communities around the country. Before the pandemic, they focused on primary health care and disease prevention campaigns (i.e. dengue, rabies, malaria). Overall, this key feature has to do with the long-term focus on preventive medicine in Thailand's public health system, which has been the country's strength (Zachary, 2020). They have been praised as "unsung heroes" for successfully tackling HIV, SARs, and now COVID-19 (Narkvichien, 2020). They fill in the gaps for inadequate general medical care at the very local level in Thailand. Thus, most people do directly to hospitals even for minor medical care. During the pandemic, CHWs helped to prevent the overflow of people in hospitals.

During the pandemic these CHWs fulfill the tasks of collecting data, contact tracing, health screening and monitoring community members, answering queries from citizens, and providing accurate information. This is in addition to solving immediate problems like shortage of masks and alcohol and delivering food and drugs to patients or those under quarantine (Tejativaddhana et al., 2020). They used discretion and made decisions during the initial stages of uncertainty to help ease public concerns. This was when the government also did not have definite answers about transmission and cure. Due to the fact that these community health workers are also community members, they are likely to be trusted and welcomed by locals. They would have direct contact with individuals at the sub-district and village level, which helps with direct communication and helps to spread the right information.

9.3.4   *Consensus on Health Issues*

The last key feature in the Thai context is the high level of consensus on health issues. There were limited debates and arguments regarding the health threat of COVID-19. The anti-government rallies were focused on political issues, as mentioned above. None were directly about COVID-19 measures. This is in contrast to other countries where people demonstrated against lockdown and social distancing measures. Moreover, unlike the United States and some countries in Europe, Thais are much less concerned with "human rights" or "liberty rights" with regard to lockdown measures or wearing masks. Thailand's lockdown measures were led by technocrats, specifically medical experts who are backed by a military-led government. The financial handouts, subsidies, and recovery packages were designed and decided by politicians and financial technocrats. The execution of the quarantine measures was led by the Ministry of Health and Ministry of Defence, in addition to provincial governors from the Ministry of Interior. This is in addition to the fact that all communication was centralized through CCSA. Thus, aligned with being a highly centralized state and Thai culture toward medical doctors, the work of medical doctors and other technocrats was not contested. As mentioned in the culture section, there is high trust in medical professionals.

Thailand belongs to the group of countries that flattened the increase in COVID-19 cases relatively well. This is an outcome of the combination of the abovementioned elements: politically, decisive and stringent pre-existing non-pharmaceutical interventions (NPIs) and social policies; socially, utilization of CHWs in Test, Trace, Isolate, Support (TTIS) and healthcare policies; and culturally, norms in social greeting, trust in health experts and common value on public health shared among politicians and the general population.

9.4 Lessons for Other Countries and Further Research

Based on these four Cs, the authors would like to offer the following two lessons for other countries. First, the centralized response is key but could be a long-term obstruction of democratic development. In addition, digital platforms provide opportunities to streamline services and consolidate data. At the same time, there is also the threat of control and further strengthening authoritarianism by the government. Second, the community-level health volunteer system is a model worth exploring for countries with inadequate health professionals. The volunteer system helps to mainstream health issues to be given importance by all and not just health professionals. Volunteers also help to integrate health services to households and individual levels, without overwhelming the hospitals. Lastly, they are important connectors to bring up information from the local level up to the national level.

Amidst the political upheaval and economic downturn, despite being quite successful in COVID-19 control, the government continues to be held accountable for its policies by its citizens. The current military junta-linked government used a combination of strict and innovative responses (World Health Organization & Ministry of Public Health (Thailand), 2020, p. 6) during the COVID-19 pandemic with the twin goals to curb the virus and the swelling of political protests around the country throughout the year 2020. Hence, overall Thailand has demonstrated mixed results in its policy responses to COVID-19. The pandemic is over (as of November 2022). COVID-19 is now the "new normal" and the country is slowly picking up on its tourism industry. The same Prime Minister, the same cabinet members, and the same political parties are still in power. A general election is due in 2023. Only then will we know what Thais think about the performance of this government.

Governance in times of crisis is an important capacity for all actors in the policy process. Further research should be conducted to compare how volunteer health worker systems work differently in different countries. Furthermore, post-pandemic economic recovery policies can also be studied and compared. Last but not least, it would be useful to understand how governments use or not use data collected during the pandemic, and how it has enhanced its political and administrative powers and capacities in any way.

References

Bangkok Post. (2020a). Samut Sakhon locked down as new cases top 500.Retrieved from https://www.bangkokpost.com/thailand/general/2038103/samut-sakhon-locked-down-as-new-cases-top-500

Bangkok Post. (2020b). Ban on mass gatherings. Retrieved from https://www.bangkokpost.com/thailand/general/2040775/ban-on-mass-gatherings

Bangkok Post and Reuters. (2020). Human transmission of coronavirus confirmed in Thailand. *Bangkok Post.* Retrieved from https://www.bangkokpost.com/thailand/general/1847884

BBC Thai. (2020). Virus Corona: Naksueksa Thai Nai Tang Daen Fong San Pokkrong Hai Rath Yokluek Khamsang Ko Bairabrongpad Kon Kao Thai [Coronavirus: Thai students abroad filed a petition with administrative court to rescind medical certificate before entering Thailand] (in Thai). Retrieved from https://www.bbc.com/thai/thailand-52057969

BBC Thai. (2021). Perd Seri Truad ATK Raka Taorai-Krai Tong Chai Bang Lang Klai Lockdown Rob 1 Tulakom [Liberalization of ATK Test Kit: What is the price-who have to use after lockdown relaxation on October 1] (in Thai). Retrieved from https://www.bbc.com/thai/thailand-58408009

Bello, W. (2020). "How Thailand Contained COVID-19." *Foreign Policy in Focus.* Retrieved from https://fpif.org/how-thailand-contained-covid-19

Boosabong, P., & Chamchong, P. (2020). Coping with COVID-19 in a non-democratic system: Policy lessons from Thailand's centralized government. *International Review of Public Policy* 2(3), 358–371. Retrieved from https://journals.openedition.org/irpp/1382

British Embassy Bangkok. (2020). Ministry of Public Health, Siam Bioscience, SCG and AstraZeneca join forces on COVID-19 vaccine manufacturing for Thailand and Southeast Asia. *GOV.UK.* Retrieved from https://www.gov.uk/government/news/thailand-joins-forces-with-astrazeneca-on-covid-19-vaccine-manufacturing–2

Chulalongkorn University. (2022, September 29). FAQs – Find out what to do and how the chula community should be prepared for when COVID-19 is declared a communicable disease under surveillance on October 1, 2022. Retrieved from https://www.chula.ac.th/en/news/87143/

Department of Disease Control of Thailand. (2021). Naew Taang Gaan Hai Vaccine COVID-19 Nai Sathanagarn Rabad Pi 2564 [Covid-19 vaccination guidelines for Thailand's outbreak situation in 2021] (in Thai). Retrieved from https://tmc.or.th/covid19/download/pdf/covid-19-public-Vaccine-040664.pdf

Department of Disease Control of Thailand. (2022). *Department of Disease Control Situational Reports.* Retrieved from https://covid19.ddc.moph.go.th/en

Ekvittayavechnukul, C. (2021). Thailand to join COVAX, acknowledging low vaccine supply. *The Diplomat.* Retrieved from https://thediplomat.com/2021/07/thailand-to-join-covax-acknowledging-low-vaccine-supply/

Emergency Operations Center, Department of Disease Control (Thailand). (2021a). *The Coronavirus Disease 2019 Situation.* Ministry of Public Health. Retrieved from https://ddc.moph.go.th/viralpneumonia/eng/file/situation/situation-no484-070564.pdf

Emergency Operations Center, Department of Disease Control (Thailand). (2021b). Thailand situation update on 10 April 2021. Retrieved from https://ddc.moph.go.th/viralpneumonia/eng/file/situation/situation-no457-100464.pdf

Geissler, P., & Prince, R. (2020). Layers of epidemy: Present pasts during the first weeks of COVID-19 in western Kenya. *Centaurus*, 62(2), 248–256. doi:10.1111/1600-0498.12295

Gleason, G., & Baizakova, K. (2020). COVID-19 in the central Asian region: National responses and regional implications. *Connections, Spring 2020, The Security Impacts of the COVID-19 Pandemic*, 19(2), 106–110.

Hfocus. (2021). Rerm Laew Prachachon Truad COVID Dai Duay Tua Eng Lang Aor Yor Keun Tabien Chud Antigen Test Kit Ha Dai Nai Ran Khai Ya [Start from now! Civilians can now have a COVID test by themselves after Food and Drug Administration approved Antigen Test Kit for sale at pharmacies] (in Thai). Retrieved from https://www.hfocus.org/content/2021/07/22287

Huaxia. (2021). Thailand receives 1st batch of COVID-19 vaccines from China's Sinovac. *Xinhuanet*. Retrieved from http://www.xinhuanet.com/english/2021-02/24/c_139763953.htm

Jaskiewicz, W., & Tulenko, K. (2012). Increasing community health worker productivity and effectiveness: A review of the influence of the work environment. *Human Resources for Health*, 10(38). doi:10.1186/1478-4491-10-38

Khaosod. (2020). Prawat kan sang Sor Bor Kor [History of CCSA creation]. *Khaosod Online*. Retrieved from https://www.khaosod.co.th/newspaper-column/general-knowledge/news_4535059

Kishimoto, M. (2021). Thai king-owned biotech starts production of AstraZeneca vaccine. *Nikkei Asia*. Retrieved from https://asia.nikkei.com/Spotlight/Coronavirus/COVID-vaccines/Thai-king-owned-biotech-starts-production-of-AstraZeneca-vaccine

Krusarnpisit, S. (2022). Garn Cheuam Yong Khomun Khaosarn Lae Karn Prachasamphan Khong Krom Prachasamphan [News, data and public relations linkages of the government public relations department] (in Thai). Retrieved from https://www.prd.go.th/th/content/category/detail/id/31/iid/102210

Kuhakan, J. (2020). Thai traffic back to gridlock as coronavirus measures ease. *Reuters*. Retrieved from https://www.reuters.com/article/us-health-coronavirus-thailand/thai-traffic-back-to-gridlock-as-coronavirus-measures-ease-idUSKBN22U0EV

Macan-Markar, M. (2020). Thailand seeks to extend COVID emergency despite no new cases. *Nikkei Asia*. Retrieved from https://asia.nikkei.com/Politics/Turbulent-Thailand/Thailand-seeks-to-extend-COVID-emergency-despite-no-new-cases

Mastercard. (2019). Global destination cities index 2019. Retrieved from https://newsroom.mastercard.com/wp-content/uploads/2019/09/GDCI-Global-Report-FINAL-1.pdf

Ministry of Interior (Thailand). (2021). Open data. Number of hospitals and hospital beds by region and province from BE 2557 to BE 2561 (in Thai). Retrieved from https://spd.moph.go.th/public-health-statistics/Mohpromth. (2021). "Mohpromt" Platform Rabob Boriharn Jadgan Vaccine COVID-19 Peua Tuk Kon Bon Paendin Thai ["Mohpromt": Platform for COVID-19 vaccination management system for everyone in Thailand] (in Thai). Retrieved from https://mohpromt.moph.go.th/mpc/mp-about/about/

Narkvichien, M. (2020). *Thailand's 1 million village health volunteers – "unsung heroes" – are helping guard communities nationwide from COVID-19.* World Health Organization. Retrieved from https://www.who.int/thailand/news/feature-stories/detail/thailands-1-million-village-health-volunteers-unsung-heroes-are-helping-guard-communities-nationwide-from-covid-19

Nation Thailand. (2020, July 30). Govt's tourism package nears target in less than 15 days. *Nation Thailand*. Retrieved from https://www.nationthailand.com/in-focus/30392164

National News Bureau of Thailand. (2021, January 29). CCSA sets up new criteria & color coding for provinces for COVID-19 control as situation improves. Retrieved from https://thainews.prd.go.th/en/news/detail/TCATG210129164610730

Online Reporters. (2021a). Brain swelling killed mixed-vaccine recipient. *Bangkok Post*. Retrieved from https://www.bangkokpost.com/thailand/general/2153767/brain-swelling-killed-mixed-vaccine-recipient

Online Reporters. (2021b). October delivery of Moderna 'still possible'. *Bangkok Post*. Retrieved from https://www.bangkokpost.com/thailand/general/2191371/october-delivery-of-moderna-still-possible

Online Reporters. (2021c). GPO sues THG chairman over Moderna vaccine comments. *Bangkok Post*. Retrieved from https://www.bangkokpost.com/business/2148683/gpo-sues-thg-chairman-over-moderna-vaccine-comments

Our World in Data. (2022). WHO Covid-19 dashboard – processed by our world in data. WHO Covid-19 Dashboard [original data]. Retrieved from https://ourworldindata.org/covid-cases

PEMANDU Associates. (2021). The Global Covid-19 index (GCI). Retrieved from https://covid19.pemandu.org/Thailand

Pornbanggird, S., & Angskul, T. (2020). WHO praises Thailand for COVID-19 effort. *National News Bureau of Thailand*. Retrieved from https://thainews.prd.go.th/en/news/detail/TCATG201115175046592

Post Reporters. (2021). Thanathorn hit with 2 more Lèse-majesté charges. *Bangkok Post*. Retrieved from https://www.bangkokpost.com/thailand/politics/2167967/thanathorn-hit-with-2-more-lese-majeste-charges

Princess Maha Chakri Sirindhorn Anthropology Center. (2021). Prasob Karn Chak Samut Sakhon: Karn Kae Punha COVID-19 Kab Miti Sangkhom Wattanatham [Experience from Samut Sakhon: COVID-19 solution and socio-cultural dimension] (in Thai). Retrieved from https://www.youtube.com/watch?v=q7jlBTR9WS8

Rajan, S., Cylus, J., & McKee, M. (2020). Successful find-test-trace-isolate-support systems: How to win at snakes and ladders. *Eurohealth*, 26(2), 34–39.

Reuters. (2020, December 30). Thailand bans New Year gatherings to contain virus outbreak. *Reuters*. Retrieved from https://www.reuters.com/article/us-health-coronavirus-thailand-idUSKBN2940CP

Reuters. (2020). Second Chinese tourist found infected with coronavirus. *Bangkok Post*. Retrieved from https://www.bangkokpost.com/thailand/general/1838009/second-chinese-tourist-found-infected-with-coronavirus

Reuters. (2021). Princess allows new vaccine imports. *Bangkok Post*. Retrieved from https://www.bangkokpost.com/thailand/general/2122619/princess-allows-new-vaccine-imports

Reuters. (2022). Thai king's medical firm reports record profit after vaccine deal with AstraZeneca. *Reuters*. Retrieved from https://www.reuters.com/business/healthcare-pharmaceuticals/thai-kings-medical-firm-reports-record-profit-after-vaccine-deal-with-2022-08-25/

Royal Thai Government. (2020). Rai Ngan Khao Tid Chua Virus Corona 2019 (COVID-19) Pracham Wan Ti 16 Kumphaphan 2563 [News report on the coronavirus disease 2019 (COVID-19) case on 16 February 2020] (in Thai). Retrieved from https://www.thaigov.go.th/news/contents/details/26532

Sager, F., Thomann, E., Zollinger, C., van der Heiden, N., & Mavrot, C. (2014). Street-level bureaucrats and new modes of governance: How conflicting roles affect the implementation of the Swiss Ordinance on Veterinary Medicinal Products. *Public Management Review*, 16(4), 481–502. doi:10.1080/14719037.2013. 841979

Setboonsarng, C. (2021). Thais resell private COVID-19 vaccination slots as free supplies build. *Reuters*. Retrieved from https://www.reuters.com/world/asia-pacific/thais-resell-private-covid-19-vaccination-slots-free-supplies-build-2021-12-20/

Smith, C. (2020). The structural vulnerability of healthcare workers during COVID-19: Observations on the social context of risk and the equitable distribution of resources. *Social Science & Medicine*, 258, 113–119. doi:10.1016/j.socscimed.2020.113119

Social Protection Toolbox. (n.d.). Facilitating COVID responses: Rao Mai Ting Gun (no one left behind) scheme. Retrieved from https://www.socialprotection-toolbox.org/practice/facilitating-covid-responses-rao-mai-ting-gun-no-one-left-behind-scheme

Sopranzetti, C. (2016). Thailand's relapse: The implications of the May 2014 coup. *The Journal of Asian Studies*, 75(2), 299–316. doi:10.1017/S0021911816000462

Sriring, O., & Thepgumpanat. (2021). Thailand defends decision not to join COVAX vaccine alliance. *Reuters*. Retrieved from https://www.reuters.com/article/us-health-coronavirus-thailand-idUSKBN2AE0CZ

Statista Research Department. (2021). Mobile phone internet user penetration in Thailand from 2017 to 2020 with a forecast through 2026. Retrieved from https://www.statista.com/statistics/974995/thailand-mobile-phone-internet-user-penetration/

Strangio, S. (2021). Thailand to cease using Sinovac vaccines after supplies are exhausted. *The Diplomat*. Retrieved from https://thediplomat.com/2021/10/thailand-to-cease-using-sinovac-vaccines-after-supplies-are-exhausted/

Sudhipongpracha, T., & Poocharoen, O. (2021). Community health workers as street-level quasi-bureaucrats in the COVID-19 pandemic: The cases of Kenya and Thailand, *Journal of Comparative Policy Analysis: Research and Practice*, 23(2), 234–249. doi: 10.1080/13876988.2021.1879599

TAT Newsroom. (2020, May 18). Thailand launches 'Thai Chana' online platform to retain effectiveness in COVID-19 control measures. *TAT Newsroom*. Retrieved from https://www.tatnews.org/2020/05/thailand-launches-thai-chana-online-platform-to-retain-effectiveness-in-covid-19-control-measures/

TAT Newsroom. (2021a). Thailand announces lockdown in 13 dark-red zone provinces. *TAT Newsroom*. Retrieved from https://www.tatnews.org/2021/07/thailand-announces-lockdown-in-13-dark-red-zone-provinces/

TAT Newsroom. (2021b). Bangkok extends COVID-19 control measures until 31 August 2021. *TAT Newsroom*. Retrieved from https://www.tatnews.org/2021/08/Bangkok-extends-covid-19-control-measures-until-31-august-2021/

Tejativaddhana, P., Suriyawongpaisal, W., Kasemsup, V., & Suksaroj, T. (2020). The roles of village health volunteers: COVID-19 prevention and control in Thailand. *Asia Pacific Journal of Health Management*, 15(3), 18. doi:10.24083/apjhm.v15i3.477

TERRABKK. (2020). Safe haven: How Thailand outperformed other countries in combating COVID-19. Retrieved from https://www.terrabkk.com/en/articles/198197/safe-haven-COVID-19

Thai PBS World. (2022, September 23). Thailand's emergency decree to end on September 30th. *Thai PBS World*. Retrieved from https://www.thaipbsworld.com/thailands-emergency-decree-to-end-on-september-30th/

Thai PBS. (2022a). Bangkok opens six walk-in vaccination facilities ahead of Songkran holiday. *Thai PBS World*. Retrieved from https://www.thaipbsworld.com/bangkok-opens-six-walk-in-vaccination-facilities-ahead-of-songkran-holiday/

ThaiEmbassy.com. (n.d.). Thailand special tourist visa. Retrieved from https://www.thaiembassy.com/thailand-visa/special-tourist-visa-thailand

Thailand Convention and Exhibition Bureau. (2022). TCEB situation update: COVID-19 situation on 30 September 2022 - termination of emergency decree & lowering status of COVID-19 to communicable disease under surveillance. Retrieved from https://www.businesseventsthailand.com/en/press-media/news-press-release/detail/1499-tceb-situation-update-covid-19-situation-on-30-september-2022-termination-of-emergency-decree-lowering-status-of-covid-19-to-communicable-disease-under-surveillance

Thairath. (2022). Yoklerk application "Thai Chana" 1 Tulakom Mai Truad Ekgasarn COVID-19 Phuderntang Kao Thai [Dismissal of "Thai Chana" application, travelers to Thailand do not have to show COVID-19 travel document from 1 October] (in Thai). Retrieved from https://www.thairath.co.th/news/politic/2514971

Tham, S. Y. (2022). 2022/29 "The Race to Produce Covid-19 Vaccines in Southeast Asia" by Tham Siew Yean. ISEAS Yusof Ishak Institute. Retrieved from https://www.iseas.edu.sg/articles- commentaries/iseas-perspective/2022-29-the-race-to-produce-covid-19-vaccines-in-southeast-asia-by-tham-siew-yean/

Thansettakij. (2020). Meun kortormor yokleuk khao pid hang 22 wan [Confusion ensues as Bangkok authorities "cancel" news release of 22-day mall shutdown] (in Thai). Retrieved from https://www.thansettakij.com/general-news/425772

The Government Public Relations Department (Thailand). (2020). Thailand ranks first in the global COVID-19 recovery index. Retrieved from https://thailand.prd.go.th/ewt_news.php?nid=9902&filename=index

The Oxford COVID-19 government response tracker (OxCGRT). (n.d.). The nine metrics used to calculate the Stringency Index are: school closures; workplace closures; cancellation of public events; restrictions on public gatherings; closures of public transport; stay-at-home requirements; public information campaigns; restrictions on internal movements; and international travel controls. Retrieved from https://ourworldindata.org/covid-government-stringency-index. For more information see https://www.bsg.ox.ac.uk/research/research-projects/covid-19-government-response-tracker

The Secretariat of the Prime Minister. (n.d.). Soon Boriharn Sathanakarn COVID-19 [Center for COVID-19 Situation Administration (CCSA)] (in Thai). Policy and

Strategy Coordination Division, The Secretariat of the Prime Minister. Retrieved from https://www.mfa.go.th/en/content/1177x?page=5f22514b78568958aa0d5 b85&menu=5f2253d49864ad7325088af4Theparat, C. (2019). Prayut: Zones vital for growth. *Bangkok Post.* Retrieved from https://www.bangkokpost.com/ business/1753349/prayut-zones-vital-for-growth

Thepgumpanat, P., & Wongcha-um, P. (2021). In first, Thailand to Mix Sino-vac, AstraZeneca vaccine doses. *USNews.* Retrieved from https://www.usnews. com/news/world/articles/2021-07-12/thailand-starts-tighter-coronavirus-lockdown-around-capital

United Nations Thailand. (n.d.). Thailand's COVID-19 response: An example of resilience and solidarity. Retrieved from https://thailand.un.org/sites/default/ files/remote-resources/c96776a1413af9a681b01cde157e8409.pdf

World Health Organization. (n.d.). WHO coronavirus (COVID-19) dashboard data explorer. Retrieved from https://covid19.who.int/more-resources

World Health Organization & Ministry of Public Health (Thailand). (2020). Joint intra-action review of the public health response to COVID-19 in Thailand: 20–24 July 2020. Retrieved from https://www.who.int/docs/default-source/searo/thailand/ iar-covid19-en.pdf

Zachary, A. (2020). Explaining successful (and unsuccessful) COVID-19 responses in Southeast Asia. *The Diplomat.* Retrieved from https://thediplomat.com/2020/04/ explaining-successful-and-unsuccessful-covid-19-responses-in-southeast-asia

10 Vietnam's Responses to COVID-19

Local Governance and Bureaucratic Coordination

Trang (Mae) Nguyen

10.1 Introduction

This chapter analyzes Vietnam's particularly successful early pandemic response in 2020, during a critical period where little was known about the coronavirus and the development of a vaccine was uncertain. Without consistent or time-tested best practices, each country had to act fast to deal with a rapidly evolving pandemic situation on its own border. As the COVID-19 pandemic rapidly spread throughout the globe in 2020, the prospects for Vietnam, the fifteenth-most populous country in the world, with 96 million people and extensive borders with China, did not look bright. It, however, managed to beat the odds (Oxford University Nuffeld Department of Medicine, 2020). As of year-end 2020, Vietnam reported just under 1,500 confirmed cases of COVID-19 and 35 deaths (Johns Hopkins University of Medicine, 2021). According to public health data from John Hopkins University, which has been tracking COVID outbreaks worldwide, Vietnam's single-party state was, by 2020, the second safest place on earth during the pandemic, just behind Taiwan, and about 3,000 times less deadly than either the United States or the United Kingdom (ibid.). Having earned high praise for its early pandemic response, Vietnam was one of the first countries able to ease social distancing measures and reopen its society, ahead of many more developed peers (Nguyen & Malesky, 2020; Fleming, 2020; Sang Minh Le, 2020). The effective public health response further enabled quicker economic recovery. The World Bank, for example, forecasted that Vietnam was among a rare group of countries that managed to experience positive economic growth in 2020 (World Bank, 2021a, 2021b).

A non-democratic regime ranked high on the Corruption Perception Index, with an underdeveloped healthcare system and not typically known for strong state capacity, Vietnam's effective pandemic response during 2020 was a surprise to many. Commentators generally attributed its success to a host of factors, including the government's early and decisive

DOI: 10.4324/9781003362760-10

actions to close schools and borders, extensive contact tracing and mass quarantine, past experience with SARS and MERS, and coercive and surveillance measures. A puzzle, however, still remained: What enables compliance with these restrictive measures in a non-democratic state that is otherwise notorious for difficulty in rule enforcement (Malesky & Taussig, 2019)?

This chapter argues that Vietnam's early effective government and public response in 2020 was enabled by the country's ongoing efforts to improve governance, both locally and in central-local policy coordination. The strength of Vietnam's state capacity was not born overnight but resulted from decades-long efforts to improve governance and responsiveness at local levels. Vietnam's story, as illustrated through its early pandemic response in 2020, thus moves beyond the simple distinction of regime type to challenge us to think deeper about bureaucratic capacity and responsiveness within all forms of government.

10.2   Vietnam's Pandemic Response: Mass Mobilization and Unprecedented Transparency

This section summarizes Vietnam's regulatory responses to the COVID-19 pandemic during 2020 and highlights two central features of its regulatory narrative: mass mobilization of civil society and unprecedented transparency from the ruling Vietnamese Communist Party (VCP or Party-State).

Vietnam discovered its first COVID-19 cases, at a time the disease was still unnamed, in late January 2020, just days before the Lunar New Year (Phan et al., 2020). Six days later, Vietnam's Prime Minister Nguyễn Xuân Phúc issued a directive declaring "fighting the epidemic is fighting the enemy" ("chống dịch như chống giặc") (Office of the Government of the Socialist Republic of Vietnam, 2020a). Vietnam was the second country affected by SARS, after China, in 2003 (WHO, 2003). This experience made Vietnam wary of developments in Wuhan, especially as the Lunar New Year triggered waves of cross-border travel by migrant workers and tourists (Le & Nguyen, 2020). Referred to as the "Tet offensive of 2020" to reminisce the military campaigns against South Vietnam during the 1968 Lunar New Year ("Tet" in Vietnamese), the call to arms against COVID-19 evoked an ethos of patriotism and sacrifice that characterized the country's long decades of warfare (NPR, 2020; Office of the Government of the Socialist Republic of Vietnam, 2020a, 2020b). Tapping into this historical and cultural context was thus an important strategy of the government's response. Without South Korea's widespread testing (Fisher & Choe, 2020) or Taiwan's highly developed healthcare system (Chang, 2020), Vietnam's so-called "low-cost" method of contact tracing hinged on the Party-State's ability to track and quarantine potentially infectious individuals before COVID-19's spread could overwhelm the country's already-crowded hospitals (Nguyen et al., 2018).

In praising Vietnam's actions, the World Economic Forum noted the government's "proactive efforts" including once-controversial measures such as early school closures (VOA News, 2020), mass quarantines (Pearson & Nguyen, 2020), and border closings (O'Connor, 2020). After China, Vietnam became the second country to implement forced quarantine, both locally and centralized (Reed, 2020). Provincial authorities were allowed to seal off whole geographic areas and quarantine travelers from other provinces (Vu & Tran, 2020). Suspected cases, whether due to international or domestic travels, were sent to centralized military camps overseen by army personnel (all provided free of charge) (Nguyen, 2020c). By the time the World Health Organization declared COVID-19 a pandemic in March 2020, an estimated 50,000 people had undergone quarantine in Vietnam, half of whom through centralized facilities run by the military (Pearson & Nguyen, 2020). In response to periodic local outbreaks, the central government swiftly imposed a nationwide social distancing order and imposed fines on those who ventured outside without masks (Office of the Government of the Socialist Republic of Vietnam, 2020b; Nguyen, 2020a). Violations of COVID-19 regulations are punishable by criminal law. For example, a 2020 Supreme People's Court's guidance letter interpreted the 2015 Penal Code to include violations of quarantine regulations and business suspension orders (Judges' Council, 2020). It also deemed the spreading of misinformation relating to the pandemic a criminal offense. The Ministry of Public Security's local police offices have started prosecuting cases on allegations of fake news dissemination and quarantine violations (Nguyen & Pearson, 2020; Ministry of Public Security News, 2020). In anticipation of looming economic effects, Prime Minister Phúc reiterated that "economic sacrifice" must be accepted to save lives (VietnamNews, 2020).

Central to Vietnam's regulatory response to COVID-19 has been the launching of a mobilization campaign redolent of wartime exigency. Similar to China, individuals and households are tasked with becoming the state's eyes and ears to detect infections and monitor quarantine violations. Neighborhood committees (tổ dân phố)—a staple of socialist grassroots administration—act as a combination of state agents and community organizers. Comprised usually of local Communist Party bureaucrats and retired army personnel, these committee members knock on doors to relay official policies, explain social distancing, collect households' health and travel history, and measure people's temperatures. Mass civic organizations, once suffering from declining budgets (Vietnam Economic Times, 2016), regained new purposes through anti-coronavirus fundraising campaigns (Vietnam News, 2020) and community outreach (Kinh Te Do Thi [Urban Economy Magazine], 2020). Notably, the Vietnamese leadership also called for unity and support from overseas Vietnamese immigrants, many of whom fled Vietnam as refugees and remain critical of the Communist state—signaling the government's view that the protection of national health should transcend political and ideological differences.

A second critical aspect of Vietnam's response to COVID-19 is an unprecedented display of transparency. The Vietnamese leadership appears to have learned from China's cover-up debacle by taking a more open approach (Wadhams & Jacobs, 2020; Hutt, 2020). Notwithstanding its past record of heavy-handed internet censoring, the regime has leaned heavily on social media sites such as Facebook and Twitter to keep netizens up to date on rapidly changing regulations and social programs relating to the pandemic.[1] The Office of the Government's Facebook portal regularly publishes information about individual COVID-19 patients, including their initials, general locations, detailed timelines of their travels and whereabouts, actions taken to keep them isolated, and updates on their health. When news broke in early March 2020 about "Patient 17"—a positive case after over two weeks with no new infections nationwide—news outlets blasted videos and images of government trucks spraying disinfectants and closing down the patient's neighborhood (VNExpress, 2020b, 2020c). These information campaigns facilitated contact tracing and boosted public confidence in the Party-State's capacity (Nguyen & Malesky, 2020). However, Vietnamese netizens have expressed divided opinions about privacy violations, bullying, and discrimination, especially when patients belong to vulnerable groups such as ethnic minorities (Pham, 2020).

10.3   The Long Road Toward Improved Governance

From legal and regulatory perspectives, this section explores what enabled Vietnam's successful early pandemic response in 2020, when information about the coronavirus was still scant and the development of a viable vaccine was uncertain.[2] As students of Vietnam well know, the implementation of central policies is anything but automatic. Rather, successful implementation that induced compliance was part of a carefully calibrated central-local relationship (Malesky, 2008). Mass mobilization of civil society, including the use of neighborhood committees, and transparency in Vietnam's single-party state cannot be taken for granted. I argue that these features were the fruit of Vietnam's decades-long efforts to improve governance and responsiveness at local levels, and that this long-term effort was foundational in inducing compliance with restrictive pandemic measures.

First, Vietnam's efforts to professionalize its administrative state dated back to the 1986 reforms to open up its economy, culminating in the mid-1990s with the Public Administration Reform program to overhaul the legal system and improve the public sector's performance (Chau, 1997).

Since 2007, with help from various international aid agencies, Vietnam launched several indices, including the Provincial Competitiveness Index and the Provincial Administrative Performance Index, where teams of experts collected survey data from businesses and citizens around the country to rank provincial leaders based on measures such as transparency, competency, and responsiveness to business and public concerns. Data from these indices show that Vietnamese provinces have made steady improvements in various public service measures, including healthcare, information access, and corruption control (Nguyen & Malesky, 2020). Notably, access to health insurance has grown rapidly over time, with 90% of Vietnamese citizens insured today (Nhan Dan News, 2019). Additionally, hospital quality has improved continuously at the same time that demands for hospital bribes have declined. Taken together with the government's policy to cover the cost of mass quarantine, at least in the early months of the pandemic, Vietnamese citizens did not have to worry about costs of COVID-19 testing, associated hospitalization, and centralized quarantine, thereby increasing their willingness to comply with extensive contact tracing and strict quarantine measures.

Second, building on the first, this increased responsiveness at local levels enabled effective central-local coordination when it mattered most. Immediately after it discovered the first COVID cases, the Vietnamese government formed a national COVID-19 response committee in January 2020, led by the deputy prime minister but located within the Ministry of Health, comprised of leaders from agencies ranging from science and agriculture to information and public security (Office of the Government of the Socialist Republic of Vietnam, 2020c). As it does with other party-state administrative functions, this COVID-19 response committee replicates itself at all levels of government, down to the towns and wards. Key decisions on rationing ventilators and protective gears were coordinated and streamlined. As noted below, this mattered for the economy, too, once early outbreaks were contained. It is worth pointing out, however, that these government actions occurred through a system of administrative documents, not through formal law.[3]

Third, returning to the point about transparency, as noted above the Vietnamese government was remarkably transparent in its COVID-19 efforts. Survey data from the Provincial Competitiveness Index—a project funded jointly by the Vietnamese government and the United Nations Development Program—documented a turnaround, albeit a slow one, in citizens' perception of government transparency at both national and provincial levels (Nguyen & Malesky, 2020). This is consistent with a general trend toward open access, as Vietnam's 2018 Access to Information Law and Vietnamese courts' web portal enable citizen access to a range of government documents, including land maps, budgets, and court judgments. Though some suspect political motives (Nguyen & Dobuzinskis, 2018), the ongoing anti-graft campaign led by Nguyễn Phú Trọng, General Secretary of the Vietnam Communist Party, generally received favorable responses from Vietnam watchers and international audiences. The anti-graft campaign also intersected with the pandemic response. The head of Hanoi's Center for Disease Control, for example, was indicted on a charge of collusion to inflate COVID-19 test kit costs.

Transparency efforts also mitigated skepticism toward the Party-State's COVID-19 reporting. The Ministry of Health posted all reported cases on its website, enabling deeper analysis by data scientists and bloggers, and gaining endorsement from public health experts. Vietnam's online network of activists, while still critical of privacy violations and the lack of freedom of speech, did not raise the alarm on widespread fatalities or cover-ups. When a patient who earlier tested positive for COVID-19 died from liver failure, the government's Facebook portal publicly discussed the reasoning for not counting his death, due to the patient's advanced liver dysfunction and a series of negative COVID-19 tests premortem. Thus, while under-counting was possible, public disclosures opened space for discussion and allowed for corrections if needed.

In sum, Vietnam's strengthened state capacity during 2020 showed evidence of a deliberate, sustained effort to improve governance starting at local levels. While it is too early and difficult to attribute causality, Vietnam's upward trends in healthcare access, transparency, and overall local governance suggest that effective local-central coordination plays an important role implementing national policies. Beyond the simple distinction between authoritarian and democratic regimes, this narrative deserves further attention as part of a larger, global account of the administrative state in times of crisis. As national focus shifted to the reopening of the economy, the official slogan likewise shifted from "fighting the enemy epidemic" in early 2020 to "live peacefully with the pandemic" by year-end (TuoiTre News, 2020a, 2020b). Yet, even for an early success story like Vietnam, COVID-19 wreaked havoc on its economy. A survey by the Provincial Competitiveness Index documented the operational difficulties local firms faced in 2019: even then, 63% reported difficulty in finding customers, 35% in getting credit, 34% in recruiting employees, 28% in finding business partners, and 27% in market downturns (Nguyen & Malesky, 2020). A survey in 2020 showed that most firms, whether foreign, private, or state-owned, projected losses and lay-offs due to declining consumption markets, lack of capital and cash flow, and anticipated lack of work (VNExpress, 2020a, 202b). Transparency, reduced corruption, and increased government responsiveness thus are all critical for healthy businesses to emerge from the lockdown.

Concurrently with the above pandemic response efforts, to promote Vietnam's domestic market, particularly firm survival, Vietnamese leaders also issued a host of relief measures including freezing business obligations to pay costs such as retirement and life insurance contributions, providing quick-access loans for wage payments, and increasing social welfare for laid-off workers (Vietnam Business Forum, 2020a, 2020b). The Access to Information Law enabled citizens and businesses to better monitor these transactions. Government responsiveness was also critical, as business advocates have voiced dissatisfaction with slow access to relief. As the country started to open up by the end of 2020, the government shifted its strategy to focus on promoting the domestic market and repositioning Vietnam for opportunities in shifting global supply chains (Abrami, 2020).

By one example, local leaders in Hanoi have put forth a plan, coordinated with other provinces, to promote linkage in the domestic market, including in tourism, agriculture, and seafood. Among other actions, this required reorienting businesses toward high-demand areas, for example from growing decorative plants to consumable produce (McKinsey, 2021). This coordination became increasingly important as foreign consumption disappeared overnight. While eager to restart its economy, provinces also made clear that economic revitalization must be balanced with public health goals by imposing limited hours for businesses, crowd control, and continued enforcement of social distancing and face-covering requirements. Compliance with these measures will further hinge on continued public trust. National and local leaders are also exploring ways to reposition Vietnam for opportunities in shifting global supply chains (Vietnam Briefing, 2020). While Vietnam likely stands to benefit from countries' desire to diversify away from China (Rapoza, 2019), its domestic businesses themselves heavily depend on China for raw materials and components. As a result, Vietnamese leaders have advocated for boosting supporting industries, particularly manufacturing, technology, and textile sectors. Cities like Hanoi have also promised economic incentives such as extended land leases and preferential loans to attract investment (Hanoi Times, 2020).

Despite the clear challenges Vietnam faces, the country's strong growth trajectory and swift COVID-19 response positioned it to be one of the world's few economic bright spots. The World Bank, for example, projected that Vietnam would be one of the few countries to experience positive economic growth in 2020 (World Bank, 2021a, 2021b).

10.4   Conclusion

As this chapter details above, Vietnam's improving local governance and central-local policy coordination have helped it weather the COVID-19 pandemic through the mass mobilization of its civil society and unprecedented transparency from various levels of government. These key features will likely remain critical for Vietnam as its new, recently elected leaders grapple with balancing the need to open up borders and the economy while protecting public health. As we collectively and continually glean lessons from the global efforts to combat the pandemic, Vietnam's story serves as a reminder to move beyond the simple distinction of and assumptions associated with regime type. It further challenges us to think deeper about bureaucratic capacity and responsiveness within all forms of government.

Notes

1 The Vietnamese government maintains active Facebook and Twitter accounts. *See* Thong Tin Chinh Phu [Government News], https://www.facebook. com/thongtinchinhphu; Vietnam Government Portal, https://twitter.com/ VNGovtPortal.
2 This section is adapted from a previous work published with the Brookings Institute. *See* Trang (Mae) Nguyen & Edmund Malesky, *Reopening Vietnam: How the Country's Improving Governance Helped It Weather the COVID-19 Pandemic*, Brookings Institution, https://www.brookings.edu/blog/ order-from-chaos/2020/05/20/reopening-vietnam-how-the-countrys-improving-governance-helped-it-weather-the-covid-19-pandemic/ (May 20, 2020).
3 This is in contrast to Taiwan, where an extensive legal framework was created to delegate authority to the executive body.

References

Abrami, Regina. The geopolitics of post-COVID-19 supply chains, *Perry World House*, https://global.upenn.edu/perryworldhouse/news/geopolitics-post-covid-19-supply-chains (Apr. 30, 2020).

Chang, Wen-Chen. Taiwan's fight against COVID-19: Constitutionalism, laws, and the global pandemic, Verfassungsblog on matters constitutional, https://verfassungsblog.de/taiwans-fight-against-covid-19-constitutionalism-laws-and-the-global-pandemic/ (Mar. 31, 2020).

Chau, Dao Minh. Administrative reform in Vietnam: need and strategy, *Asian Journal of Public Administration*, 19:2 (1997): 303–320.

Corruption Perception Index, https://www.transparency.org/en/cpi/2020.

Fisher, Max & Sang-Hun, Choe. How South Korea flattened the curve, *New York Times* (Apr. 10, 2020).

Fleming, Sean. Viet Nam shows how you can contain COVID-19 with limited resources, *World Economic Forum*, https://www.weforum.org/agenda/2020/03/ vietnam-contain-covid-19-limited-resources/ (Mar. 30, 2020).

Hanoi Times, Hanoi plans to have 900 firms in supporting industries by end-2020, http://hanoitimes.vn/hanoi-plans-to-have-900-enterprises-in-supporting-industries-by-end-of-2020-311999.html (May 7, 2020).

Hutt, David. The Coronavirus loosens lips in Hanoi, *Foreign Policy*, https:// foreignpolicy.com/2020/04/15/coronavirus-vietnam-communist-party-hanoi/ (Apr. 15, 2020).

Johns Hopkins University of Medicine, Coronavirus Resource Center, https://coronavirus.jhu.edu (last visited Feb. 1, 2021).

Judges' Council, Vietnam Supreme People's Court, Circular 45/TANDTC-PC on adjudicating criminal sanctions relating to the prevention of the COVID-19 pandemic, https://www.toaan.gov.vn/webcenter/portal/tatc/chi-tiet-chi-dao-dieu-hanh?dDocName=TAND114227 (Mar. 30, 2020).

Kinh Te Do Thi [Urban Economy Magazine], Đoàn thanh niên phường Kim Liên tổ chức trắc nghiệm kiến thức dịch Covid-19 [Kim Lien District's youth group organized a community quiz on pandemic prevention knowledge], http://kinht-edothi.vn/doan-thanh-nien-phuong-kim-lien-to-chuc-trac-nghiem-kien-thuc-dic h-covid-19-380924.html (Apr. 12, 2020).

Le, Trien & Nguyen, Huy. How Vietnam learned from China's Coronavirus mistakes, *The Diplomat*, https://thediplomat.com/2020/03/how-vietnam-learned-from-chinas-coronavirus-mistakes/ (Mar. 17, 2020).

Malesky, Edmund. Straight ahead on red: How foreign direct investment empowers subnational leaders, *Journal of Politics* 70:1 (Jan. 2008)

Malesky, Edmund & Taussig, Markus. Participation, government legitimacy, and regulatory compliance in emerging economies: A firm-level field experiment in Vietnam, *American Political Science Review* 113:2 (2019): 530–551.

McKinsey, Reimagining tourism: How Vietnam can accelerate travel recovery, https://www.mckinsey.com/featured-insights/asia-pacific/reimagining-tourism-how-vietnam-can-accelerate-travel-recovery (Mar. 19, 2021).

Ministry of Public Security News, "Bo Cong An So Ket Cong Tac Phong, Chong Dich COVID-19 Trong Luc Luong Cong An Nhan Dan Nam 2020" [The ministry of public security reviews 2020 tasks on COVID-19 preventions and management], Dec 21, 2020.

Nguyen, Ha. Vietnam imposes hefty fines for going maskless, *VOANews*, https://www.voanews.com/science-health/coronavirus-outbreak/vietnam-imposes-hefty-fines-going-maskless (Apr. 1, 2020a).

Nguyen, Kai. Quarantined in Vietnam: Scenes from inside a center for returning citizens, *NPR*, https://www.npr.org/sections/pictureshow/2020/04/06/823963731/quarantined-in-vietnam-scenes-from-inside-a-center-for-returning-citizens (Apr. 6, 2020b).

Nguyen, Sen. Coronavirus: life inside Vietnam's army-run quarantine camps, *South China Morning Post*, https://www.scmp.com/week-asia/health-environment/article/3076734/coronavirus-life-inside-vietnams-army-run-quarantine (Mar. 24, 2020c).

Nguyen, Tran. COVID-19 - What do we know about the situation in Vietnam? A deep dive into Vietnam COVID-19 patient data, *Towards Data Science*, https://towardsdatascience.com/covid-19-what-do-we-know-about-the-situation-in-vietnam-82c195163d7e (May 2, 2020d).

Nguyen, Mi & Dobuzinskis, Alex. At Vietnam's biggest corruption trial, some skeptical views, *Reuters*, https://www.reuters.com/article/us-vietnam-security-trial/at-vietnams-biggest-corruption-trial-some-skeptical-views-idUSKBN1EZ0E7 (Jan 10, 2018).

Nguyen, Phuong & Pearson, James. Vietnam introduces 'fake news' fines for coronavirus misinformation, *Reuters*, https://www.reuters.com/article/us-health-coronavirus-vietnam-security/vietnam-introduces-fake-news-fines-for-coronavirus-misinformation-idUSKCN21X0EB (Apr. 15, 2020).

Nguyen, Suong Thi Thao et al., Waiting time in the outpatient clinic at a national hospital in Vietnam, *Nagoya Journal of Medical Science* 80:2 (2018): 227–239.

Nguyen, Trang (Mae) & Malesky, Edmund. Reopening Vietnam: How the country's improving governance helped it weather the COVID-19 pandemic, *Brookings Institution*, https://www.brookings.edu/blog/order-from-chaos/2020/05/20/reopening-vietnam-how-the-countrys-improving-governance-helped-it-weather-the-covid-19-pandemic/ (May 5, 2020).

Nhan Dan News. Phat trien ben vung, tien toi bao hiem y te toan dan [Developing sustainably to lead to health insurance for all people], https://perma.cc/UJ5A-D57B (Dec. 30, 2019).

NPR. There have been fewer than 300 COVID-19 cases and no deaths. Here's why, In Vietnam, https://www.npr.org/sections/coronavirus-live-updates/2020/04/16/835748673/in-vietnam-there-have-been-fewer-than-300-covid-19-cases-and-no-deaths-heres-why (Apr. 16, 2020).

O'Connor, Tom. China's neighbors close borders as country's Coronavirus cases surpass last major outbreak, *Newsweek*, https://www.newsweek.com/china-neighbors-close-borders-coronavirus-sars-1484978 (Jan. 30, 2020).

Office of the Government of the Socialist Republic of Vietnam, Directive 05/CT-Ttg on Preventing, Combatting the respiratory disease caused by a new strain of the Coronavirus, Jan. 28, 2020a.

Office of the Government of the Socialist Republic of Vietnam, Viet Nam to go into 15-day nationwide social distancing to curb COVID-19, http://news.chinhphu.vn/Home/Viet-Nam-to-go-into-15day-nationwide-social-distancing-to-curb-COVID19/20203/39472.vgp (Mar. 31, 2020b).

Office of the Government of the Socialist Republic of Vietnam, Decree No. 170/QD-Ttg on the creation of the national steering committee to prevent, manage a respiratory infection disease caused by a new Coronavirus, Jan 30, 2020c.

Oxford University Nuffeld Department of Medicine, Centre for Tropical Medicine and Global Health, How Vietnam managed to keep its coronavirus death toll at zero, https://www.tropicalmedicine.ox.ac.uk/news/coronavirus-how-overreaction-made-vietnam-a-virus-success (June 1, 2020).

Pearson, James & Nguyen, Phuong. Vietnam quarantines tens of thousands in camps amid vigorous attack on coronavirus, https://www.reuters.com/article/us-health-coronavirus-vietnam-quarantine/vietnam-quarantines-tens-of-thousands-in-camps-amid-vigorous-attack-on-coronavirus-idUSKBN21D0ZU (Mar. 26, 2020).

Pham, Linh. Vietnam reports 67th Covid-19 case, linked to mass Muslim gathering in Malaysia, *Hanoi Times*, http://hanoitimes.vn/march-18-vietnam-reports-67th-case-linked-to-mass-muslim-gathering-in-malaysia-311398.html (Mar. 18, 2020).

Phan, Lan T. et al., Importation and human-to-human transmission of a novel Coronavirus in Vietnam, *New England Journal of Medicine* 382 (2020): 872–874.

Rapoza, Kenneth. China Trade War updated: Global supply chain shifting, but Asia not easy winner, *Forbes*, https://www.forbes.com/sites/kenrapoza/2019/06/27/china-trade-war-update-global-supply-chains-shifting-but-asia-not-easy-winner/?sh=16b28449df56 (June 27, 2019).

Reed, John. Vietnam's coronavirus offensive wins praise for low-cost model, *Financial Times*, https://www.ft.com/content/0cc3c956-6cb2-11ea-89df-41bea0557 20b (Mar. 23, 2020).

Sang Minh Le. Containing the coronavirus (COVID-19): Lessons from Vietnam, World Bank Blogs, https://blogs.worldbank.org/health/containing-coronavirus-covid-19-lessons-vietnam (Apr. 30, 2020).

TuoiTre News, Chung sống an toàn với COVID-19 [Co-exist safely with COVID-19], https://tuoitre.vn/chung-song-an-toan-voi-covid-19-20200421084052951.htm (Apr. 21, 2020a).

TuoiTre News, Who have been in close contact with Vietnam's 17th COVID-19 patient?, https://tuoitrenews.vn/news/society/20200307/who-have-been-in-close-contact-with-vietnams-17th-covid19-patient/53347.html (Mar. 7, 2020b).

Vietnam Briefing, COVID-19 and the effects on supply chains in Vietnam, https://www.vietnam-briefing.com/news/covid-19-effects-supply-chains-vietnam.html/ (Apr. 10, 2020).

Vietnam Business Forum, Doanh nghiệp vẫn loay hoay tìm cách tiếp cận nguồn hỗ trợ [Businesses continue to struggle to find support], https://vccinews.vn/news/28237/doanh-nghiep-van-loay-hoay-tim-cach-tiep-can-nguon-ho-tro.html (May 12, 2020a).

Vietnam Business Forum, Urgently making economic recovery scenarios, https://vccinews.com/news/38018/urgently-making-economic-recovery-scenarios.html (Apr. 20, 2020b).

Vietnam Economic Times, Budget for mass organizations becoming a burden, https://vneconomictimes.com/article/banking-finance/budget-for-mass-organizations-becoming-a-burden (June 14, 2016).

Vietnam News, Over $12 million raised to support COVID-19 efforts, https://vietnamnews.vn/society/653911/over-12-million-raised-to-support-covid-19-efforts.html (Mar, 20, 2020a).

Vietnam News, Vietnam willing to sacrifice economic benefits for public health, https://vietnam.vnanet.vn/english/vietnam-willing-to-sacrifice-economic-benefits-for-public-health-pm/439705.html (Mar. 13, 2020b).

Vietnam Office of the Government's Facebook portal, https://www.facebook.com/thongtinchinhphu/photos/a.914137021996819/2936406939769807?hc_location=ufi (last visited Feb. 1, 2021).

VNExpress, COVID-19 could bankrupt 50% of Vietnamese enterprises: VCCI, https://e.vnexpress.net/news/business/economy/covid-19-could-bankrupt-50-pct-of-vietnamese-enterprises-vcci-4081637.html (Apr. 9, 2020a).

VNExpress, Hanoi CDC chief arrested for graft in coronavirus test kit purchase, https://e.vnexpress.net/news/news/hanoi-cdc-chief-arrested-for-graft-in-coronavirus-test-kit-purchase-4088948.html (Apr. 23, 2020b).

VNExpress, Vietnam confirms 17th Covid-19 patient, https://e.vnexpress.net/news/news/vietnam-confirms-17th-covid-19-patient-4065517.html (Mar. 7, 2020c).

Vu, Minh & Tran, Bich. The secret to Vietnam's COVID-19 response success: A review of Vietnam's response to COVID-19 and its implications, *Diplomat*, https://thediplomat.com/2020/04/the-secret-to-vietnams-covid-19-response-success/ (Apr. 18, 2020).

Wadhams, Nick & Jacobs, Jennifer. China concealed extent of virus outbreak, U.S. Intelligence says, *Bloomberg News*, https://www.bloomberg.com/news/articles/2020-04-01/china-concealed-extent-of-virus-outbreak-u-s-intelligence-says (Apr. 1, 2020).

World Bank, Vietnam overview, https://www.worldbank.org/en/country/vietnam/overview (last visited Mar 15, 2021a).

World Bank, Vietnam: country profile, https://www.worldbank.org/en/country/vietnam/overview (last visited Feb. 1, 2021b).

World Health Organization, Severe Acute Respiratory Syndrome (SARS) - Multi-country outbreak update 39 (Apr. 25, 2003), https://www.who.int/csr/don/2003_04_25/en/.

11 Conclusions and Policy Implications

M. Jae Moon and Dong-Young Kim

11.1 Summary of Chapters

This book compares the major issues and policy responses of nine countries when mitigating COVID-19. The nine countries were carefully selected based on two criteria: regional representation and unique characteristics of COVID-19 policies. Geographically speaking, there are three in Europe (Sweden, Finland, Germany), one in North America (United States), one in Oceania (New Zealand), and four in Asia (Japan, Korea, Thailand, and Vietnam). In terms of political system, five countries (Japan, Thailand, Finland, Germany, Sweden, New Zealand) are parliamentary systems, while Korea and the United States are presidential systems. Only Vietnam is a socialist republic system. Five Asian-Pacific countries (South Korea, Japan, Thailand, Vietnam, and New Zealand) are basically unitary systems, while others are federal systems.

As the Table 11.1, there are wide variations in the total number of confirmed cases and deaths per million. As of May 28, 2021, for example, the total number of confirmed cases per million ranged from 66 in Vietnam to 100,422 in the United States, while the total deaths per million ranged from 0.5 in Vietnam to 1,794 in the United States.

Ko and Cho investigate the Korean government's policy responses to COVID-19. He first reviews the response of South Korea to COVID-19, focusing on adaptation and learning frameworks. Although South Korea was heavily hit by COVID-19 in February 2020, the Korean government and citizens showed remarkably successful control of COVID-19. The success was not because of a heavy lockdown, as China adopted in response to the Wuhan crisis. Rather, the libertarian approach that was based on citizens' compliance, technologies, and systematic testing, tracking and treatment is a key success factor. The accumulated disaster response experiences have enabled the Korean government to realize the importance of shared information, risk cognition, and collaboration needs. The series of revisions of laws and guidelines can be seen as attempts to find a

DOI: 10.4324/9781003362760-11

Table 11.1 Selected countries

Region	Country	Political system	Centralization	Total confirmed cases (per Mill)	Total death per million
Asia	Korea	PRS	Unitary	2,720	38
	Japan	PAL	Unitary	5,842	101
	Thailand	PAL	Unitary	2,106	13.7
	Vietnam	SOC	Unitary	66	0.5
Oceania	New Zealand	PAL	Unitary	554	5.4
Europe	Finland	PAL	Federal	16,648	171
	Germany	PAL	Federal	43,924	1,054.7
	Sweden	PAL	Federal	10,5797	1,430.9
N. America	USA	PRS	Federal	100,422	1,794.4

* PRS: Presidential System; PAL: Parliamentary System; SOC: Socialist Republic System.
Source: Created by the authors from https://ourworldindata.org/covid-cases.

more effective way to communicate and coordinate actors in the disaster response network. Korea's whole community approach highlights communication and coordination rather than command and control capacity. Therefore, the most important lesson learned from Korea is that no single factor or actor can explain or underpin disaster response success or failure. The whole-community approach should be valued over the myth of the effectiveness of the strong command and control of the government-driven approach.

Suzuki and Sakuwa explore how Japan responded to and mitigated the spread of COVID-19. Despite several unfavorable conditions controlling the pandemic, Japan seems to have managed the pandemic more effectively than several other industrialized democratic countries in terms of its numbers of COVID-19 infection cases and fatalities. However, Japan does not seem to have been as successful in containing the disease as other Asia Pacific countries. Japan's pandemic measures appear relatively loose, based on citizens' self-restraint behaviors and without a clear legal basis, when compared to other industrialized democracies and several Asia-Pacific countries. We argue that Japan's approach is characterized as a cautious and self-restraint-based approach that relies on citizens' self-restraint behavior and personal hygiene practices rather than on enforcing strict, legally binding measures and proactively testing and tracing potentially infected individuals. Unlike many other industrialized democratic countries, Japan never implemented a strict lockdown, a process that requires enforced mobility and activity restrictions and mandatory quarantines with financial penalties for violations. Instead, Japan implemented "mild lockdowns" using nonbinding request-based approaches to reduce mobility and certain types of public activities and relying on citizens' self-restraint behaviors to control the pandemic. In this chapter, we show several performance indicators of governments' responses to the pandemic and examine Japan's response to the pandemic from a broader comparative perspective. Then, we explain three institutional factors that may have been associated with the distinctive characteristics of Japan's pandemic approach. These factors include (1) institutional constraints on the prime minister's leadership, (2) limited administrative capacity and pandemic unpreparedness, and (3) bureaucratic professionalism and closedness. The institutional and political settings in Japan with respect to the COVID-19 response are characterized by stronger restrictions upon the administration and the prime minister's leadership. Finally, we outline Japan's COVID-19 containment policy by examining several phases of Japan's response from January 2020 to early 2021.

Poocharoen and Chattragul provide a description and analysis of policy responses to COVID-19 in Thailand from March 2020 to February 2021. The current military junta-linked government used a combination of strict and innovative responses during the COVID-19 pandemic with the twin goals of curbing both the virus and the swelling of political protests around the country throughout 2020. The author offers four features of the Thai context that explain the policy results – the 4Cs. These include a culture of greeting and respecting doctors; centralized government; community health workers; and consensus on health science. First, the culture in Thailand is such that there is very little physical contact when greeting and interacting. People normally do not shake hands, kiss, or hug as a way of greeting. Thais respect doctors and their advice. Second, the government, which was already highly centralized, responded in a swift and coordinated manner from the beginning. There were no competing narratives or instructions. Early on, the Prime Minister set up a central coordinating body to give advice, make decisions, and communicate. Third, Thailand has a strong and long history of 1 million community health workers on the ground. These semivolunteers played crucial roles in conducting contact tracing, providing accurate information, observing community members, and making initial diagnoses. Fourth is the consensus in Thai society on health issues. There were very few debates related to freedom of movement or freedom of choice, which was observed in other countries. There are two lessons for other countries. The first centralized response is key but could be a long-term obstruction to democratic development. Second, community-level health volunteers are a model worth exploring for countries with inadequate health professionals. They can disseminate health information and provide necessary services on the ground.

Nguyen examines how Vietnam, a nondemocratic regime and a developing country, effectively mitigated COVID-19. Vietnam's single-party state was, by 2020, the second safest place on earth in regard to the pandemic, just behind Taiwan; moreover, the virus was approximately 3,000 times less deadly than in either the United States or the United Kingdom. Vietnam's effective pandemic response was in fact a surprise to many. According to reports, its success can be attributed to a host of factors, including the government's early actions to close schools and borders, extensive contact tracing and mass quarantine, past experience with SARS and MERS, and coercive and surveillance measures. In this chapter, Nguyen argues that Vietnam's effective response is enabled by the country's ongoing efforts to improve governance and central-local government policy coordination. The strength of its state capacity was not born overnight but resulted from decades-long efforts to improve governance and responsiveness at local levels. Vietnam's story thus moves beyond the simple distinction of regime type to challenge us to think deeper about bureaucratic capacity and responsiveness in all forms of government.

With respect to New Zealand's comparatively successful management of the pandemic, Henderson and Withers in Chapter 6 examine how distinctive situational and institutional factors combined to produce a policy environment conducive to staunch public health interventions. New Zealand was, in many ways, the most striking performer among OECD countries. As of January 2021, there had been only 460 confirmed cases per million people and 26 fatalities. Having acted relatively swiftly, decisively and with a clear prioritization of public health over economic concerns or the preservation of civil liberties, New Zealand was able to 'flatten the curve' of COVID-19 infections during the early stages of the pandemic and thereafter pursue a strategy of elimination that few others have been able to emulate. The chapter prefaces its analysis with an overview of aspects of New Zealand's geographic, political, and demographic context relevant to the pandemic, emphasizing policymaking propensities associated with being a small and remote island nation with a unitary system of governance and a history of regional stewardship. We then provide an in-depth assessment of the government's public health and economic policy responses during critical phases of the COVID-19 timeline – assessing how key policies were informed, formulated, communicated, and implemented – before linking these interventions to an underlying matrix of political, analytical and operational capacities informed by the current and previous governments. Importantly, we identify that these capacities (or lack thereof) not only enabled New Zealand's highly restrictive response but also constrained the ability to pursue alternative measures that may have attained similar outcomes with fewer shortcomings. Finally, we consider these drawbacks with respect to the ongoing social and economic challenges arising from unilateral border closures and periodic lockdowns, noting that disadvantaged Māori and Pasifika populations are disproportionately affected by associated hardship and identifying sector-specific impacts for industries of national importance.

Ahonen examines how the Finnish government handled the pandemic crisis by focusing on the roles of local governments and health communities. He also discusses the Finnish politics of COVID-19. Health care in Finland is essentially a responsibility of the self-governing municipalities, which draw the bulk of their revenue from the local income tax, although there is also statutory occupational health care, a system of health care for students at universities and in polytechnic higher education, and commercial health care providers. During the pandemic, the capacity of Finland's health care sufficed reasonably well in terms of COVID-19 testing, COVID-19 care at homes, COVID-19 care in the inpatient clinics of municipal health centers, analogous care in the central hospitals and university hospitals both run by associations of municipalities, and intensive COVID-19 hospital care and COVID-19 vaccinations. In the fight against the pandemic, the Finnish municipal sector, including its clinical professionals and its health care managers, worked remarkably independently, supported by major government funding paid to the municipal sector in the capacity of a major extraordinary grant. However, the pandemic has also revealed important fault lines in Finnish politics and society. Socially isolated people have been hit hard, as have many of those working in such vulnerable sectors as hotels, restaurants, and transportation. Recently, one of Finland's four parties with the most seats in Parliament has been the right-wing populist party called the Finns. Generally, those who indicated that they supported the Finns also indicated the lowest willingness to obey COVID-19-related restrictions and follow COVID-19-related recommendations. However, regarding reluctance to take a COVID-19 vaccination, the supporters of Finns, typically males, have been tailed by supporters of Greens, typically females.

Franzke and Kuhlmann analyze how German public administration has coped with COVID-19 intergovernmental coordination, federal, Länder, and local policy responses to the pandemic and the issues of scientific policy advice, institutional trust, and the population's support of containment measures. After some basic statistical information about COVID-19 in Germany is presented, the institutional setup of crisis management in the German federal system is introduced, and the preparedness and capacities of the health system for a pandemic are assessed. Focusing on the developments in 2020, four major phases of German pandemic governance can be differentiated: Phase I: reliance on local management; Phase II: unitarization and centralization; Phase III: reemphasis on local discretion and variance; and Phase IV: intergovernmental centralism. The responses and measures adopted by the federal, Länder and local governments in these phases are outlined, and the (changing) coordination mechanisms at play are characterized. The chapter also shows that while this country was well prepared in terms of health capacities (ICUs, hospitals, etc.) and (local) public health services, numerous shortcomings and deficits became apparent during the crisis; some of these, such as understaffed hospitals and care facilities, originated in the policy decisions of previous years. Furthermore, the analysis reveals multiple problems that have occurred over the course of the crisis, such as insufficient interdisciplinary policy advice, weakened parliamentary control mechanisms, poor digital preparedness of local health authorities, shortcomings in data transmission, and (partially) shrinking support levels of the German government's crisis management by the population. Regarding intergovernmental coordination, a general trend toward more unitarization and centralization in pandemic-related decision-making up to what we label "intergovernmental centralism" worked out, while at the same time, the increasingly overburdened local levels were still responsible for major implementation and management functions.

Dahlström and Lindvall examine Sweden's public health policies in the twelve-month period between January 2020, when Swedish authorities took the first steps to prepare the country for the new epidemic, and December 2020, when Sweden found itself in the middle of the epidemic's second wave and new, more restrictive policies were being prepared and enacted. The chapter aims to uncover why Sweden adopted public health policies that were markedly different from those of most other Western European states. It begins with a brief overview of the spread of COVID-19 within Sweden. It then describes the public health policies Sweden put in place during the COVID-19 crisis in 2020 before turning to an analysis of the social and political factors that explain Sweden's distinctive approach to public health policy during the pandemic. We reject a few common interpretations of Sweden's distinctive policies. Our own analysis emphasizes continuity, not change, and suggests that long-standing views within the public health community were allowed to prevail due to the autonomy Swedish civil servants typically enjoy as long as they act within their remits.

Using a theoretical framework of complex adaptive systems, Comfort traces the interactions among decision processes at federal, state, and local levels that led to fragmented perceptions of threat, partisan rhetoric advancing uncertain science, and responsibilities for action shifted from the national to subnational governments that enacted scattered and disparate policies. The challenge of managing an unknown, deadly virus during a presidential election year significantly affected the social and political dynamics that altered the capacity of the nation to achieve a coherent consensus for collective action to suppress the virus. The outcome of the November 2020 election produced a change in presidential leadership, management strategy, and evidence-based reporting on the status of the pandemic to the public. The scientific discovery of two vaccines reversed the trajectory of failed, uncoordinated management to the threat of COVID-19 over the preceding months of 2020 and placed the United States in a leading position among nations of the world in the production of vaccines and in vaccinating its population. The experience of the United States shows that three factors are essential for developing the capacity for global cooperation and collaboration in addressing problems, such as the pandemic, that no one country can solve alone. These factors include the role of science, the power of information technologies, and the development of national information infrastructures that can be linked together to form a global knowledge base to develop an interdisciplinary, international program of continuous learning and adaptation for the global community of nations. The goal of sustaining a healthy, humane world is clear; the means are available; and the challenge is building the level of understanding and commitment to enact the goal in practice.

The final chapter summarizes the core findings and policy lessons by integrating the policy responses and outcomes of selected countries from a comparative perspective. This chapter also discusses directions for future comparative policy studies in the post-COVID-19 era when governments are expected to face similar but more wicked policy problems in the future.

11.2   Discussions and Policy Implications

COVID-19 has been one of the most compelling and challenging wicked problems that pushed all governments nearly equally to an edge of cliff. Arguably, no other social and economic problems put the same level of challenges to governments in terms of geographical and chronical scope. After the first confirmed case was identified at the end of 2019 in Wuhan, COVID-19 quickly spread globally and reached the pandemic stage, which was officially confirmed on March 11, 2020. As of March 6, 2021, the numbers of infected patients and deaths reached 117 million and 2.6 million, respectively.

While the epidemiological challenges were similar across different countries, there is a wide discrepancy in terms of the contents, processes, and outcomes of the policy responses of different nations to the pandemic. Why did some countries, such as New Zealand and Vietnam, quickly decide to implement strong and restrictive border controls, while others did not? Why did some countries, such as South Korea, proactively introduce centralized and coordinated policy responses to COVID-19, while other countries, such as Japan and Sweden, took somewhat cautious and decentralized responses? Why did some countries effectively mitigate COVID-19 while others mitigated it in a somewhat ineffective way?

Observing variations in the outcomes of government responses to COVID-19, the same kind of global external shock and risk, we aim to examine why and how different countries ended up with different policy positions and responses by surveying a sample of countries that are geographically, politically, and culturally diverse. This study includes nine different countries, including Finland, Germany, the United States, Japan, New Zealand, South Korea, Sweden, Thailand, and Vietnam, and then carefully reviews the developments of the policy responses of each country and investigates how the policy responses led to different outcomes in terms of the spread of the virus and fatalities. Based on the survey of policy responses and outcomes of selected countries, we conduct a comparative assessment and draw lessons from those experiences (success or failure) that can be shared with many other countries.

11.3 The Spread of the COVID-19 as a Pandemic

Despite the continuing debate on the origin of COVID-19, recent research by Beyer and his colleagues (2021) suggests that the emergence of the virus is closely related to the change in bat diversity ultimately caused by climate change. After the first confirmed patient was reported in Wuhan, China, at the end of 2019, the virus swiftly spread over different parts of the world, which ultimately led to the announcement of the global pandemic by the World Health Organization on March 11, 2020. In particular, the initial exponential surge in Europe beyond Asia shocked the world and sent strong and serious signals of danger and potential public health as well as economic and social impacts to the global community.

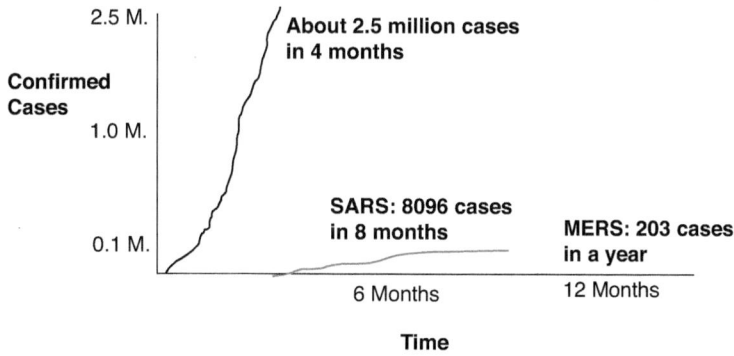

Figure 11.1 Comparison of SARS, MERS, and COVID-19.

Source: Moon (2020), Modified from Wu and Chow (2020).

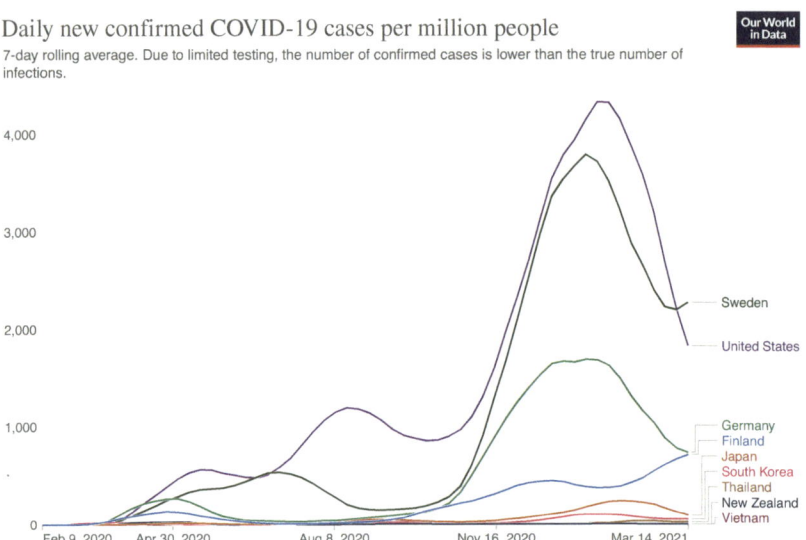

Figure 11.2 Changes in the number of COVID-19 confirmed cases per million for selected countries as of March 12, 2021.

Source: OurWorldInData.org/coronavirus, CC BY.

COVID-19 reportedly originated in Wuhan, Hubei, China. Initially, COVID-19 appeared to be similar to Middle East respiratory syndrome (MERS) and particularly severe acute respiratory syndrome (SARS). However, the new virus is more contagious and impactful in provoking economic and social instability and igniting more psychological fears among individuals than previous infectious diseases. For example, as Figure 11.1 suggests, the number of infected patients grew much faster than that of patients with previous diseases, reaching more than 234,000 (with 9,840 deaths) as of March 20, 2020[1]; by comparison, SARS and MERS caused 8,437 infections (with 813 deaths) and 2,499 infections (with 861 deaths), respectively (Wu and Chow, 2020). In addition to the number of infected patients, COVID-19 spread much faster and wider, reaching the pandemic stage in nearly all countries compared to SARS and MERS, which limitedly affected 26 and 27 countries, respectively.

Although many countries often share similar epidemiological challenges and policy problems as they follow similar waves of COVID-19 spread, there are some variations in the spread of COVID-19 among different countries. The variations might be caused by different policy responses of countries, such as coercive tools (border control, school closure, movement constraints), incentive tools (emergency assistance, economic boosting assistance), and informative and facilitative tools (public information campaigns for social distancing, mask wearing). In addition to policy responses, there are many other contributing factors, including national healthcare systems, applications of digital technology, institutional arrangements and governance systems, and political and civic culture. Figure 11.2 shows daily newly confirmed cases (per million) of nine selected countries, including five Asian Pacific countries, three European countries, and the United States. The figure suggests that the numbers of daily newly confirmed cases of five Asia-Pacific countries (Japan, New Zealand, South Korea, Thailand, and Vietnam) are contrastingly much smaller than those of the other countries.

11.4 Policy Responses to COVID-19: Does Policy Matter?

Although they all have the same goal of mitigating and containing COVID-19, different countries have a wide range of policy responses. The variation in policy responses among countries is attributed to various factors, such as leadership styles, risk assessment, and risk perception regarding COVID-19, policy learning and policy styles, and political culture. In the course of mitigating COVID-19, each country has developed its own policy positions and introduced policy actions in terms of introducing alternative policy tools, including coercive, remunerative, and informative measures. Policy positions and policy actions are somehow a product of various variables at different levels, including policymakers at the individual level, and healthcare systems and government systems at the institutional level as well as the domestic and global spread of the virus at the national and global levels.

As a common policy response, coercive policy tools have been widely adopted by governments as direct and immediate forceful public actions to reduce the mobility of the public and to contain the virus through different policy instruments, including school closings, workplace closings, cancellations of public events, restrictions on gathering size, public transportation closures, home stay requirements, and restrictions on domestic and international travel. Remunerative policy instruments have also been introduced to provide public assistance to those who suffer from the negative economic impacts (i.e., unemployment, reduced incomes) of the pandemic. In addition to coercive and remunerative policy measures, governments have employed public information campaigns and other alternative technology-based and public health-related instruments, such as contact tracing, testing policy, and vaccination policy. According to the COVID-19 policy stringency index provided by the Oxford COVID-19 Government Response Tracker (OxCGRT), as Figure 11.3 suggests, there is wide variation in terms of the degree of stringency of policy responses by countries. In some countries, of course, governments are likely to take

COVID-19 Containment and Health Index, Mar 13, 2021

This is a composite measure based on thirteen policy response indicators including school closures, workplace closures, travel bans, testing policy, contact tracing, face coverings, and vaccine policy rescaled to a value from 0 to 100(100 = strictest). If policies vary at the subnational level, the index is shown as the response level of the strictest sub-region.

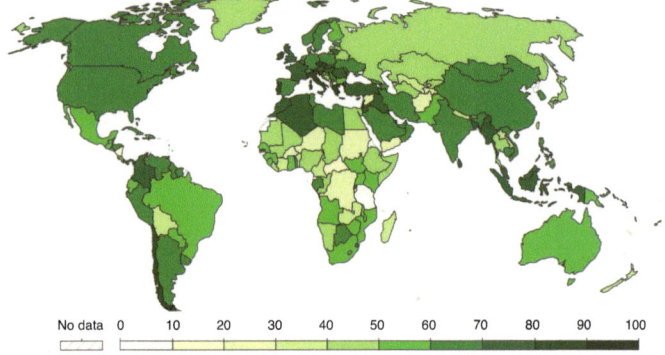

Figure 11.3 A global map on policy stringency index.
Source: OurWorldInData.org/coronavirus, CC BY.

more stringent policy responses when the pandemic situation worsens, which is reflected in increasing numbers of confirmed cases and deaths. In fact, there is a positive correlation between the spread of the virus and policy stringency simply because of growing societal and political pressure for aggressive and often restrictive policy measures. Of course, political systems and citizens' acceptance of restrictive measures affect the extent to which governments can stretch their policy arms in choosing their own policies among different policy options of different degrees of restriction.

Although Vietnam is a relatively low-income country, it was able to mitigate the pandemic effectively from the early stage, particularly with its immediate restrictive actions, such as border closure and school closure, as well as close central-local policy coordination, which is characterized as a low-cost model (Nguyen, 2025). Similarly, the Thailand case also suggests how strongly the Junta-linked government could introduce proactive and highly restrictive measures to mitigate COVID-19 (Poocharoen and Chattragul, 2025). While centralized policy responses might lead to effective mitigation of the pandemic, they often constrain individual freedom and fringe democratic values, as noted in Thailand, where some restrictive measures, such as the prohibition of mass gatherings, are often used to suppress political protests (Poocharoen and Chattragul, 2025).

In contrast, it took a long time for Sweden to take restrictive measures even during the rapid spread of the virus and the growing number of deaths among elderly and fragile individuals in elder care centers (Dahlström and

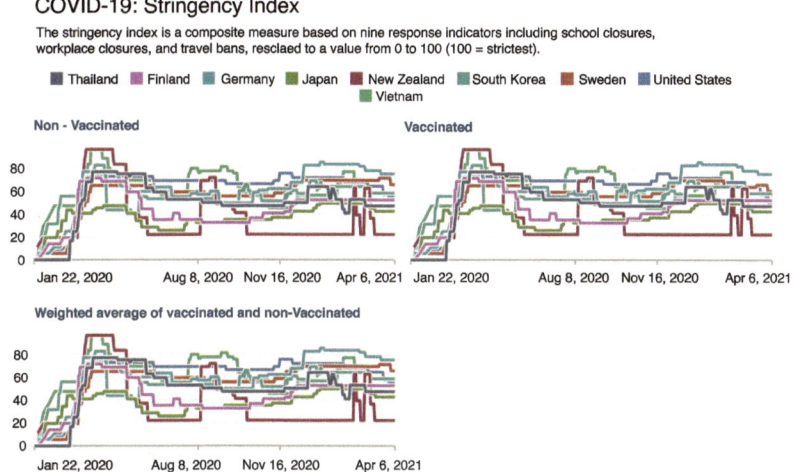

COVID-19: Stringency Index

The stringency index is a composite measure based on nine response indicators including school closures, workplace closures, and travel bans, resclaed to a value from 0 to 100 (100 = strictest).

■ Thailand ■ Finland ■ Germany ■ Japan ■ New Zealand ■ South Korea ■ Sweden ■ United States ■ Vietnam

Figure 11.4 Policy stringency index of nine selected countries by time.

Source: OurWorldInData.org/coronavirus, CC BY.

Lindvall, 2025). The failure to coordinate restrictive policies in a decentralized and democratic political system often leads to detrimental policy failure, particularly in managing nonroutine crises such as pandemics. Among Western countries, New Zealand took very restrictive measures earlier than other Western countries (Henderson and Withers, 2025). For example, the stringency index for New Zealand was 96.3, while those of other Western countries were much lower, as seen in Germany (79.6), the United States (72.7), Finland (64.8), and Sweden (37.9), as of March 23, 2020. Among Asian countries, Japan had the least restrictive policy measure, as it implemented loose and self-restraint policies rather than proactive policy responses (Suzuki and Sakuwa, 2025).

The policy response to COVID-19 is not solely determined by epidemiological factors. Policymakers often consider political, economic, social, and international factors when considering various policy alternatives. Policymakers often lift coercive policy tools such as school closure, workplace closure, or travel restrictions because of growing political pressure from citizens and businesses who want to have a high level of mobility among people. Furthermore, policymakers often make policy response decisions based on the severity and prediction of the pandemic, the voices of citizens and businesses, and domestic and international factors.

Figure 11.4 shows possible variations in the policy responses of different countries over time. As the figure suggests, a government makes a different set of policy actions as a response to its own COVID-19 situation. For example, Sweden's stringency index began to rise in October 2020 and then to drop and rise again in January and March, respectively. That of the United States had three peaks in March, August, and December 2020 in response to three waves of the pandemic and then began to drop from the beginning of 2021 when the national vaccine program for COVID-19 accelerated (Comfort, 2025). In contrast, in early 2021, four Asian-Pacific countries, including Japan, Korea, Thailand, Vietnam, and New Zealand, were overall much lower than the Western countries (Germany, the United States, and Sweden) except Finland. Starting in the beginning of 2021, the policy stringency of the United States began to substantially drop, particularly because of the effect of wide vaccination, while that of some Asian countries, such as Vietnam and Thailand, began to sharply rise.[2]

11.5   Policy Coordination and Quality of Governance: Does Governance Matter?

There is a wide range of government performance in mitigating COVID-19 among countries as the pandemic opened up a series of tests for governance quality and performance in fighting COVID-19 again. Poor quality governance and leadership tend to cause rapid spread of the virus as well as a high fatality rate. Many believe that policy failure is largely attributed to incompetent public leadership and poor policy capacity, which is closely associated with ineffective policy coordination among related policy actors. Many attempts have been made to identify political and institutional factors as primary explanatory variables for the successes and failures of COVID-19 policies in countries. These factors include public leadership and intragovernmental relationships: intergovernmental relationships, intersectoral relationships, and others.

An uncommon editorial entitled "Dying in a Leadership Vacuum" was written collectively by editors of the New England Journal of Medicine in October 2020. The editorial argues that tardy, irresponsible, and inconsistent policy actions taken by incompetent government and poor leadership led to a fatal failure in mitigating COVID-19. Failures of policy actions could occur at various stages, such as disseminating warning and public health information, conducting tests, tracing infection paths and networks, treating infected patients, providing financial assistance, and recovering the resilience capacity of society. Public leadership failure is not only caused by poor judgment and inability of individual political leaders such as presidents but also caused by ineffective policy coordination and the overpoliticization of policy issues, which are often expected to be managed based on scientific evidence.

While some countries took immediate and agile responses to the initial outbreak of COVID-19, others failed to make initial responsive actions because of decentralized political systems and politicization of the pandemic issue. For example, Sweden could not handle COVID-19 through centralized and highly coordinated policy packages; instead, it had to work through decentralized and voluntary mechanisms because of its decentralized administrative system for intergovernmental relations, which bestows only limited administrative and policy power to the central government, particularly when it restrains individual rights (Dahlström and Lindvall, 2025). Germany also experienced an initial delay because government responses often undergo administrative procedures and long-standing scrutiny of the legislative body, although they have shifted from local government responses toward intergovernmental centralism for effective policy coordination between the federal government, Länder, and local governments (Franzke and Kuhlmann, 2025). In contrast, Finland responded to the pandemic without much delay, although its administrative system is also decentralized (Ahonen, 2025).

Countries with unitary government systems, such as Korea, Thailand, Vietnam, and New Zealand, were able to adopt relatively agile and centralized policies to combat the pandemic. Demonstrating a low-cost model, Vietnam and Thailand show how highly centralized political systems could introduce highly restrictive measures in an earlier stage, which helps them mitigate the pandemic in a cost-efficient way, although some restrictive actions could be misused and abused, as they limit individual freedom and democratic values in an excessive way. For example, Vietnam often places the violation of COVID-19 regulation subject to criminal law (Nguyen, 2025), whereas the Thai military government uses strong and restrictive measures both to mitigate COVID-19 and curb political protests against the regime (Poocharoen and Chattragul, 2025).

In fact, this is closely related to the centralization thesis, which is a long-standing debate with respect to crisis management. The centralization thesis is a question concerning whether a centralized governance structure is more effective than a decentralized governance structure. As Hart, Rosenthal, and Kouzmin (1993) note, there are three major elements of a crisis: severe threat, time pressure, and high uncertainty. In other words, a crisis can be worsened if it occurs in an uncertain, dynamic, and complex environment. Hart et al. (1993) suggest that the role of the government and centralized crisis management should be based on a small group with strong decision-making power, a central institution with embedded and highly concentrated decision-making power, and powerful leadership rather than decentralized decision-making mechanisms.

The centralization thesis can be divided into four dimensions of centralization schemes, including social, political, administrative, and structural decentralization. As seen in Table 11.2, social centralization represents the transfer of leadership roles from the market to the

Table 11.2 Key issues of centralization thesis

Dimension of centralization	Nature of the centralization	Key players
Social centralization	From market to government	Social demand for an active governmental role, social involvement
Political centralization (executive centralization)	Shifting toward the executive branch and the top executives (e.g., president)	Executive branch plays the major role rather than the legislative branch
Administrative centralization	Shifting toward the central government and the top decision-makers	Key agencies and top decision-makers play a significant role
Structural centralization	Shifting toward a small policy group	Small decision-making group for timely policymaking

Source: Created by the authors from Moon (2019). Unpublished paper.

government based on social demand for an active governmental role and social involvement. Second, political centralization is a synonym for executive centralization, which is related to centralization dynamics among three different branches. Under politically centralized circumstances, decision-making power often shifts toward the executive branch, centered around the president, rather than the legislative branch, particularly under emergency circumstances, which often require immediate actions. Third, administrative centralization implies a shift toward the central government and the top decision-makers within the executive branch. In other words, the key agencies and top decision-makers play a significant role in administrative centralization. Finally, structural centralization represents the shift of decision-making power toward a small policy group. In this type, the major key player is a small, informal decision-making group.

A centralized governance system is effective, particularly when agile policy decisions are critical, as in the COVID-19 crisis. However, it might face some challenges when the crisis is complicated, uncertain, and changing, which requires the governance system to become an adaptive system (Comfort, 2025). Notably, a decentralized system is not necessarily an adaptive system either. As experienced in the United States, Sweden, and Germany, decentralized systems often face difficulty in reaching policy coordination not only among different units of the government but also between central and local governments. Strong political leadership and a sense of urgency based on scientific evidence are essential to make decentralized systems agile, adaptive, and effective (Moon, 2020).

11.6 Science and Politics: Does Politics Matter?

Evidence-based decisions are critical, particularly when governments make policy decisions to handle wicked problems, which are often characterized as uncertain, borderless, complex, and multiplicative. Theoretically, it is easy and normative to make decisions based on evidence. However, it is not challenging and often difficult, particularly when scientific evidence is not clear. For example, there were intense debates on whether wearing facial masks was necessary in the early pandemic stage in 2020.

Crisis management is often doomed to fail when governments put politics/policy over science (Comfort, 2007, 2025). A great policy problem such as COVID-19 easily becomes a salient policy issue that is often naturally politicized. For example, the initial policy failure of the United States is partially because of hyper partisanship on the issue during the presidential election. The politicization of COVID-19 was often intensified thanks to the uncertainty of the issue, the limited influence of scientific evidence, and the lack of expert involvement, among others reasons, which eventually led to poor evidence-based policy (Comfort, 2025). The COVID-19 issue was also politically handled in Japan with some concerns about the possibility that the spread of COVID-19 might affect the schedule of the Tokyo Summer Olympic Games (Moon et al., 2021). The politicization of crisis management often widens the gap between cognition/interpretation of the crisis and policy actions. The overpoliticization of the pandemic with excessive partisanship caused the public's frustration with policy failures, which eventually led to power changes from the Abe administration to Suga administration in Japan and from the Trump administration to the Biden administration in the United States.

As Dahlström and Lindvall argue in their chapter, interestingly, a lack of politicization might cause a timely response to the pandemic, particularly when scientific evidence is not available and is still controversial. To make an agenda salient and shape timely policies, a certain level of politicization is inevitable and necessary. Excessive deference to scientific evidence might delay timely actions under uncertain policy environments, as does simple delegation of political leadership to administrative authorities, as indicated in Sweden's case (Dahlström and Lindvall, 2025). This suggests that the active role of political leadership with an open and flexible position on scientific evidence is quite challenging but clearly necessary in handling wicked problems such as COVID-19.

11.7 Policy Learning and Experiences: Does Policy Learning Matter?

While COVID-19 was novel to every country, some countries have been more exposed to similar infectious diseases, such as SARS or MERS, than other countries. For example, many Asia-Pacific countries, including Japan, Korea, Thailand, Vietnam, and New Zealand, experience SARS frequently, so both governments and citizens have a higher level of awareness than other Western countries, which might make some differences in the government's initial responses. SARS experiences and societal acceptance of mask-wearing have helped to mitigate the pandemic in Asian countries.

In particular, the MERS experience in South Korea is noteworthy in that it prepared this country to handle the pandemic in terms of separating confirmed patients in hospitals from other patients, developing testing kits, contact tracing, preparing negative pressure rooms, transparent information sharing to citizens, etc. In fact, many civil servants in the Korean CDC were those who experienced the MERS case with pains and developed institutional memories and policy learnings (Ko and Cho, 2025; Moon, 2020). As noted in the MERS Whitepaper (MSWH, 2016), the following key lessons and policy recommendations from the MERS experience were applied to handling COVID-19.[3]

Based on these policy recommendations, the South Korean government upgraded the KCDC to a deputy ministerial-level agency and strengthened its autonomy and professional specialties by increasing the number of epidemiological surveyors. The MERS experience was costly but a great learning experience for the South Korean government, as it led to reevaluation and reform that enhanced the KCDC's autonomy and capacity as well as established procedural protocols to control and prevent new infectious diseases such as COVID-19.

Of course, it should also be noted that past experiences are not enough since we experience new challenges. Despite many benefits from policy learning from the MERS experiences in South Korea, the South Korean government had many unexpected difficulties because COVID-19 had different characteristics, such as asymptomatic patients, the emergence of variants, and the high scale and speed of spread, among others. These require governments to be much smarter, more flexible and open learners. As Lee, Hwang, and Moon (2020) argue in their study on policy learning, governments need to be equipped with quadruple-loop learning, which includes traditional learning as well as context-based learning and continued learning, in dealing with the uncertainty and complexity of wicked problems.

11.8　Citizen Participation and COVID-19: Does Communitarian Citizenship Matter?[4]

Considering the significance of nonpharmaceutical interventions (NPIs), such as social distancing and mask-wearing, citizen participation is critical to coping with the pandemic (Ko and Cho, 2025; Moon, 2020; Moon et al., 2021). It has been argued that many communitarian countries are handling the pandemic better than most individualistic countries (Etizioni, 2020). While this statement has not necessarily been empirically proven, scholars and practitioners need to revisit the roles of socially responsible citizens and their social duties from a communitarian and civic perspective rather than considering only traditional rights-bearing individualism.

The public health literature has often stressed that to combat infectious diseases, selfish individualism needs to be shifted to responsible and communitarian citizenship simply because no one can be fully free from a highly infectious disease, and mutual concerns for community members and social benefits are critical for the safety of the community (Wiseman, 1998). Similarly, public interest and mutual concerns are the fundamental basis of social citizenship (i.e., the provision of merit goods such as health services), which highlights the rationale for providing minimum social support and security to protect individual members and ensure the stability and prosperity of the whole community (Musgrave, 1957; Wiseman, 1998).

Communitarianism is somehow located in the middle ground where individual and communal concerns intersect and individual rights and the common good overlap. For example, wearing masks is important to individual health but also to public health because of the contagious nature of infectious diseases. Communitarian citizenship is different from individualistic libertarian citizenship, in which liberty is an absolute and unnegotiable value.

Countries with high-level communitarianism under the influence of Confucian values such as group consciousness and face savings seem to easily promote citizen participation in social distancing and other NPI measures. However, the nature of citizenship differs among countries. It is closely related to cultural background (Confucian versus Western), political systems (socialist versus democratic), and sense of community and urgency. The pandemic experience at least reminds the people of the significance of communitarian values. Communitarian citizenship and citizen participation for coproduction is essential for solving future wicked problems such as various public health issues and environmental issues such as climate change.

11.9   Transparency and Public Trust: Does Transparency Matter?

Transparency seems to be an important factor in the effective management of the pandemic, particularly because citizens tend to be fearful and uncertain about the pandemic. They often rely on governments' official announcements and other related information obtained from both legacy and new media. The 2020 Global E-government Survey of the United

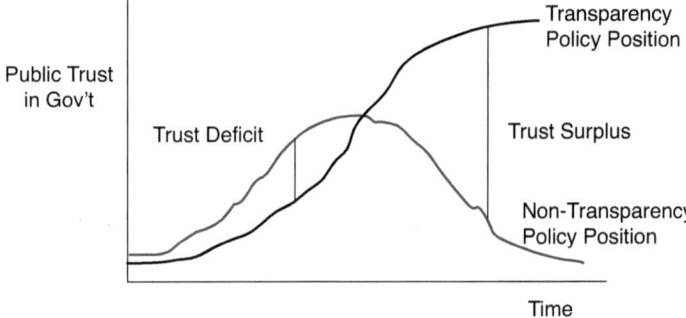

Figure 11.5 Impacts of transparency and nontransparency positions on public trust.

Source: Adapted from Moon (2020).

Nations suggests that most countries appear to provide citizens with COVID-19-related information, such as daily confirmed cases and deaths, as well as public campaigns on public health through their own e-government systems, such as dashboards and mobile apps, in addition to legacy media. The literature on risk communication emphasizes the timeliness, credibility, and transparency of information. The quality of risk communication often affects public trust in government actions.

Transparency policy and nontransparency policy might affect public trust in government and public perception of policy responses to COVID-19 from short-term and long-term perspectives. Some citizens might have unnecessary fear concerns about COVID-19 when governments provide any COVID-19-related information to citizens, which often tempts the government to provide information selectively to avoid or minimize unnecessary fear. As Figure 11.5 suggests, for example, a transparency policy position might have a trust deficit from a short-term perspective because the growing number of new infected patients or deaths might cause citizens' frustration with poor government performance during the pandemic and lead to decreased public trust in government. However, a policy of transparency eventually leads to a trust surplus from the long-term perspective because it helps make governments reliable and trustworthy (Moon, 2020). The transparency policy position helps to gain public trust not only in developing countries such as Vietnam (Nguyen, 2025) but also in developed countries. Intended or unintended nontransparency practices often cause growing public anger and distrust in government even in developed and democratic countries such as the United States, where the number of nursing home deaths was reportedly undercounted in New York (Siemaszko, 2021). This later forced Cuomo, governor of New York, to issue public apologies for nontransparency practices.

This report offers a comprehensive review of policy responses to COVID-19 in different countries. This enhances our understanding of both similarities and differences in policy responses and then offers a comparative analysis of various factors that determine differences in policy responses and outcomes. Since COVID-19 continues to evolve, we do not know how different governments respond to the pandemic in the future. Of course, vaccination and economic recovery are expected to be focal policy attention. Some dimensions, such as political systems, science and evidence-based policymaking, public participation, and transparency policy, will remain key determining factors for future policy choices.

Notes

1 WHO data from the situation report by WHO. https://www.who.int/docs/default-source/coronaviruse/situation-reports/20200320-sitrep-60-covid-19.pdf?sfvrsn=8894045a_2 (accessed on March 20, 2020).
2 The stringency indices are Germany (75.0), Vietnam (69.1), Sweden (65.7), Thailand (59.3), South Korea (58.3), US (56.9), Finland (52.3), Japan (49.1), and New Zealand (22.2).
3
  1. Strengthening the capacity of the Korea Centers for Disease Control and Prevention (KCDC)
  2. Building the capacity of local governments for infection control and securing organizational capacity
  3. Strengthening the capacity of medical institutions for infection control and establishing the government's management system
  4. Building infection control networks among central government, local governments, and medical institutions
  5. Establishing a monitoring system for infectious diseases and upgrading infection disease information systems
  6. Preparing for new infectious diseases and stocking necessary resources with strategic national stockpiles
  7. Creating isolated areas for treatment and establishing test and treatment protocols
  8. Promoting R&D for new infectious diseases
  9. Securing national budget for responding to public health crises
  10. Strengthening risk communication capacity in the new infectious diseases era
  11. Improving the ethics of infectious diseases and strengthening psychological support for infected patients

4 This part of the chapter is partially an excerpt of the author's unpublished manuscript (Moon and Cho, 2021).

References

Ahonen, P. 2025. Finland's responses to COVID-19: Uneven, fairly effective, and craving to return to the normal. In Moon and Kim(Eds.), *International Comparative Analysis of Early COVID-19 Responses* (pp.98–123). Routledge. DOI: 10.4324/9781003362760-4

Beyer, R.B., Manica, A., and Camilo, M. 2021. Shift in global bat diversity suggest a possible role of climate change in the emergence of SARS-CoV-1 and SARS-CoV-2. *Science of the Total Environment*. 767. 145413. https://www.sciencedirect.com/science/article/pii/S0048969721004812

Comfort, L.. 2007. Crisis management in hindsight: Cognition, communication, coordination, and control. *Public Administration Review*, 67 (special issue). s1 pp.189–97.

Comfort, L. 2025. The United States' responses to COVID-19: Sciences, uncertainty, and partisanship. In Moon and Kim(Eds.), *International Comparative Analysis of Early COVID-19 Responses* (pp.124–152). Routledge. DOI: 10.4324/9781003362760-5

Dahlström, D. and Lindvall, J. 2025. Sweden's responses to COVID-19 crisis. In Moon and Kim(Eds.), *International Comparative Analysis of Early COVID-19 Responses* (pp.72–97). Routledge. DOI:10.4324/9781003362760-3

Etizioni, A. 2020. COVID-19 tests communitarian values. *The Diplomacy*. July 14. 2020. https://thediplomat.com/2020/07/covid-19-tests-communitarian-values/

Franzke, J. and Kuhlmann, S. 2025. Germany's responses to COVID-19: Crisis governance in a multilevel system. *International Comparative Analysis of Early COVID-19 Responses* (pp.10–71). Routledge. DOI: 10.4324/9781003362760-2

Hart, P., Rosenthal, U., and Kouzmin, A. 1993. Crisis decision making: The centralization thesis revisited. *Administration & Society*, 25(1), 12–45.

Henderson, S. and Withers, M. 2025. Aotearroa New Zealand's policy responses to the COVID-19. *International Comparative Analysis of Early COVID-19 Responses* (pp.153–181). Routledge. DOI:10.4324/9781003362760-6

Ko, K. and Cho, Y. 2025. South Korea's responses to COVID-19. *International Comparative Analysis of Early COVID-19 Responses* (pp.182–208). Routledge. DOI: 10.4324/9781003362760-7

Lee, S., Hwang, C., and Moon, M.J. 2020. Policy learning and crisis policymaking: Quadruple-loop learning and COVID-19 responses in South Korea. *Policy and Society*. 39(3). 363–381. https://www.tandfonline.com/doi/full/10.1080/14494035.2020.1785195

Ministry of Social Welfare and Health. 2016. *MERS Whitepaper: Learning from MERS Experiences*.

Moon, M.J. 2019. The centralization thesis revisit in crisis management. Unpublished manuscript.

Moon, M.J. 2020. Fighting COVID-19 with agility, transparency, and participation: Wicked policy problems and new governance challenges. *Public Administration Review*. 80(4). 651–656. https://doi.org/10.1111/puar.13214.

Moon, M.J. and Cho, B. 2021. Bring citizens back-in for wicked policy problems. Unpublished manuscript.

Moon, M.J., Suzuki, K., Park, T.I. and Sakuwa, K. 2021. A comparative study of COVID-19 responses in South Korea and Japan: Political nexus triad and policy responses. *International Review of Administrative Sciences*. 87(3). 651–671.

Musgrave, R. 1957. A multiple theory of budget determination. *FianzArchiv, New Series*. 25(1). 33–43.

Nguyen, T. 2025. Vietnam's responses to COVID-19: Local governance and bureaucratic coordination. *International Comparative Analysis of Early COVID-19 Responses* (pp.274–285). Routledge. DOI:10.4324/9781003362760-10

Poocharoen, O. and Chattragul, P. 2025. Thailand's responses to COVID-19 and acceleration of public sector reform. *International Comparative Analysis of Early COVID-19 Responses* (pp.239–273). Routledge. DOI:10.4324/9781003362760-9

Siemaszko, C. 2021. New York Gov. Cuomo facing calls to apologize for undercounting Covid-19 nursing home death. *NBC News.* https://www.nbcnews.com/news/us-news/new-york-gov-cuomo-facing-calls-apologize-undercounting-covid-19-n1258053 (Feb. 17, 2021)

Suzuki, K. and Sakuwa, K. 2025. Japan's responses to COVID-19. *International Comparative Analysis of Early COVID-19 Responses* (pp.209–238). Routledge. DOI:10.4324/9781003362760-8

Wiseman, V. 1998. From selfish individualism to citizenship: Avoiding health economics' reputed "Dead End." *Health Care Analysis.* 6. 113–122. https://link.springer.com/article/10.1007/BF02678117

Wu, J. and Chow, D. 2020. Coronavirus diseases: Comparing COVID-19, SARS and MERS by the number. *NBC News* (March 5, 2020). https://www.nbcnews.com/health/health-news/coronavirus-diseases-comparing-covid-19-sars-mers-numbers-n1150321

Index